RESOLVING IMPASSES IN THERAPEUTIC RELATIONSHIPS

Resolving Impasses
in
Therapeutic Relationships

Sue Nathanson Elkind

THE GUILFORD PRESS
New York   London

© 1992 Sue Nathanson Elkind
Published by The Guilford Press
A Division of Guilford Publications, Inc.
72 Spring Street, New York, N. Y. 10012

Printed in the United States of America

This book is printed on acid-free paper.

Last digit is print number: 9 8 7 6 5 4 3 2 1

Library of Congress Cataloging-in-Publication Data

Elkind, Sue Nathanson
    Resolving impasses in therapeutic relationships / by Sue Nathanson
Elkind.
        p. cm.
    Includes bibliographical references and index.
    ISBN 0-89862-892-X
    1. Impasse (Psychotherapy)   2. Psychotherapist and patient.
3. Psychotherapy—Complications.   I. Title.
    [DNLM: 1. Counseling.   2. Professional–Patient Relations]
3. Psychotherapy.   WM 55 E43r]
RC489.I45E45   1992
616.89′14—dc20
DNLM/DLC
for Library of Congress   92-1692
                                                                    CIP

❖ *Acknowledgments* ❖

This book would not have come to fruition without substantial help from many individuals. I am indebted beyond measure to the patients and therapists, whose privacy I will preserve at the expense of personal recognition, who have joined me in venturing forth on the new pathway of consultation to therapeutic dyads. I am also grateful to the many patients and therapists who shared their painful experiences with impasses and ruptures in therapy. They will undoubtedly recognize their contributions.

Diane Cleaver, my agent, shepherded the manuscript safely to its home with Guilford. Kitty Moore, Senior Editor, seasoned it with her unwavering infectious energy, enthusiasm, and humor added to a perceptive understanding of psychotherapy. My gratitude to the entire Guilford staff for their talented and skillful contributions to the final product.

With her talents as a therapist, consultant, and writer, Kim Chernin sustained a vision of the book and its value throughout the ups and downs of working on it, as she did for my first book, *Soul-Crisis*.

For their concept and provision of an expanded relational network in support of my endeavor to provide consultations, I thank the women of the Stone Center: Judith Jordan; Alexandra Kaplan; Jean Baker Miller; Irene Stiver, who is well-known for providing consultations; and Janet Surrey.

The following colleagues and friends generously shared their experience, insight, and ideas: Alice Abarbanel, Claire Allphin, Mary Boyvey, Linda Cozzarelli, Neil Kostick, Joyce Lindenbaum, Ruth Parker, Ellen Siegelman, Barbara Stevens Sullivan, and Jeffrey Trop.

Hilde Burton, Marjorie Nathanson Keeler, Frances Tobriner, and Julie Patrusky carefully read and edited different versions of the manuscript and supplied honest, pointed, and thoughtful comments. Jane Lewin's sharp mind and pencil were always available. Dorothy Witt refined the final draft with her special gift for simplicity and precision of language.

Family relationships have been sustaining: my parents, Milton and Maria Nathanson; my mother-in-law, Vera Elkind; and my children, Lauren, Perrin, and Ethan, who continually remind me of the irreducible diversity in point of view on virtually every subject, and that loving relationships call for knowing and respecting the vulnerabilities and strengths, similarities and differences, of each person.

Above all, I thank my husband and life-partner, Peter, not only for his diverse and (usually) good-humored contributions, but for his constant presence and for the relationship we keep creating.

❖ *Author's Note* ❖

In the case examples throughout the book, I refer to patients by first name and to therapists with the formal title of "Dr." In practice, patients and therapists address each other in different ways for different reasons. My particular choice both highlights an inherent imbalance in authority and power, and enables readers to distinguish patient and therapist easily in the text.

Each case example is a fictionalized composite based upon actual therapeutic relationships and consultations. In addition to the fictionalized features of the cases, identifying characteristics of therapists and patients have been significantly altered to protect confidentiality. However, when possible I have also worked on these fictionalized case representations with the individuals involved, obtaining their permission and assistance.

The process of working on the vignettes with the patients and therapists who participated in consultations with me was unexpectedly rewarding. At the outset, I focused simply on obtaining their permission. I was concerned about the impact of contacting patients and therapists without warning, sometimes after several years had passed since we had met. I did not know whether I would reopen past wounds to no avail, or whether patients and therapists would feel exposed or exploited, despite the careful fictionalization. Yet I did not want to bar them from choosing to omit the vignette, deleting parts of it, or from knowing about their contribution if the example were included. Above all, I wanted to honor the relationship we had forged in the consultation. The possibility of receiving their help in accurately conveying the experiences of impasses and wounding had not occurred to me.

My contact with the patients and therapists I had worked with quickly became more than a simple matter of obtaining permission. Without exception, they were responsive and helpful. They grappled with their feelings about both what I had written and how they would convey their responses to me. They were honest, thoughtful, articulate, focused upon preserving the psychological accuracy of the experiences presented, and interested in helping others who might have similar experiences in therapy. Consequently many of the vignettes are a seamless composite of their contributions and my own. Some were preserved intact, and others were edited in minor ways. But all of them are a product of the same integrity, mutuality, respect, and empathy that characterized our initial effort to make constructive use of the impasses, wounding, and ruptures that occurred.

In my experience, case vignettes that are a joint effort of the therapist, patient, and consultant (even if few changes result) rather than the product of one individual working alone are unusual. Certainly they constitute a radical departure from the traditional approach in books and articles, and as such represent a move toward including the different subjective experiences of each participant in therapeutic relationships.

❖ *Contents* ❖

RESOLVING IMPASSES IN THERAPEUTIC RELATIONSHIPS

❖ *Introduction* ❖

I had an impasse with a therapist three years ago that was just devastating. We terminated abruptly. I feel damaged by the experience and don't know if I'll ever be able to recover. I've barely been able to talk about it.

—MARK

Sometimes I think Freud was right—psychotherapy is an impossible profession. I read, go to workshops, get consultation, and still there are patients I can't help and patients that I get into stalemates with.

—DR. W.

A patient recently terminated abruptly after I misunderstood her and there was nothing I could do. I wonder how she is doing, I ruminate about what I might have done to help her remain in therapy. I think about her often.

—DR. R.

I feel stuck with my therapist and I don't know why I'm stuck or how to get out of it or even whether I'm with the right therapist for me. He can't seem to help us. I guess it's up to me. I don't know where else to turn.

—STEVE

At the heart of this book lies the uniquely human striving for experiences of intimacy, connection, and attachment with others despite the impossibility of sustaining them. In the face of the impermanence and imperfection of all human relationships, we yearn and strive for sustaining, harmonious, satisfying connections. But intimate relationships, whether between marital partners, lovers, parent and child, siblings, or close friends, are like double-edged swords. They expose us not only to exquisite experiences of loving and being loved, of giving and receiving empathic understanding, but also to indescribably painful times of betrayal, hurt, and loneliness. At pivotal junctures they bring us to a crossroad, offering either an opportunity for psychological transformation or the danger of wounding without gain. Depth psychotherapeutic[1] relationships are no exception, even though the relationship is established with the prescribed purpose of facilitating healing and positive change in the patient, and even though the roles of each participant are carefully structured. I have written this book because I would like to bring some light to this hidden and uncharted, but nonetheless real, problematic side of the healing profession of psychotherapy.

Patients[2] in therapy hope to and do come to understand and transform their deepest wounds as well as have new experiences of themselves and others. Therapists[3] anticipate and do enjoy the gratifying experiences of being helpful and feeling competent and skillful. But more often than we imagine to be the case, as my clinical work and that of other therapists document, painful predicaments serious enough to rupture the relationship can and do arise, leaving both patient and therapist vulnerable to profound wounding and immediate and often prolonged feelings of failure and despair. If the therapeutic relationship ends painfully in a rupture, both participants must manage a complex set of feelings and come to some understanding of how the impasse and abrupt termination came about.

I have written this book from the dual perspective of therapist and patient, drawing upon twenty years of experience as a therapist in private practice, my accumulated knowledge of different theoretical perspectives, and my experiences as a patient in therapy during these years. Although I have the advantage of having occupied both positions within the therapeutic relationship, my experiences are processed through the particular filters provided by being a Caucasian, middle-class, married woman with children. I offer my background to help readers locate and clarify my unavoidable biases and gaps. I have written the book for patients and therapists, including in each the therapist-in-the-patient and the patient-in-the-therapist.

Within the medical model that has traditionally provided the framework for the therapeutic relationship, therapists have been viewed simplistically as experts who are psychologically healthy. Patients have been regarded equally simplistically as individuals who suffer and need help. But virtually all psychotherapists have also been patients in psychotherapy, often more than once. Many therapists have been patients in therapeutic relationships that ruptured in the face of unresolvable dilemmas. Because ruptured terminations (as distinct from negative therapeutic reactions in which patients repeatedly destroy therapeutic relationships) are rarely talked about, either by therapists or patients, we have no information as to how therapists have assimilated and integrated these experiences, nor about how their disturbing personal experiences as patients have affected their attitude toward their work.

Analogously, patients often have accurate perceptions of the vulnerabilities of their therapists (and of themselves) that go unacknowledged or disconfirmed because psychological health tends to be located exclusively in the therapist. Many of the problems that bring patients to psychotherapy have resulted from their efforts to heal and maintain the psychological stability of others, despite the personal cost involved. I emphasize the importance of recognizing the therapist-in-the-patient and the patient-in-the-therapist because, as the ensuing chapters will illustrate, predicaments in therapeutic relationships have the best chance of being worked with constructively when the strengths and vulnerabilities of both participants, regardless of their role as patient or as therapist, are acknowledged and explored. *A major challenge facing the profession of psychotherapy consists of finding constructive ways of including the vulnerabilities of psychotherapists, without discrediting their capacity to help patients, as well as those of patients in understanding the experiences that occur within the therapeutic relationship.* The most problematic impasses, wounding, and ruptures occur when patients' and therapists' vulnerabilities intersect in problematic ways.

I initially became interested in the topic of therapeutic impasses and ruptured terminations because of two experiences I had as a patient during the time that I was also a therapist. In both relationships, one that lasted six years with a psychoanalytically oriented therapist and one that lasted four and a half years with a Freudian psychoanalyst, I reached a stalemate that led to an experience of profound wounding that could not be integrated into the relationship. Both therapeutic relationships eventually ended in a rupture, leaving me with the profoundly disturbing feeling that I had been harmed rather than helped. I was also left with other difficult feelings, including anger, frustration, grief, shame, failure, and a fear of being beyond help as a patient. In addition, I had grave concerns about my chosen profession of therapy. Two subsequent experiences as a patient with analysts of both genders were positive. The therapeutic relationships that ended with predominantly positive feelings and an experience of mutual empathy also included impasses and wounding, but the difficult phases were negotiated successfully.

I wanted to learn from these equally intense and contrasting experiences as a patient both to enhance my personal self-awareness and professional skills, and to convey to other therapists and patients what I had learned. Beginning in 1986, I began giving presentations to groups of therapists on the topic of impasses and ruptured terminations. The therapists who attended the talks were interested, receptive, and eager to share their personal experiences. I began to receive requests to provide consultation to therapists and patients who were in the midst of impasses or who had terminated in a rupture as a consequence of an impasse. The individuals who contacted me wanted help in understanding what had transpired as well as an orientation toward working constructively with the situation. The following chapters synthesize what I have learned over the years from the multiple perspectives of patient, therapist, and consultant about how therapeutic impasses, wounding, and ruptured terminations come about and how they can be worked with constructively by therapists and patients.

In an effort to find out how common impasses and ruptured terminations of therapeutic relationships might be among other psychotherapists, I conducted a survey in 1986. I sent a questionnaire (see Appendix A) to the 330 therapist-members of the Psychotherapy Institute in Berkeley, California inquiring whether they had been patients in long-term therapy that ended in an impasse with accompanying feelings of rage, disappointment, or sense of failure. The rate of return of the questionnaires was consistent with that for other mailings, suggesting that the therapists who responded were representative of a group of active members-at-large rather than of a special subgroup of therapists who had experienced impasses and ruptures in personal therapeutic relationships.

A table containing the results of the research can be found in Appendix B, but I will summarize them here. I found no statistically significant difference in whether the ruptured termination occurred with the same or opposite sex therapist-dyad or within specific age categories, indicating that ruptures cannot be attributed to simple, visible factors such as gender and age differences. The source of impasses and ruptured endings to therapeutic relationships is more complicated, residing in the interaction of the individual psyches and subjective experiences of the patient and therapist.[4]

As many as 87.5% of the therapists who responded reported that they had had patients leave them in a state of impasse. Although the percentage is high, the finding itself is not surprising. Most therapists have had the troubling experience of patients leaving them abruptly in a state of distress. Even when the abrupt and angry departure of patients is attributed to their psychopathology or their lack of readiness to confront their issues, the experience is nonetheless disturbing for therapists.

I had anticipated that a small percentage of the therapists who responded might have been patients in therapeutic relationships that ended in a rupture. I thought that ruptured terminations would be unusual in a sample of therapists, who presumably constitute a highly motivated, psychologically minded group of patients. I was therefore startled to find that as many as 53% had been patients in a therapy that ended in a rupture. Of these therapists, 19% had been patients in two or more therapy experiences that terminated in an impasse. Perhaps the most striking and intriguing additional finding was that *72% of the therapists who as patients terminated psychotherapeutic relationships in an impasse were left feeling harmed by their experience.* The recognition that I was working in a helping profession that had an underestimated and unacknowledged potential to leave patients feeling harmed was particularly distressing. I had inadvertently stumbled on an area of exploration that would preoccupy me for some time: What could have happened in the therapeutic relationship that left such a large number of patients feeling not only that the experience was a waste of time and money, but that they had actually been hurt? What could have happened to leave a large number of therapists not only concerned about their professional skills but doubtful of the value of their chosen work?

Findings on the resolution of the experience of a negative ending were hopeful. Some respondents (20%) reported that they had resolved the experience on their own. Others (58%) reported that they had resolved it in another therapy, suggesting that individuals are not completely discouraged from seeking help from a new therapist after having a problematic experience with a past therapist. Another group (22%) reported that they had resolved the experience both on their own and in another therapy. Nearly one fifth of the respondents (17%) reported that the ending still felt unresolved, indicating that it can take a long time to arrive at an understanding of a ruptured termination experience. Impasses, wounding, and ruptured terminations are intense, powerful experiences that, if not ignored or repressed, can offer a special opportunity for new awareness of their vulnerabilities and defenses for both patients and therapists.

In addition to the statistical findings of my survey of Institute members, the comments that forty-five of the therapists who responded wrote on the questionnaires added substance and texture to the numbers. The comments, although brief, transform abstract numbers into actual people who have suffered and have intense feelings about their painful experiences in psychotherapy, regardless of whether they are in the role of patient or of therapist.

Comments written by therapists who were troubled by the experience of having had patients terminate abruptly in an unresolvable stalemate indicate that therapists are clearly vulnerable to being wounded by patients. The comments, submitted anonymously, describe feelings of anger, hurt, and especially disappointment. Most therapists are invested in their work with patients and want the relationship to be positive and beneficial. One therapist wrote the following comment about two patients who decided to terminate abruptly in the midst of an impasse: *One ended suddenly over the phone. The other patient "did it right" and terminated over a period of several weeks. With both of them I felt and still feel unfinished. I have a sense of failure, I'm angry at them, still wondering what were my needs and what were theirs.* Once patients leave, therapists have no further access to them. They are left to ponder alone how their patients might be working with the problematic ending and to speculate endlessly about how they might have worked differently with them.

Comments from therapists who were patients in therapeutic relationships that ended in a rupture, like the tip of the proverbial iceberg, provide a sense of the wide range of experiences and the amount of emotional pain that often remains out of sight, hidden beneath the surface. One patient wrote about her abrupt termination: *The ending was very devastating to me. The therapist would not deal with issues between us. I dreamed of her for more than a year after we stopped meeting. Many dreams indicated that her wounding was similar to mine. After eight years I am angry still.* A man who had two severed therapeutic relationships with therapists wrote: *My disappointment and rage with my therapies, particularly the first one, took a long time to ease after the relationships ended.* The tone of the comments suggests that given an opportunity, individuals are eager and relieved to be able to share their experiences, want to learn from them, and when possible, repair them.

As my survey indicates, along with findings from other research studies that are summarized in Appendix C, impasses and ruptured terminations are not limited to therapeutic relationships with patients who would be considered to have serious psychological disturbances or who have a compelling psychological need to end the relationship in a rupture, as in negative therapeutic reactions. They occur in relationships between experienced and skilled therapists and patients who are not only effective in managing their lives, but who are motivated and introspective. But the prevailing view of psychological "health" has been firmly grounded in the ideal image of a rational person who does not have psychological vulnerabilities. Therapists as well as patients have resisted talking openly about impasses and ruptures because these experiences have been regarded as failures that could have been avoided if the patient were less disturbed or the therapist more skillful.

The new perspective that I am emphasizing in this book views the unresolvable dilemmas—mismatches, impasses, and wounding—that can lead to ruptures, not as avoidable failures, but rather as *common, inevitable occurrences that present us with a special opportunity for new awareness and change as well as for the dangerous possibility of a wounding and disillusioning setback.* Mismatches occur when the vulnerabilities and defensive modes of patient and therapist intersect in problematic ways. Impasses, wounding, and ruptures occur when the primary vulnerabilities of both patient and therapist cannot be accessed, are being avoided, or once activated cannot be managed.

When our central vulnerabilities come to the surface in a therapeutic relationship, we have a rare opening to work with them that cannot occur when they lurk in the background. By viewing mismatches, impasses, wounding, and ruptures as failure experiences that can be avoided, by locating the source exclusively in the patient's psychopathology or patient-induced countertransference, and by backing away from the difficult task of describing them in words, we pass by the special opportunity that they provide to work constructively with our most central vulnerabilities.

When mismatches, impasses, wounding, and ruptures are regarded as uncharted territory rather than as problems that can be solved or avoided, we embark on a risky exploration that we have resisted undertaking because it challenges both the viability of our healing profession and our desire for certainty. Once we contemplate these relatively unexplored dilemmas with interest and curiosity rather than with preconceptions based upon a fear that our fundamental beliefs and assumptions will be irrevocably disrupted, we begin to see the vast store of information that they hold. *A second major challenge faced by the profession thus consists of including the silent voices of patients and therapists who have experienced unworkable impasses, wounding, or ruptures.*

The resistances on the part of both patients and therapists to moving toward these troubling experiences are not difficult to understand. Both therapists and patients wish to appear competent and fear exposing vulnerabilities or inadequacies. Our culture values highly the capacity to put painful experiences behind us. As human beings, we know that we must continue on with our lives in the face of the painful losses that are part of the human condition. We fear becoming mired in grief or immobilized by despair. No wonder that we have difficulty holding opposites in consciousness simultaneously: the possibility of being both competent and vulnerable, the healer and the wounded, strong and weak, rational and irrational.[5] In therapeutic relationships, these pairs of opposites have been split. The patient has carried one side and the therapist the other. Patients have assumed the role of the irrational, vulnerable, weak, wounded member of the dyad, whereas therapists have assumed the role of the rational, invulnerable, strong healer. Both patients and therapists have been limited by these constricted roles, and more importantly, the potential for what can be included in the therapeutic relationship has been curtailed.

Even for those patients and therapists who overcome the resistance to sharing painful experiences, describing in ordinary language the intense emotions that are an essential part of mismatches, impasses, wounding, and ruptured terminations of therapeutic relationships is a daunting task. How can the patient who could not tolerate a scheduling mishap and demanded to have his session at the time he thought was his, even though his therapist was with another patient, communicate the depth of his rage and pain without appearing to be disturbed? How is he to explain his temporary loss of self-control as more than an overreaction? How can the ordinarily compassionate therapist communicate the full extent of his distress, his annoyance at his vulnerable patient for being incapable of agreeing to return for the extra session he offered?

Not only is it difficult to find language to fit these experiences, which are more common than we realize, but patients and therapists also feel considerable shame about the intensity of their responses to them. Patients who reveal their response to wounding in therapy know that they are apt to appear naive, childish, and psychologically undeveloped. Their emotional responses to the behaviors of their therapists can seem extreme to others, leaving them at risk of pathological judgments. The events that triggered the impasses, wounding, and ruptures often do seem ordinary or trivial to those who are outside the relationship and outside the context of the personal meaning to the patient. Therapists also resist experiencing themselves or being seen by others as inadequate and incompetent, as overreacting to a trivial mishap, and experiencing the despair that can arise from facing the impossibility of avoiding experiences of wounding in therapy.

Despite these resistances and difficulties, I have been persisting in an exploration of therapeutic impasses and ruptured terminations in therapy because of my conviction that they contain a rich source of information, one that is just as valuable as the personal accounts of successful psychotherapy experiences. Mirroring a culture that prizes rational understanding, the profession of therapy has overvalued our theories of therapy and has emphasized primarily the personal experiences that support these theories. By excluding and silencing the voices of patients and therapists who have endured impasses, wounding, and ruptures that fall outside the realm of successful therapeutic relationships, we have lost access to the knowledge that might be gained from the experiences that do not fit our models.

The major founders of the profession—Freud, Jung, Klein—relied on self-analysis of difficult personal states as the basis for the theoretical concepts that are their legacies.[6] Over time their theoretical contributions have been elevated in stature, while their human qualities and experiences have been pushed into the background or brought forth in sensationalistic rather than respectful and compassionate ways.[7] The gap between life experience and theory has increased accordingly, as has the rigidification of theory that renders it unresponsive to new experiences.

Psychotherapists are currently making an effort to shift our reliance upon a medical model to a relational model that encompasses the interaction of both therapist and patient and their mutual impact upon each other.[8] But paradigm shifts occur over time, and an expanded paradigm of therapy has not yet become widely accepted. An extensive literature is evolving and incorporates concepts that can be employed in explaining impasses and ruptures in therapeutic relationships. The professional literature includes such concepts as transference and countertransference dilemmas, projective identification (whereby patients communicate nonverbally to the therapists by inducing in them painful affect states and experiences that cannot be conveyed in descriptive language), and empathic failures.

Although each of these concepts is useful, particularly when applied in individual cases, the inclusion of the enduring personal vulnerabilities of therapists that are not reducible to difficult states their patients induce has not yet become widely accepted. Moreover, the language of relevant concepts, including such terms as "countertransference" and "projective identification," is highly technical and consequently inaccessible to many patients. The abstract terminology implies that if we can label a mechanism or occurrence, we can understand and master it, and that "pathological" or undesirable responses can be avoided, reinforcing the illusion that impasses and ruptures can be avoided by individuals who have acquired sound psychological skills and who are psychologically "healthy."

But intimate human relationships, like nature and life itself, cannot be fully understood or controlled. Mismatches, impasses, wounding, and ruptures occur in relationships just as thunderstorms and fires occur in nature and unexpected events happen in life. I have worked toward evolving a conceptual frame, couched in ordinary language, that encompasses the many different kinds of mismatches, impasses, wounding, and ruptured terminations that inevitably occur and that includes the psychological vulnerabilities of both therapist and patient without pathologizing or judging either individual. The following chapters will provide examples of the kinds of predicaments that occur in therapeutic relationships and will suggest ways of working with them when possible, enduring them, and healing from them if necessary. In addition to providing a wide range of clinical examples, I will return throughout the book to two extended cases in order to consider them from different theoretical perspectives. With a differentiated conceptual understanding of the variety of the dilemmas that can occur, those that herald a necessary although painful change can be distinguished from those that signal a fundamental problem in the therapeutic relationship.

For the purpose of organization, even though there are overlaps between and within categories, I have found that predicaments in therapy that lead to ruptured terminations fall into three categories. One includes relationships in which problems arise as a result of *a lack of fit or mismatch* between patient and therapist. Mismatches arise around a number of factors that range from visible characteristics of patients and therapists, such as gender, age, and theoretical orientation, to more complex and elusive qualities, such as the patients' and therapists' personalities, core vulnerabilities, and empathic capacities.

The second category consists of impasses in which the therapeutic relationship is caught in a stalemate. In these impasses, patients and therapists are stuck in an entrenched mode of relating and are unable to shift to a different or more expanded mode that would enable a wider range of issues to be brought into the therapeutic relationship. Patient and therapist might participate, for example, in a comfortable, familiar, superficially gratifying mode of relating that prevents both of them from tripping into areas of vulnerability that need to be entered if the therapy is to progress. Although a sense of control and stability is preserved, nothing new and informative can occur and an impasse results. Patient and therapist may also become trapped in agonizing deadlocks in which the patient experiences the therapist as dangerous and harmful and the therapist cannot restore a working alliance with the patient. Impasses can also occur at the beginning of a new developmental phase when the needs of the patient shift and a different response from the therapist is required, or conversely, when the therapist's needs change and a different response from the patient is required.

Painful ruptures can occur when either the patient or the therapist attempts to break out of an entrenched mode of relating and the other individual frantically resists the change and struggles to restore the old, familiar alliance.[9] If a rupture of the therapeutic relationship occurs at this juncture instead of the establishment of a new relational mode, and if the patient and therapist try to move on and put the ruptured termination behind them, the opportunity is lost to understand what might have been opened up had a new phase of therapy begun.

The third category consists of patients who have been wounded, either by an outside life event or by an action of the therapist, in what I have called *areas of primary vulnerability*. Patients in this category are the ones most likely to feel that they have been injured or harmed by the experience. I have used the term "primary vulnerability" despite the fact that analogous concepts exist (e.g., psychotic or primitive core, basic fault, or borderline part of the personality), because it avoids the pathological connotations of the other terms and because the other terms have been used only in reference to patients and not to therapists as well. The unbalanced focus on patients has consequently been perpetuated, leaving the impression that therapists qualitatively differ from them rather than emphasizing the reality that patients and therapists alike are human beings and as such grapple with psychological issues, more or less successfully, as a fundamental part of being human.

The concept of primary vulnerability, which will be addressed at length in a subsequent chapter, refers to an area of central sensitivity in the patient and therapist. When patients are wounded in an area of primary vulnerability by their therapists, or when therapists are wounded in an area of primary vulnerability by their patients, painful impasses can ensue. Therapists, thrown off by the intense and seemingly extreme responses of their wounded patients, are in danger of responding to the patients in a manner that creates an additional level of wounding and places the therapeutic relationship in jeopardy. When the relationship is at risk, the threat of a rupture of the important attachment bond that patients form with their therapists creates additional anxiety and fear of loss that in turn escalate the problems in the relationship.

Therapists embroiled in turmoil with patients are understandably apt to overlook the extent to which their patients are attached to them, particularly when the patients are behaving as if the relationship is worthless. When therapists feel devalued and discounted, their capacity to empathize with their patients is thwarted because their psychological energy is directed toward the preservation of their sense of a therapist-self, and their need for empathic understanding and appreciation is heightened. The intense affects that patients and therapists experience, their defensive reactions in relation to each other, and their diminished capacities for empathy and psychological reflection need not diminish the value of psychotherapy as a tool for understanding and change nor constitute manifestations of psychopathology or incompetence in the patient or therapist.

In addition to being useful in orienting patients and therapists who are caught in painful predicaments, an in-depth understanding of the kinds of dilemmas I have outlined has opened up challenging new territory: the possibility of providing special consultation to therapists and patients who are at the pivotal juncture of one of these dilemmas. *A third major challenge to the profession of psychotherapy lies in exploring the risks and benefits of providing an expanded relational context in the form of consultation for therapeutic dyads that are being stretched to their limit.* The continuing requests for consultation that I have been receiving as a result of giving presentations on the topic of impasses and ruptured terminations attest to the need for the special functions that a therapist-consultant can provide—functions that have not yet been formally articulated. There is no existing model for consultation of this kind, and the prospect of it gives rise to important questions and anxieties: Does consultation to therapeutic relationships or to patients by definition constitute an intrusion into an ongoing therapy, or can consultation be conducted in a manner that makes it a constructive and creative response to therapeutic relationships that are at risk? Under what circumstances does a consultant meet with the therapist, the patient, or both, and at whose request? Is it correct to assume that patients will simplistically perceive the therapist with whom they are struggling as "bad" and a consultant whom they hope will rescue them as "good?" Theoretical perspectives, which also reflect the psychological needs of the therapists who are drawn to them, have vastly different philosophical underpinnings that lead to varying conceptions of consultation. For example, consultation can be perceived by a therapists with different convictions about psychotherapy as bringing in the helpful presence of an "other," as an interference or an intrusion into the sanctity of the existing therapeutic dyad, as providing a safe holding environment for the therapeutic dyad, or as a communication to the patient that she is too much for the primary therapist or to the therapist that she is inadequate.

These questions and concerns need to be addressed explicitly, so that the pressing needs of patients and therapists who have been seeking consultation do not go unmet because of anxieties and resistances that operate individually and collectively. The chapters in Part III take up these questions and provide examples of how a consultant can function in situations of mismatches, impasses, and wounding. A consultant centered in a nonpathologizing, nonjudgmental framework, who keeps the vulnerabilities and strengths of both patient and therapist clearly in view, has an opportunity to identify unworkable mismatches and to make recommendations that enable patients and therapists to shift relational modes without feeling that they have failed or been rejected. A consultant can intervene with a new perspective when therapist–patient dyads are locked into unresolvable deadlocks, facilitating the shift that can help the therapeutic relationship move forward. In therapeutic relationships in which wounding in the realm of primary vulnerability has occurred, a consultant can humanize one individual for the other, enabling each participant to regroup psychologically, allowing the wounding to be understood within a restored therapeutic alliance or endured until a shift occurs. If the therapeutic alliance cannot be restored, the consultant can help the therapist and patient terminate without judgment or blame, with an awareness of the vulnerabilities that were exposed in the relationship and that remain to be worked on. Both participants can terminate with some sense of resolution and completion instead of with feelings of failure, self-doubt, and hopelessness. A consultant centered in this framework can help patients whose therapeutic relationships have already ended in a rupture come to terms with the experience, so that they can move on without the lingering burden of painful feelings or a pervasive sense of shame and failure.

In Part II of the book, I will draw upon aspects of different existing theoretical perspectives, singling out and explicating concepts that relate to mismatches, impasses, wounding, and ruptures in therapeutic relationships. I will also present findings from the currently proliferating research studies on infant development that shed light on the origin of our areas of vulnerability. Readers who are not already familiar with the theoretical concepts should find that they are explained in a readily accessible language that does not presume a familiarity with the theories from which they derive. I hope that readers who are familiar with the theoretical concepts and research findings will discover that considering them anew in relation to impasses, wounding, and ruptured terminations can provide a fresh understanding. For example, concepts that are analogous to the realm of primary vulnerability take on new meaning when applied to the therapist as well as to the patient. *A fourth challenge to the profession of psychotherapy—if we are to include therapeutic dyads that struggle with impasses, wounding, and ruptures among those we consider typical—resides in the need to develop theoretical concepts that further our understanding of troubled therapeutic relationships.* We need concepts that will enable us to describe the modes of relating and the modes of representing self, other, and the relationship that characterize *both* patients and therapists in therapeutic dyads that are at risk of a rupture.

I hope that an expanded consciousness of the issues involved in impasses, wounding, and ruptures in therapy will enable patients and therapists alike to be less fearful of the powerful forces that can be unleashed in therapeutic relationships. Agonizing predicaments in therapy occur at the brink of our most central psychological vulnerabilities and consequently provide an invaluable opportunity for understanding at the deepest level both ourselves and the individuals with whom we are in relationship. We then have the possibility of experiencing the intimacy and compassion that accompanies such understanding.

Throughout the book, I have attempted to weave together the knowledge that can be derived from theory with the equally valuable information gleaned from personal experience. The interweaving of knowledge derived from personal subjective truth with that derived from analytic thinking and outside authorities leads to the rich form of constructed knowledge described by the authors of *Women's Ways of Knowing: The Development of Self, Voice, and Mind*.[10]

Writing the book has given me another opportunity to construct personal knowledge from the raw material of life experience as therapist, patient, and human being, and from the conceptual knowledge abstracted from the efforts of others. I hope that the book will be of use to those individuals who wish to enter with a new orientation the relatively unexplored domain of dilemmas that put therapeutic relationships at risk and of ruptured therapeutic relationships. I hope, too, that the book will encourage other individuals who are endeavoring to construct and maintain personal knowledge and meaning to persist in their struggle. Therein, perhaps, lies the beginning of wisdom.

PART I

❖ **Mismatches, ❖
Impasses, and
Wounding**

CHAPTER ONE

❖ *Mismatches* ❖

An initial dislike may persist and grow, or an initial liking may fade.
It does not mean that this patient could not be analyzed
successfully by someone else. I have taken over and carried on the
analysis of patients referred to me by colleagues, and I know that
more than one patient with whom I failed has worked successfully
with another analyst, whom he found more compatible.

—MARGARET LITTLE[1]

I went to him [Fairbairn] because we stood philosophically on the
same ground and no actual intellectual disagreements would
interfere with the analysis. But the capacity for forming a relationship does not depend solely on our theory. Not everyone has the
same facility for forming personal relationships, and we can all form
a relationship more easily with some people than with others. The
unpredictable factor of "natural fit" enters in. Thus, in spite of his
conviction Fairbairn did not have the same capacity for natural,
spontaneous, "personal relating" that Winnicott had.

—HARRY GUNTRIP[2]

The analysis of a good fit is no doubt possible, but we experience it
as painful, even destructive. To question the good fit is not unlike
questioning the child about the reality status of his transitional
object. Implicitly we know this must not be done. Where there is a
good fit—in contrast to an apparent one produced by compliance—
the relationship itself is healing. The healing consists, in part, in the
faith that we are understood—held fast by a love to which our own
capacity for self-love will some day be anchored.

—STEPHEN KURTZ[3]

Lack of Fit

As the profession of psychotherapy expands the model of an expert
therapist working with troubled patients to a more complex model of
two individuals with separate subjectivities interacting with and
creating each other as they interact, the question of a mismatch, or a
problematic fit between patient and therapist, becomes both more

complicated and more important. In the former model, a mismatch could only be understood as a lack of fit between the particular expertise of the therapist and the problem presented by the patient, as a consequence of a patient being "too disturbed," or as the result of a therapist's lack of experience, use of faulty technique, or inadequate personal analysis. For example, a therapist specializing in working with children, with substance abuse issues, or with more disturbed patients, would refer out prospective patients whose problems were outside her range. If a patient consulted with a therapist who had expertise in the appropriate area and could be assumed to apply that expertise effectively, but the therapeutic relationship did not seem helpful to the patient, the patient could only assume that the problem resided in her and that she might be beyond the pale of psychological help.

In a model of psychotherapy in which a therapist uses her personhood, including knowledge and experience in the field, and the relationship with the patient as instruments of change, the question of how to determine compatibility between patient and therapist becomes much more difficult. In this model, theoretical orientation can no longer be viewed as separate from the therapist who relies on it. The particular theory to which a therapist is drawn, whether it be psychoanalysis, Jungian theory, Object Relations theory, Self psychology, or other frameworks such as the Self-in-Relation theory of female psychology (the Stone Center) and interpersonal psychoanalytic theory (William Alanson White Institute), or some combination of these, has to do with the psychological characteristics of the therapist. Similarly, the theoretical orientation to which a patient is drawn has to do with the psychological characteristics of the patient. Even when there is a good fit between the theoretical orientation of the therapist and that to which the patient is drawn, other variables will affect what transpires in the therapeutic relationship, as the comment at the beginning of this chapter by well-known British Object Relations theorist Harry Guntrip indicates.

With the change in model of psychotherapy from one in which authority resides in the therapist to one in which both patient and therapist are separate centers of subjectivity and initiative, we enter a realm of uncertainty and leave behind the security of objective rules. Choosing a therapist by his or her training and experience or by gender, although important, is not sufficient to protect patients and therapists from situations of mismatch. In this realm of uncertainty, mistakes in choices are inevitable: There will be dyads of patients and therapists who are not good matches but who cannot assess the fit accurately at the outset of the relationship. Others may initially seem to be a good fit but later may encounter issues that render them a mismatch. There will be still others who sense a poor fit early on. These individuals have the task and challenge of acknowledging the mismatch nonjudgmentally and honestly, and of constructively using the experience to gain new information about themselves and to facilitate making a subsequent better match.

As psychotherapy moves toward an intersubjective model, patients and therapists may begin to participate in mutually assessing the nature of the fit and in forthrightly confronting a match that does not work. Currently the burden rests too often with the patient, who is left to extricate herself from an unsatisfactory relationship without the therapist's support and encouragement. Because patients generally find it hard to hold a different opinion from that of their therapists, extricating themselves without their therapists' approval is neither simple nor easy. Therapists are only beginning to confront openly and to share explicitly with patients who are suffering the effects of a mismatch, the *inner* aspects of themselves, other than their theoretical approach or range of experience, that might be contributing to a mismatch or problematic match.

Therapists and patients may arrive at a stalemate in the therapy because of a lack of fit or mismatch that prevents the patient from making use of the therapist and the therapist from having the necessary empathy for the patient. Mismatches that block the communication and empathy that are essential ingredients of psychotherapy can surface in relation to a variety of identifiable factors, including gender, age (phase of life and level of psychological development of patient and therapist), personality characteristics, as well as in relation to the core psychological vulnerabilities of the patient and therapist. But the source of a poor fit may also remain elusive, as mysterious as the source of a good fit, as the quotation at the beginning of the chapter by Stephen Kurtz, the therapist author of *The Art of Unknowing*, suggests. Unlike the good fit, which is best left in place, unanalyzed perhaps until the end of the therapy, poor fits can provide useful information about therapists and patients alike. But until patients and therapists shift their attitude toward mismatches, the sense of failure and blame that pervades the experience of a poor fit will prevent the individuals involved from thinking about the nature of the lack of fit with benign curiosity and interest.

Most therapists wish to help every patient who comes to them. Most patients, unless caught in the grip of an unconscious destructive impulse, hope that the therapist they initially consult will be able to help them.[4] In the initial phase of therapy, both therapist and patient are apt to be enamored of the positive possibilities inherent in the relationship. These expectations are both useful and potentially dangerous. The patient's tendency to perceive the therapist as an idealized healer and the therapist's corresponding tendency to identify with the ideal of the omnipotent healer mesh harmoniously to create the foundation of a positive therapeutic alliance and fuel the special combination of love, nurturance, and compassion that engages the healing energies of both individuals. Gradually, optimally in manageable doses, reality in the guise of difficult interactions and experiences modifies the initial illusions. Patient and therapist come to recognize the impossibility of an enduring perfect fit and accept the reality of a good enough fit, one that includes both areas of connection and areas of disjunction. The innately human yearning nevertheless remains a potential, ready to be reawakened.

The therapist's and patient's hope for a good enough fit makes the acknowledgment of an unworkable match particularly hard. Both individuals are apt to struggle to make the relationship work rather than to relinquish the wish. To end a therapeutic relationship, even one that has gone on only a session or two, requires a level of consciousness that is difficult for patients and therapists to reach and maintain. For a therapist to acknowledge that she is not the best therapist for a particular patient and for a patient to acknowledge that the therapist is not the best person to help her means going against the tempting illusion that therapists should be good enough for most patients who seek their help and requires facing and accepting ordinary human limitations.

Even when therapists are unable to accept a referral because of lack of available time or limitations in area of expertise, most feel a twinge of disappointment: Who was the human being with whom I spoke? What would our relationship have been? When therapists experience a lack of compatibility with potential patients, they face the challenge of determining whether the problematic fit is part of the relational difficulties and personal issues the patient is bringing to therapy for help. If necessary, therapists have the delicate task of referring the patient to another therapist in a balanced, compassionate manner, so that the patient feels seen, understood, and helped, rather than rejected and abandoned. The wish to be helpful often obscures the recognition of inner red flags signaling the therapist that the match is problematic.

Therapists also like to give each therapeutic relationship the benefit of the doubt. A feeling of dislike or of "otherness" in relation to the patient can sometimes be a useful source of information about both the patient and the therapist rather than an indication that there is a lack of fit that will impede the therapeutic relationship. Barbara

Stevens Sullivan, in her book, *Psychotherapy Grounded in the Feminine Principle*, gives an extended case example of a patient named Betty whom she initially disliked.[5] Betty immediately became attached to the therapist in a clinging, dependent, unboundaried manner that the therapist could not tolerate. Her clinging behavior constellated rejecting feelings in the therapist, who initially did not want to face consciously how rejecting she felt. Instead, the therapist had imagined that she would welcome the patient rather than dislike her if only, for example, she would leave the office when the hour was up rather than prolong the session by blowing her nose. When the therapist finally confronted her dislike of her patient, rather than continue to wish that the patient would behave differently, the nature of their relationship changed. The therapist came to understand that her feelings of dislike were part of an attempt to manage the intense fears of abandonment and engulfment that had been activated in both herself and the patient.

When problematic matches are apparent to patients early in the relationship, they often find some reason to leave. One woman in her fifties chose not to meet with a younger therapist because she was certain she needed to see a therapist older than herself. A male patient took an immediate dislike to the office decor of a potential therapist and felt that his dislike represented a lack of mutuality with the therapist that indicated a therapeutic relationship would not work.

When therapists believe that there is an unmanageable, problematic match, they face the challenge of describing their experience of a mismatch carefully to the patient, so that the patient is not left with a feeling of being disliked or of having failed. A colleague of mine once took the risk of including in a paper for presentation a situation in which she had gently suggested to a young man she had been seeing for over a year that she was no longer the best person to help him. Eventually she was able to refer him to a male therapist who she felt would best be able to take the young man to the next phase of his psychological journey. I recall how I wondered at the time whether I would have been able to facilitate such a change.

Sometimes the best intentions and efforts on the part of the therapist to recommend a change of therapist are not sufficient to avoid wounding vulnerable patients who have taken a personal risk by initiating and investing hope in a therapeutic relationship. Recently a colleague nearing retirement age felt that he could not be psychologically available for the intensive, long-term, turbulent relationship that he knew would be necessary with a patient. When he assessed the situation with his patient, the patient became enraged and overwhelmed with suicidal and murderous impulses. He fled from the room and left telephone messages threatening to sue the therapist or kill himself. Although he had a professional and moral obligation to protect the long-term interests of the patient by ensuring that the patient was working with a therapist who could be as available to him as he needed, the therapist was beset by anxiety and fear for himself and for the patient. The telephone threats eventually subsided, but the therapist, despite having behaved responsibly and ethically, has had to live with continuing episodes of worry and uncertainty about how the patient managed his distress: Did the wounding experience drive the patient into further hopelessness and despair, or was the patient able to find a therapist who could work with him?

A sense of compatibility on the part of both participants in the therapeutic relationship is essential. If patients who are paired with incompatible therapists are unable to terminate the relationship and instead continue to struggle unsuccessfully to make the relationship work, a frustrating course of therapy and a termination laden with disappointment and negative feelings may ensue. As long as patients and therapists are burdened by the unfortunate illusion that all therapists are experts who can help any patient who comes through the door, letting go of therapeutic relationships in which there is an unmanageable match will be a struggle. This illusion prevents patients from moving on when they feel that the therapist they have chosen is not right for them. Therapists are equally inhibited from finding empathic ways of providing prospective patients with referrals to other therapists who would be a better match. Consultation to patient and/or therapist who are caught in this dilemma can be helpful in ending a painful stalemate.

Sometimes a therapist and patient try to work together in spite of an experience of an unmanageable lack of fit, either because they disavow its significance, hope to work through it to a better place, or attribute its presence to personal psychological problems that will be resolved as the therapy progresses. When effort is invested in the therapeutic relationship, patient and therapist alike find it difficult to make the decision to let go. Familiarity and inertia, as well as the psychological problems that bring patients to therapy, operate to maintain the relationship rather than to facilitate a change.

If the lack of fit between patient and therapist prevents a solid attachment bond from forming and blocks communication and empathy, the therapy cannot progress. A rupture in the relationship, although extremely painful for both individuals, can serve the positive function of ending the stalemate and enabling patients to leave. But the patients who terminate such unproductive relationships without an understanding that the relationship was not a good enough fit are vulnerable to intense feelings of frustration, anger, hopelessness, or disappointment.

Lack of Fit Due to Stage of Life

A good example of a lack of fit or mismatch due to the stage of life of the therapist is provided by Harry Guntrip, well-known British analyst and theorist. Guntrip chose W. R. D. Fairbairn as his first analyst toward the end of Fairbairn's life. Fairbairn was ill himself, as well as depressed because of the death of his wife, and consequently had less energy available for his work. Guntrip profited from the analysis but perhaps not to the extent he would have if he had come to Fairbairn earlier in his life.[6] Guntrip writes about Fairbairn in the last article he wrote during his lifetime. The article, his final legacy to us, was published posthumously:

> I went to him in the 1950s when he was past the peak of his creative powers of the 1940s and his health was slowly failing. He told me that in the 1930s and 1940s he had treated a number of schizophrenic and regressed patients with success. . . . By the 1950s when I was with him, he wisely declined to take the strains of severely regressing patients. To my surprise I found him gradually falling back on the "classical analyst" with an "interpretive technique," when I felt I needed to regress to the level of that severe infancy trauma.[7]

The regression to infancy that Guntrip sought also did not occur during a second analysis with D. W. Winnicott, despite Winnicott's remarkable intuitive understanding of Guntrip's significant early losses (his mother's emotional unavailability and his younger brother's death when Guntrip was three years old). Guntrip's yearned-for regression to an experience of his depressed and unavailable mother ironically happened at the end of his life, many years after their therapeutic relationship had ended, shortly after Guntrip learned of Winnicott's death. The regression took place in a series of dreams that permitted Guntrip to reexperience what it was like to be in the presence of his depressed, unavailable mother during the early years of his life.

Although Guntrip, from the vantage point of the end of a long and full life, was aware of the limitations of Fairbairn and Winnicott, he nonetheless expressed his gratitude and appreciation of the positive influence that both therapists had on his psychological growth. Well aware, too, of the potential for harm of any therapeutic relationship, he concluded his final article with the following sentence:

All through life we take into ourselves both good and bad figures who either strengthen or disturb us, and it is the same in psychoanalytic therapy: it is the meeting and interacting of two real people in all its complex possibilities.[8]

Lack of Fit Due to Limits of Knowledge

The profession of psychotherapy is a relative newcomer to the scene and continues to evolve rapidly. Therapists and patients are continually extending the frontiers of our understanding. One consequence of the changing state of our knowledge and experience is that certain patients bring issues to their therapy that the therapists are not yet able to understand and respond to. These patients become the teachers of their therapists, paving the way for others to come.

Margaret Little, another well-known British psychoanalyst, consulted Winnicott after completing an analysis with psychoanalyst Ella Sharpe that taught her a great deal about analysis and helped her qualify as a psychoanalyst herself. But, in Little's words, "when she [Sharpe] died, I knew that none of my real problems had been touched."[9] According to Margaret Little, Sharpe's failure to address her real problems was due to Sharpe's limitations: "Ella Sharpe didn't recognize psychotic anxiety or transference psychosis. They were beyond her limits. That wasn't her 'fault,' and it wasn't due to any lack of integrity in her; analysis had not developed that far yet."[10] In a more recent book-length account of her analyses with Sharpe and Winnicott, Little describes the mismatch:

> The overall picture of my analysis with Miss Sharpe is one of constant struggle between us, she insisting on interpreting what I said as due to intrapsychic conflict to do with infantile sexuality, and I trying to convey to her that my real problems were matters of existence and identity: I did not know what "myself" was: sexuality (even if known) was totally irrelevant and meaningless unless existence and survival could be taken for granted, and personal identity established.[11]

Little eventually began an analysis with Winnicott, whose evolving ideas on regression to a state of dependence, the facilitating environment, and the importance of psychological holding, along with his recognition of Little's psychotic anxiety, enabled her to journey in his company from a state of illness to health. When she ultimately expressed her gratitude and her wish to Winnicott that she had gotten to see him sooner, "he answered that he could not have done my analysis sooner—he would not have known enough."[12]

Lack of Fit Due to Personality Type

An extensive example of two failed therapeutic relationships because of a lack of fit due to personality type is contained in the book *Flowers on Granite: One Woman's Odyssey Through Psychoanalysis* written by Dorte von Drigalski, a female physician in psychoanalytic training.[13] Drigalski worked first with a female therapist and then with a man. In both therapies, her personality and those of the therapists were a poor fit. Without support for acknowledging the mismatch and without encouragement to make a change, both relationships ended unsatisfactorily.

Drigalski, like many patients who take for granted that the therapist is an expert who can help them, assumed that her first therapist, the woman, carried the "truth" about her. From the beginning of their relationship, she disavowed her own feelings and perceptions, accepting the therapist's interpretations even when they felt absolutely incorrect. Drigalski disliked her therapist from the beginning because of distinct differences in personality and lifestyle between them. Drigalski was an attractive young woman, oriented toward a healthy way of life. Her therapist was a small woman who continued smoking cigarettes despite a persistent, racking cough. Drigalski disavowed these differences even though they prevented the establishment of a strong positive therapeutic alliance. Instead, she tried to accept her friends' opinion that she was avoiding her positive feelings for her therapist. The fact that other patients in therapy with the same woman had positive feelings for her left Drigalski confused and in doubt as to the validity of her negative perceptions.

An example of how Drigalski accepted the therapist's interpretation of the meaning of her behavior and relinquished her own is provided by the following incident: Drigalski became interested in a man shortly after beginning analysis. The analyst interpreted her interest as a resistance to the analysis and her attraction to the man as a derivative of sexual interest in her stepfather (who, like the man, had bags under his eyes). When the relationship with the man ended (in part as a result of her interpretations), the analyst was impatient with Drigalski's mourning of its loss.

Drigalski eventually moved to another town and changed to a male analyst with whom she got off to another bad start, again the result of a lack of fit related to personality type and perhaps to theoretical orientation and gender as well. Although she experienced negative feelings about the analyst from the very beginning, his reputation and her need to complete a successful analysis in order to further her own training, as well as personal issues that caused her to blame herself for her negative feelings about him, kept her from terminating the work and finding a different therapist.

The therapist had fixed ideas and perceptions about his patient from the beginning. But Drigalski was not a compliant woman and did not accept his interpretations when she disagreed with him. She left her first session feeling as if he had not really listened to her. She continued to meet with him but quickly reached an impasse over a disagreement in their interpretations of the meaning of a particular interaction between them. This deadlock resulted in tension, which Drigalski labeled the "Westwall atmosphere" (after the Berlin Wall). The Westwall atmosphere recurred at various times throughout their relationship.

From the perspective of an outsider, Drigalski's insistence on maintaining her subjective point of view in the face of differences with her male analyst would appear to be an improvement over her passive compliance in her first therapeutic relationship with the female therapist. But her analyst did not like her resistance to his interpretations and formed a negative opinion of her state of mental health and her readiness to advance in the training institute of which they were both a part. They finally agreed to terminate the relationship after enduring repeated states of impasse that were never understood or resolved. Unfortunately, the analyst was influential in the training institute's denial of advancement for Drigalski, and she ultimately left the field of psychoanalysis altogether.

Drigalski's book describes in excruciating detail the disastrous consequences of ignoring a lack of fit due to personality type. Had either therapist been able to relinquish their inflexible viewpoints and operate from a working model of psychotherapy that includes the subjectivities of both therapist and patient, then the lack of fit arising from personality differences, including the therapists' need for power and control and their related rigid theoretical stance, might have been circumvented.

Even if a failure experience occurs, as in Drigalski's case, both patient and therapist can expand their self-knowledge by exploring it rather than avoiding the painful experience of facing it. Just as scientific experiments in which the results do not support the hypothesis can contribute important information, so, too, accounts of failed therapies can further our understanding. Scientific experiments that disconfirm hypotheses may be disappointing, but they do not constitute an indictment of the scientific field, the researchers, or diminish the significance of the problem at hand. Similarly, accounts of failed therapies need not serve as condemnations of the profession or of the competence of the individuals involved.

Unfortunately the English translation of Drigalski's book is prefaced by an introduction by Jeffrey Moussaieff Masson, an iconoclastic scholar of Freudian psychoanalysis, who uses her story to bolster his point of view that the very idea of one person seeing another in psychotherapy is dangerous and wrong. His critical comments are valuable in pinpointing specific problem areas of the profession, such as the power imbalance between therapist and patient, but his conclusions about its inherent destructiveness are as incomplete and unbalanced as those who contend that psychotherapy only heals.

Lack of Fit Due to Theoretical Orientation

The book *My Kleinian Home*, written by psychoanalyst Nini Herman, represents another unusual book-length account of unsuccessful therapeutic relationships by a patient.[14] Herman's story opens a window onto the complexity of situations in which there is a lack of fit, one that in her case was largely created by the therapist's theoretical orientation. Because many patients who seek psychotherapy are not well acquainted with the variety of theoretical perspectives that exist—Freud, Jung, Self-Psychology, British Object Relations, Interpersonal—they cannot know clearly what approach might best suit their needs before trying one out or immersing themselves in a therapeutic relationship. Many therapists practicing today draw from more than one theoretical perspective, particularly as the dialogue between practitioners of different schools increases.[15]

The lack of fit in Herman's situation is due to the misalliance between the theoretical orientation of the first two therapists that she consulted and her specific needs. Herman writes candidly about the inappropriateness of her first analysis with a Jungian therapist because she needed to come to an understanding of her early life experience before working with dreams and archetypal aspects of herself. The Jungian analyst she consulted did not work with early experiences in the family of origin, but rather concentrated on dream analysis and the archetypes. The result was a mismatch between the therapist's theoretical orientation and the patient's personal needs related to her level of psychological development.

Unfortunately, Herman could not come to know her needs without first living through the experience of failing to have them adequately met. The therapist, who knew no other mode of therapy, could not recommend an alternative method as more appropriate. The Jungian analyst was clearly devoted to Herman and did her best to be helpful with all the resources she had available. In fact, she was able to urge Herman to return to analysis at a critical crisis point in Herman's life. Herman is able to describe in retrospect the theoretical lack of fit between the two of them:

> Jung was never much concerned with the infant struggling to get out in the course of psychotherapy. His genius overlooked this funda-mental ABC, which it scorned as "reductive" in its search for higher truths and transcendental nourishment. This the infantile mind cannot digest or utilize, where it has failed to solve its earlier conflict situations.[16]

> [referring to the archetypes] "the Shadow" and "the Personal," "the Human Types" and "the Mandala"; these constitute a luxury. But the sick and starving mind gasps for deeper understanding the infant can assimilate.[17]

After the death of Herman's child and the ensuing dissolution of her marital relationship, Herman's Jungian analyst urged her to return to analysis in the town to which she had moved. Herman took the Jungian analyst's advice and consulted a retired therapist, a Freudian, who served as a bridge that carried her eventually into a Freudian analysis. Herman writes eloquently about this "fine man," affirming that theoretical orientation "does not a therapist make." Personal wisdom, culled from life experience through the fire of suffering, is what makes a therapist:

> Eclectic in a home-brewed sweep, he was basically a Freudian, and gradually instilled in me a taste for that great edifice I had been skirting to my cost. I would not presume to judge just how competent he was by the later standards I acquired, based upon concepts of their own, for this remarkable old man was largely outside categories, thanks to the accomplishment of an integral and well-seated soul, as is all too rarely found in the orthodox professional ranks.
>
> I went to see him twice a week, lay on his simple, generous couch, felt contained by his staunch support and started thinking that perhaps I had a future once again, instead of nothing but a broken past.[18]

Herman then entered training to become a Freudian analyst, for which a personal training analysis was required, as it had been for Drigalski.

Recognizing only in retrospect that she should not have relinquished responsibility for the important choice of an analyst, Herman allowed the training program superiors to choose for her. She writes about the experience that ensued:

> Always readily seduced by outermost appearances, I was instantly entranced by the Freudian therapist to whom they had allocated me. . . . His ambience of the "wise old man" linked him to my Jungian days on this unknown Freudian path. . . . It was the ambience of this gracious family home [where the analyst had his office] that eventually proved to be the enduring benefit of this Freudian therapy. Not the analytic work.[19]

Herman realized in retrospect that the analyst was taken in by her competent persona and did not recognize the fragmented child-self that she had brought to him for help. Consequently he did not focus upon the earliest months of her life. To classical Freudian analysts, the Oedipus Complex, predominant around five years of age, is central to psychological difficulties. To make matters worse, as Herman brought her primitive anxieties and intense affect states of hostility to her therapist, he lost confidence in himself. Herman, sensing his crisis of confidence, became increasingly fearful. Only later did she recognize that the analyst had never worked with the transference issues that would have helped both of them understand the impasse they eventually reached.

Like Drigalski, Herman was not only caught in a deadlock with her analyst, but she was trapped in a similar outer life dilemma as well. If she disrupted her analysis by terminating, she risked being expelled from her training institution and jeopardizing her goal of working in the profession. Fortunately, albeit with great difficulty, an inner voice prevented her from carrying on with the analysis and blaming herself for its failure to help her:

> As the second training year bumped along this rutted course some inmost oracle began increasingly to prophesy complete disaster if I continued to ignore its warnings to break off this so-called psychotherapy, to go in search of expert help as an absolute priority, even if I was expelled from the unbending training course.[20]

Herman learned from a new colleague about Kleinian analysis, which was then becoming popular in England. Melanie Klein's major contribution, one that has been affirmed by findings from recent research on infant development, was to focus attention upon earliest infancy as having great significance for fundamental psychological difficulties. By giving names to the profound anxieties, wishes, and fears that she believed to be characteristic of this stage, Klein made it possible to include these anxieties in a therapeutic relationship. But even though Herman intuitively sensed, quite accurately, that a Kleinian analysis would help her, ending her Freudian analysis was not easy. She puts into words the dilemma patients face who know they are with the wrong therapist:

> I learnt [sic] that it can be easier to transplant oneself across whole worlds, than to find the courage it requires to terminate a therapy, with all the self-doubt that this implies and the paranoid anxieties that are inevitably multiplied by such a unilateral step. I could not find a precedent for this particular divorce, however ardently I searched.[21]

She began to borrow books from her therapist, a practice he permitted rather than analyzed,[22] thus confirming her worst fear that he was out of his depth and could not help her. When he finally suggested that she ask the training institution to permit her to shift to a Kleinian analysis, Herman was "terror-stricken to see this gentle warrior lay his empty rifle down."[23] Her worst fears—that she had drained and depleted him and that, having had three therapists, she was beyond help—seemed to have been realized. Fellow students, meanwhile, were encouraging her to stick it out with the Freudian analyst, given that she had come so far. Finally, Herman extricated herself from the Freudian analysis with great difficulty, able to accomplish an ending only by leaving a note in her analyst's mailbox.

Through sharing in Herman's experience, we can come to understand that patients are not always able to behave in ways that our theories prescribe as "correct." Herman, grappling with the painful inner and outer (expulsion from the training program) aspects of terminating, could not make herself attend the "appropriate" final termination sessions. Her therapist, who we can imagine felt frustrated and defeated, could not facilitate a cordial and supportive ending.

Fortunately for Herman, she eventually reached the office of a Kleinian therapist whose theoretical orientation and personal presence offered exactly what she needed. Her analyst was unafraid of her wildest feelings and fears and of her love: "I shall give you an awful time . . . I fear," she told him, and he replied calmly, "That is alright."[24] Indeed, her analyst was to survive onslaughts of anguish, rage, grief, and love. His calm and patient stance in the face of her feelings enabled Herman to make sense of her early experiences, to place her affect states in the context of a narrative structure, and, finally, to believe that internal storms can be weathered and good feelings can prevail.

A review of Herman's book in a respected psychoanalytic journal exemplifies the mistrusting attitude that many therapists have toward patients' subjective accounts of their experiences of failure in therapy.[25] Patients who do not want to risk being misunderstood and misperceived have good reason to keep their painful experiences in therapy hidden. The reviewer of Herman's book shares the doubts he had both before and after reading the book: "how much of the account can the reader simply believe, given how difficult it is to differentiate the real person of the analyst from his phantasy aspects?"[26]

Unable to accept Herman's subjective experience as valid and true from her perspective, he assumes that his analytic perception of her is correct. He writes, "It is a great temptation to make fun, as she does, of her Jungian and Freudian therapies. But I found myself feeling somewhat skeptical about the author's objectivity."[27] But his view of Herman as making fun of her Jungian and Freudian therapies is in itself a subjective understanding. From my different and equally subjective vantage point, Herman in no way made fun of or devalued her Jungian and Freudian therapies. She clearly states that she valued both of them for specific and clearly expressed reasons.

As our model of psychotherapy in which the therapist is an objective and expert observer shifts to one that includes the interaction of the subjective worlds of both patient and therapist, the patient need not claim to have an "objective" point of view. In fact, an objective point of view within a relational and intersubjective model of psychotherapy simply does not exist. Within the latter model, all we have to work with is the subjective viewpoint of the patient, therapist, or outside observer.

The reviewer's description of Herman's account of her experiences in therapy is less an "objective" review than an account of the reviewer's subjective understanding of the book. That is, the review reveals more about the reviewer's subjective world than it provides an objective assessment of Herman's experiences to potential readers of her book. The reviewer assumes, in accordance with a conception of psychotherapy in which the psychoanalyst has the objective and valid point of view, that the patient's perception is distorted by her unconscious fantasy. Instead, we might consider the possibility *that the theoretical perspectives of Herman's therapists were not right or wrong in and of themselves, but that they were not well suited to the developmental stage of the patient or to the psychological realm that the patient needed to work with and explore.* Yearning for solid ground, we continue to be drawn toward a model of psychotherapy in which theoretical perspectives hold objective truth rather than provide a language to articulate subjective experience. Consequently we are not apt to think of theories flexibly—for example, in terms of their validity for the particular stage of psychological growth of the patient, the function they serve for the therapist, and their place in history and culture. Herman's book substantially contributes to the possibility of considering psychodynamic theory in terms of its fit with the stage of psychological development and particular psychological needs of the patient as they intersect with the psychological needs and characteristics of the therapist.

Drigalski's stories of her two failed psychotherapies and Herman's of her four experiences provide us with examples of stalemates that arise from a lack of fit or mismatch between therapist and patient. They also serve as reminders that the patient's subjective experience is of primary importance in determining the extent to which the ongoing experience of psychotherapy, and its ultimate outcome, is positive or negative. Had Drigalski been less burdened by the conception of psychotherapy that views the doctor as the expert, she might have trusted her reactions and been able to extricate herself sooner from unhelpful therapeutic relationships. But without access to therapists who rely on a different working model of psychotherapy, one in which theoretical concepts enhance the communicability of the patient's experience instead of determining it, she would have had nowhere else to turn. Herman was fortunate in being able to persist through three therapeutic relationships until she could find the right match for herself, and fortunate, too, that a diverse group of therapists was accessible to her.

Lack of Fit Related to Personal Issues

Perhaps the most elusive source of stalemates resulting from mismatches between patient and therapist are those that arise at the intersection of the personal vulnerabilities of each individual. The sensitivities and modes of psychological functioning of patient and therapist are invisible to outside observers. Whether core vulnerabilities become available to consciousness for the patient and therapist depends upon the reflective capacity of the individuals who grapple with them and the amount of psychological work they have completed. Patients and therapists have a better chance of appreciating problematic intersections of personal issues when they are conscious of them, but awareness of them is often out of reach at the beginning of psychotherapy. Stalemates in this category are beginning to be addressed within the domain of psychoanalytic inquiry.[28]

Stalemates of this nature may also arise when the psychological issues of patient and therapist mesh harmoniously as well as when they clash. When they mesh harmoniously, neither individual recognizes that a psychological problem rather than "objective reality" is at issue. Atwood, Stolorow, and Trop (1989) provide the example of Peter, whose complaints about the mechanization and depersonalization of American life meshed with the world view of the therapist. Consequently the therapist did not explore Peter's perceptions, viewing them as realistic, and the conflicts concerning intimacy and attachment underlying the perceptions that patient and therapist shared were not addressed.[29]

Stalemates also arise when there are disjunctions or disharmony between the personal issues of patient and therapist. These may produce repeated and painful interactions between therapist and patient in which the patient feels misunderstood. When the interactions occur in the patient's realm of primary vulnerability (see Chapter Five), the patient is often retraumatized in the areas that she sought therapy in order to understand. These patients are the ones who are left with the subjective experience of being harmed. When the interactions occur around issues that are less central, the therapeutic relationship is nonetheless doomed unless the reflective capacities of the patient and therapist can become constructively engaged. Atwood, Stolorow, and Trop provide the example of Robyn, who desperately needed positive regard from her therapist in order to feel alive.[30] Her family of origin had been consistently nonresponsive to her, except for her father's sexual interest, which began when she was nine. Her therapist was a man who had strong needs for power and control; his mother had been tyrannizing, leaving him resistant to relinquishing his autonomy. Robyn's demands for mirroring from him elicited a resistance that caused him to be withholding and unresponsive. His style of relating drove Robyn to more and more extreme efforts to elicit the responses she urgently needed. Their reactions reinforced each other in an intensifying downward spiral until the patient broke off the therapy and attempted suicide.

A recent book by Stephen Kurtz eloquently describes an aspect of the "fit" between the unconscious issues of therapist and patient that we rarely attend to. He focuses on the nature of the analyst's space, the fit between the psychological space that the analyst provides (embodied in the couch or chair) and the psychological space the analyst occupies, which Kurtz poetically describes as the symbolic childhood corner of the analyst, the place to which the analyst as a child retreated for solitude. The fit between the couch or chair that the patient needs and the space the analyst provides eludes description in words. Kurtz writes:

> The analyst who has become the embracing corner, and the patient who comes for sanctuary there, find one another in the analytic space.... The ideal analyst would be a corner capable of molding and remolding itself to fit the shape of each new patient. In actuality, his flexibility is limited, so that some fits are impossible, many are adequate, and a few are nearly perfect. ... Analysis is possible and necessary in the large number of instances where the fit is good enough to support the relationship but impeded in discrete, manageable ways by discontinuities.[31]

When stalemates occur that are related to the harmony or clashing of personal issues or, in Kurtz' language, to the lack of a good enough fit, therapists are obliged to focus attention on their personal areas of psychological sensitivity in order to transcend the collusion that results. Although considerable attention has been paid to the aspect of therapists' countertransference that is elicited by the patient, for example, in which the therapist experiences herself as like the patient or as like the patient's mother or father, little attention has been paid to the impact of the personal vulnerabilities the therapist brings to the relationship. As therapists feel more comfortable acknowledging areas of personal sensitivity, viewing them as lifespan issues rather than as problems they ought to have fully resolved and eliminated as patients themselves in therapy, our perspective on mismatches in therapeutic relationships will broaden accordingly.

In a model of therapy in which the psyches of two individuals have an impact on each other in visible and invisible ways, unmanageable matches between certain therapists and certain patients are both inevitable and unpredictable. Once they have occurred, they may only be partially and imperfectly understood. Like all relationships, therapeutic relationships are fraught with mystery, comprised of moments of healing and perfect attunement as well as moments of wounding and misunderstanding that seem to arrive unbidden, beyond the conscious control of either participant. Yet the fact that mismatches occur need not be taken as a condemnation of the profession of psychotherapy nor of either the therapist or the patient (although incompetent therapists and patients caught in a self-destructive unwillingness to risk change certainly exist). In a model that conceives of therapy as a relationship between two individuals formed for the purpose of an enhanced awareness of self and other so that problematic self representations and representations and modes of being in relationship can be modified, unmanageable matches can be recognized as a valuable source of information, although perhaps a more painful source than therapeutic relationships in which there is a good enough fit.

CHAPTER TWO

❖ *Impasses* ❖

In one case, a man patient who had had a considerable amount of analysis before coming to me, my work really started with him when I made it clear to him that I recognized his non-existence. He made the remark that over the years all the good work done with him had been futile because it had been done on the basis that he existed, whereas he had only existed falsely. When I had said that I recognized his non-existence he felt that he had been communicated with for the first time . . .

—D. W. Winnicott[1]

I've been in an impasse with my patient Lori for months. When she comes for her sessions, she sits in an anguished silence, either unable to talk to me or else critical and rejecting of me. I've tried everything I can think of with her: sitting in silence too, occasionally sharing what I feel as I sit with her, sometimes gently asking her to describe what she is experiencing, and other times asking her specific questions about her life. Even though we sit only a few feet from one another, I feel as if we're separated by a dense fog. I can't penetrate the opaque grey mist and find her, much as I know she wants to be found. I know she feels terrified and alone—she calls me in between her sessions and leaves panicked messages—but when I try to reach her back, she's never there. I don't know what will end the stalemate.

—Dr. R.

I don't know what to do. I'm so angry at my therapist that I can't bear sitting in her office but I'm too attached to her to leave. She's the one person in my life that I've ever been able to love. She led me on to believe I mattered to her and then she betrayed me. I can't forgive her and I can't leave.

—Josie

T herapeutic relationships rarely progress steadily and painlessly toward an expanded sense of self and other. At times they can persist indefinitely in a state of impasse. The patient and therapist may have a vague sense of being "stuck," of treading water, but they may not know what to do about it. Or the patient and therapist may suffer in painful impasses, like Dr. R. and Josie, whose comments begin this chapter, but not know how to extricate themselves. In other therapeutic relationships the therapist and patient continue to meet, unaware that they are perpetuating an entrenched mode of relating to each other that is comfortable for both but that protects them from the anxiety and risk taking that leads to new experiences of self and other and to new understandings. The comfortable relationship needs to change if something new is to happen. In most therapeutic relationships, as the example in Chapter Three illustrates, a number of factors interact simultaneously.

Both Freud and Winnicott, without using the concept of an impasse, addressed theoretically the problem of therapies that persist interminably. Their contributions provide both historical reference points and an understanding of therapeutic relationships in which, metaphorically speaking, patient and therapist seem to be treading water rather than moving into new areas. Following a brief review of their contributions, examples are given of representative types of impasses in which the therapeutic relationship is stalemated. The cases evoke the quality of the patient's and therapist's experience of a stalemate as well as typical contributing factors. Lori and Dr. R. illustrate a therapeutic relationship that remains in an impasse in which the patient is unable to begin making use of the therapist. The case of Josie and Dr. M. exemplifies a relationship deadlocked in a negative, angry relational mode that signals an urgent need for a shift in the structure of the relationship. The story of Josie and Dr. M. will be picked up again in Chapter Thirteen with the intervention of consultation. The concluding example, Martin and Dr. F., conveys the quality of impasse that results when the patient's and therapist's different modes of managing anxiety impedes the therapist's capacity to respond adequately to the needs of the patient.

Freud: Interminable Therapies

Freud recognized that psychotherapy could continue on interminably if the participants set unrealistic goals or if they lacked the necessary capacities. In his paper "Analysis Terminable and Interminable," Freud pondered the obstacles within the patient that could contribute to an interminable therapy.[2] He concluded that the key factors in the patient that determine whether an analysis will work are the traumatic etiology of the problem, the relative strength of the patient's instincts that would have to be controlled, and the state of the patient's ego (i.e., the patient needs to have enough ego to enable the therapist to align with it). He believed that an analysis could not be successful if any one of these factors was too extreme.

Freud also considered the characteristics of the analyst that contribute to an interminable psychoanalysis: "Among the factors which influence the prospects of analytic treatment and add to its difficulties in the same manner as the resistances, must be reckoned not only the nature of the patient's ego but the individuality of the analyst."[3] Unlike a medical doctor who can treat patients even if her own body is diseased, an analyst's psychological "defects" do interfere with her ability to assess the patient accurately and to respond to the patient in useful ways. Freud alluded to the possibility that analysis might become the third "impossible profession"—the other two being education and government—if we demand perfection of the analyst rather than ordinary humanity.[4] He believed that analysis would not continue interminably if the analyst made an accurate determination of the patient's qualifications and if the analyst had been analyzed sufficiently.

The third factor in an interminable analysis, according to Freud, has to do with the nature of the goals that the patient and therapist establish. Basically, Freud asserted, the termination of analysis is a practical matter. He wrote:

> Our aim will not be to rub off every peculiarity of human character for the sake of a schematic "normality," nor yet to demand that the person who has been "thoroughly analysed" shall feel no passions and develop no internal conflicts. The business of the analysis is to secure the best possible psychological conditions for the functions of the ego; with that it has discharged its task.[5]

But many patients hope to accomplish more than the circumscribed goals of Freud, and when therapists strive to accompany them and avoid imposing limits, they create fertile ground for interminable therapies.

To summarize Freud's view, interminable analyses may be avoided if the patient has the necessary capacities for analysis, if the analyst has been well analyzed, and if the analyst and patient set reasonable goals and are content to exchange neurotic misery for the ordinary problems of being human. But as psychotherapy is practiced today, Freud's preconditions no longer prevail. Patients who have the "necessary capacities" to which Freud referred may nevertheless remain in interminable therapies, while patients who lack them may have positive experiences in therapy. Individuals can be "well analyzed" after years of therapy and yet still be plagued by the problems that initially brought them for help. Therapists regularly meet with patients who have suffered severe trauma, who at times lack access to the ego functions that enable them to cope, or who need to relinquish ego functions that are strangling their potential, and whose uncontrollable instincts are not only perceived as problematic but are appreciated for the vitality they bring. Therapists, even if "sufficiently analyzed," can be catapulted by their patients into unexpected and perhaps previously unknown areas of vulnerability.

Many therapists today, like many patients, are able to value the experience of being propelled into areas of vulnerability as much as they fear it. The potential for personal growth is part of the gratification of being a therapist, although it is not the primary aim of the relationship as it is for patients. Patients and therapists who seek to extend the boundaries of their personalities and who consequently stand at the cutting edge of the field, are not content to set and reach specific goals. And, as Freud appreciated so well, neurotic misery or maladaptive coping mechanisms are inextricably linked to the problems inherent in being human that arise throughout life. As we move away from the medical model, we are freer to relinquish our wish for certainty, for reachable goals, and to acknowledge that there is no static, fixed state of psychological well-being.

Winnicott: Analyses of the False Self

British psychoanalyst D. W. Winnicott labeled those therapeutic relationships that continue on interminably with no apparent progress or a worsening of the patient's psychological state as "analyses of the False Self."[6] By False Self, Winnicott referred to a personality organization that develops in infancy within the mother–infant unit that exists before and after birth. Infants who must comply with their mothers' needs and are unable to have their own spontaneous gestures accepted and appreciated become compliant and reactive. They develop a False Self that reacts and conforms to environmental pressure, while their True Self, embodying their unique human potential, remains hidden and protected beneath the false facade. Winnicott, who valued creativity and spontaneity above all else, believed that only the True Self of an individual can be creative and feel real. Individuals who negotiate the world with a False Self personality organization lack a sense of aliveness, even though to all outer appearances they seem to be functioning with great success.

Winnicott cautioned therapists to be on the lookout for a False Self personality organization in their prospective patients. He understood that when psychotherapy with these patients begins, the therapist makes the necessary arrangements with the False Self personality that "brings" the individual for help. He warned of the treacherous transition time that ensues when the therapist encounters the long-hidden True Self of the patient. In this critical transition stage, the patient falls into a state of extreme dependence upon the therapist until a new organization of self, one that integrates aspects of both the True and False Selves that have formerly been split apart, can form. Therapists who confuse a False Self adaptation with a True Self will avoid the treacherous transition-regression with their patients and will fall into an interminable therapy that leaves patients with a greater sense of futility than they had when the therapeutic relationship began.

Winnicott attributed interminable therapies to the therapist's failure to recognize a False Self adaptation in her patients: "In psycho-analytic work it is possible to see analyses going on indefinitely because they are done on the basis of work with the False Self."[7] The therapist, in order to recognize and extricate herself and her patient from the collusion, must notice that the central element of creative originality (Winnicott's phrase) is missing from the patient and must comment upon it. Winnicott gives the example of a patient who had gone through a great deal of futile analysis in collusion with former therapists. The patient said to Winnicott, "The only time I felt hope was when you told me that you could see no hope, and you continued with the analysis."[8]

Winnicott believed that False Self adaptations exist on a continuum, so that they are a matter of degree rather than an all-or-nothing personality configuration. At the healthy end of the spectrum, a False Self adaptation resembles the persona that most of us have in the outer world. Each of us has a False Self adaptation to some degree, although we might use a different descriptive label for it. I suspect that those therapists who collude with their patients in relating only on the False Self level are therapists who are unaware of the extent of their own False Self adaptation, or in other language, their attachment to preserving a particular persona. A collusion to avoid anxiety-arousing territory is most likely to occur when therapist and patient share similar vulnerabilities, and a False Self personality organization, functioning to protect a hidden, fragile, potential True Self, certainly constitutes a shared vulnerability.[9] Such a collusion, although it protects both participants from anxiety related to risking change, is ultimately frustrating for both patients and therapists. Worse, the collusion protects a fixed, invariant sense of self that can thwart the development of an enhanced capacity for flexibility in representations of self and other.

Statements from therapists that convey to patients a recognition of their feeling of futility and of the missing element of originality are, as Winnicott indicates, experienced by patients not as harsh comments but as welcome communications to the True Self. As C. Kerenyi, a Hungarian classicist, mythologist, and philosopher, writes in his prolegomena to *Essays on a Science of Mythology* concerning the inherent compulsion toward spiritual growth in every human being, "woe to anything that wants to grow when there is nothing in the environment to correspond to it, and when no meeting can take place there!"[10]

When the Patient Cannot Use the Therapist: Lori and Dr. R.

Therapeutic relationships can remain "stuck" when the patient is unable to make use of the therapist as an object in the way she needs, either because of her perception of the therapist, which in turn is related to the issues she brings to therapy, or because the therapist is (unconsciously) resistant to being made use of in the way the patient needs. In impasses of this nature, the patient needs to be able to create the therapist into an object to be used. The therapist's task and challenge is to find a way to enable the patient to make use of her and to enable herself to be made use of. Dr. R, who commented at the beginning of the chapter on her inability to reach her patient, Lori, was the therapist in an impasse of this kind.

Lori, a gentle and shy young woman in her early twenties, came to meet with Dr. R. in the midst of a breakdown. Waiflike in appearance, with large brown eyes and dressed all in black, she seemed to disappear into the black leather couch in Dr. R.'s office. Her pale face, moonlike against the black of the furniture, and her dark hair and eyes had an eerie luminescent quality.

In the first session, Lori talked about her inner experience in a clear, articulate manner that seemed at odds with the primitive states she was describing:

A lot of the time I feel like I'm watching pieces of myself float in front of my eyes. It's worse when I'm alone in the house, which is most of the time. Sometimes I get an incredible sense of panic—my heart starts pounding so hard that I feel it beating against the wall of my chest and I can't get enough air in my lungs. I actually have to gasp for breath. Even when I try to concentrate on breathing slowly and evenly, I can't really control the panic. It comes and goes on its own and I never know why. Sometimes it goes away but other times—the ones I fear the most—it can shift into violence. When that happens I get really terrified. A tremendous energy wells up in me, a violent energy, like a tidal wave, and I feel like I could rip the furniture apart, or throw the dishes on the floor one by one, or even stab myself with a kitchen knife.

Dr. R. met with Lori every day during that first week, hoping to stave off a breakdown and hospitalization, but Lori became unable to manage on her own outside the therapy sessions. She spent several weeks in the psychiatric ward of a local hospital. During Lori's hospital stay, Dr. R. was able to continue regular sessions. Lori's frightening visual images subsided without the help of medication, and the frequent contact with Dr. R. enabled a therapeutic alliance to form.

During individual sessions while Lori was in the hospital, and through minimal contact with Lori's family, Dr. R. obtained only bits and pieces of Lori's family history and present circumstances. Lori was a middle child with two brothers who appeared to be functioning successfully in their lives. Lori had been the black sheep of the family, rebellious despite the fact that her parents were relatively permissive and always supportive. Her adolescence had been a troubled, stormy time with episodes of being out of control, drinking, and experimenting with drugs. Despite these episodes, Lori had managed to complete high school, two years of a community college, and a training program in culinary arts. Upon her graduation Lori had excellent skills in cooking and restaurant management, an area of pleasure and interest for her.

Dr. R. eventually was able to fill in a picture of the circumstances that led to Lori's breakdown. The small and cohesive group of fellow trainees that had sustained Lori during the training program in culinary arts had disbanded just before her breakdown, not only for the summer, but for good. The loss of the structured program and of the significant relational network that the fellow students had provided was a major contributing factor to Lori's state of fragmentation. In addition to these losses, Lori had returned to her family home to find that her parents had decided to end their twenty-seven-year marriage and get a divorce. The shock of discovering that her father had moved out of the home and that he had become involved with a younger woman "knocked the stuffing out" of her.

By the time Lori was discharged from the hospital, the frightening experiences of fragmentation had ended and Lori had reestablished a stronger, although still fragile, sense of self. She made plans to work part-time and found an apartment to share with two other young women. Her parents, although divorced, agreed to contribute to her financial support until Lori's therapy helped her find and maintain a solid footing. Twice-a-week therapy sessions with Dr. R. were established.

After the hospitalization, Dr. R. expected that Lori would continue to have the positive feelings both for her and the therapy that Lori had expressed during the hospitalization. Dr. R. looked forward to a continuation of the intimacy and positive alliance that had been established at the beginning. Dr. R. anticipated that she and Lori would slowly build an understanding of Lori's vulnerabilities and strengths as well as the adaptive mechanisms that she relied upon to negotiate in the world. But instead, the attachment bond between them that had seemed to be developing so well over the first few weeks virtually disappeared.

During the therapy sessions, Lori retreated inside herself, disappearing into the fog that Dr. R. described at the beginning of the chapter. Session after session she would sit in an anguished silence, appearing to Dr. R. to yearn for a connection but unable to allow one to happen. In between the twice-a-week sessions Lori would telephone Dr. R. but would then be unavailable when Dr. R. returned the calls. Vacillating between a terror both of closeness and of distance, Lori could not make use of Dr. R. As Dr. R. conceptualized Lori's dilemma, when she was in the office with Dr. R., the possibility of losing her sense of a separate self in an intimate connection with Dr. R. became terrifying, immobilizing her. When Lori was away from Dr. R., the terror of disconnection and fragmentation loomed perilously close. When Lori reached out to make contact during these episodes of terror, she could not risk allowing it. Instead of being available for a connection with Dr. R., Lori behaved in a rejecting, critical, and denigrating manner. Dr. R. recognized that Lori's sense of self was precarious enough that the possibility of closeness with Dr. R. represented as extreme a danger to Lori as the vast distance of the time between sessions. If Lori came too close to Dr. R., she could lose her fragile sense of a separate, cohesive self. When she was too far away she lost a sense of existing at all. Leaving telephone messages for Dr. R. was her means of establishing enough contact to tide her over until her next session. Caught in the treacherous field between two dangerous poles, Lori could not find her way through to Dr. R.

Dr. R. patiently conveyed to Lori her sense of the dilemma in which they were caught. She struggled to maintain a patient, consistent stance with Lori, a daunting challenge in the face of Lori's rejection and withdrawal. Lori insisted that even if she was caught in the dilemma that Dr. R. described, she would not want to resolve it with Dr. R. Someone else could do a better job. At times Dr. R. could barely hold on to the belief that she could be a good enough therapist for Lori. She hoped that reiterating the dilemma and offering a cognitive understanding of the dynamic between them would eventually enable Lori to observe herself in relation to Dr. R. and to use her awareness to risk new behaviors. But the rational interpretations, rather than bridging the gap between them, only seemed to increase it. Lori became increasingly filled with despair. Dr. R. struggled to maintain a sense of hope both internally and in occasional direct comments to Lori—"We are experiencing something important together that we will eventually need to understand"—but Lori could not seem to make use of the therapeutic relationship, and the impasse persisted. Both Lori and Dr. R. were left feeling unrelated and increasingly hopeless.

Dr. R. continued holding on to hope that a shift would take place at the same time that she tried various ways to reach and be available to her young patient. An array of psychodynamic concepts were useful in describing the troubled therapeutic relationship, but could not alter its course. Dr. R. patiently interpreted both the transference aspect of their relationship and her own feelings of hopelessness and despair as powerful nonverbal communications from Lori. But the interventions prescribed by psychodynamic theory and technique continued to fall by the wayside. Dr. R.'s interpretations such as "I feel as helpless and alone as you must have felt in your family," or "You are afraid to rely on me because if I fail, you'll be in an even worse mess," or "You must be angry at me for not helping," fell on apparently deaf ears.

Consultation did not provide a direct way out of the impasse either. The therapists that Dr. R. consulted with were in basic agreement, although they used different conceptual language, in their understanding of what was occurring in the relationship with Lori, but no one had a suggestion for what Dr. R. could say or do beyond the interpretations that Dr. R had already tried. The consensus seemed to be that Dr. R. would simply have to wait the impasse out, enduring patiently and hoping for a shift. Although the members of Dr. R.'s peer consultation group did not provide a clear idea of a new specific response that Dr. R. could make, they provided a crucially important function in enabling Dr. R. to remain psychologically present and interested in the work with Lori. Without the holding environment provided by her peers as well as the senior clinicians she met with for consultation, Dr. R. might well have become discouraged enough by the impasse that she could have subtly pushed Lori away by withdrawing psychological and emotional energy from the relationship while remaining physically present.

With no hope of using cognitive understanding and psychological theory to provide a way out of the impasse, Dr. R. gave up searching in that direction. She hoped that somehow things would shift. And eventually Dr. R. did have an inspiration that she believed to be a gift of intuitive understanding, unmediated by thought, from her unconscious. The inspiration began with Lori's criticisms and an image: As Dr. R. sat with Lori in one of the pained, silent sessions, she began to see herself visually through Lori's eyes. In her vision, Dr. R. looked like a conventional, traditional, "square" middle-aged woman dressed in prim, proper clothing. Lori, an unconventional, counterculture waiflike outsider, made a completely contrasting visual image.

Looking at the images of the two of them, Dr. R. recognized that their disparate physical appearances embodied the nature of the psychological gulf between them. Without common ground, some bond between them, no alliance or communication necessary for therapeutic work could occur. As Dr. R. sat with the images, a glimmer of a way to talk to Lori began to form. The beginning intuition grew stronger until it overrode the doubts created by Dr. R.'s training in therapeutic technique.

Dr. R. began recalling a time during her own adolescence when she had been rebellious and out of control. Her personal psychotherapy in early adulthood had enabled her to understand this phase of her life, and now settled in her own family and career, she rarely gave much thought to her turbulent adolescence. As she sat quietly in the session with Lori, who had tears streaming down her face, Dr. R. allowed herself to float mentally into that phase of her life. She remembered the desperation she felt, the utter lack of concern for her physical safety and well-being, how it was living moment to moment as if no future existed, the feeling of having left everything familiar behind, the discontinuity in her sense of self as she seemed to leap from one state of being to another without a connecting thread, the feeling of other people coming and going into and out of her life like cartoon figures.

Dr. R. began to talk to Lori, slowly at first and then with increasing passion, about that time in her life. She found herself adding details about her behavior, her feelings, some that she had not shared with anyone, because she had not remembered or given special thought to them. When Dr. R. felt "finished" with what she was saying, she fell into a silent reverie. She felt no impulse to ask Lori for her response, but she experienced a strong sense of connection to her young patient. When the allotted time for the session was up, Dr. R. ended the hour and Lori left without having uttered a word.

After the session, Dr. R. began to feel mounting anxiety. She expected to receive one of Lori's panicked telephone calls. But this time, Dr. R. feared that Lori, upset by the personal disclosures Dr. R. had made, might want to cancel all her future appointments. But no telephone calls of any kind came. As the time for the next appointment drew near, Dr. R. found herself in a state of anxiety anticipating the session. She began to believe that her self-disclosure had been inappropriate, had burdened Lori unduly, and would drive her away. In fact, Lori might not even appear for her scheduled appointment.

But Lori came in and for the first time began to talk freely about herself. She did not mention the previous session, nor did she talk about her family. Instead, she began sharing more of her history. Nor did Dr. R. allude to the preceding session. She sat and listened to Lori talk about the background of her family relationships, heartened by her awareness that a significant shift in the therapeutic relationship was now under way. Dr. R. did not disclose to her colleagues the way the shift had come about, fearing their condemnation of her unusual and uncharacteristic self-disclosure, a significant deviation from principles of technique, until several years later, after Lori had terminated the therapy.

When Patient and Therapist Need to Shift Relational Modes: Josie and Dr. M.

Therapeutic relationships that enable participants to try out new modes of relating and modified representations of self and other, like all intimate relationships, need a quality that I will call *elasticity*. The relationship must be flexible enough to change in response to the changing psychological states and developmental needs of *both* patient and therapist. None of us is a unitary, fixed entity. Impasses may occur at pivotal transition points in relationships when different self-states of the participants emerge in response to any number of factors, or when one participant is ready to move on to a different mode of relating and the other either is not able to respond in new ways, resists responding in new ways, or clings to the familiar "old" ways rather than risk change. A patient we will call Josie and her therapist, Dr. M., provide an example of such an impasse.

Josie, a single woman in her forties, worked as a court reporter. She lived a rather marginal and isolated existence, unable to tolerate the stress of intimate relationships. An only child who reported feeling lonely all her life, Josie yearned for the quality of intimate connection that she could not bear to sustain. She believed herself to be forever condemned to observe relationships secondhand through her work recording testimony in legal situations.

Josie entered into a therapeutic relationship with Dr. M., a man, when she was in her late thirties. After several years of maintaining a safe distance from Dr. M. in regular biweekly sessions, Josie increased the frequency of sessions to three times a week. As soon as she started meeting more often with Dr. M., Josie fell into a powerful positive attachment to her male therapist that was maternal, not erotic. For the first time in her life, Josie felt love for and loved by another human being. Dr. M., responding to Josie's intense yearning for closeness and nurturing, felt devoted to his patient and even lowered his fee substantially to enable Josie to afford the three sessions per week. Witnessing the revival of yearnings for relatedness in Josie and the return of a long-suppressed emotional vitality in a lonely, isolated woman awakened powerful nurturing instincts in Dr. M. For a long time the relationship continued on in a state of harmonious bliss.

The blissful state eventually came to a painful end. Dr. M., who had responded as flexibly as possible to Josie's requests for extra sessions, time changes when necessary, and telephone calls outside the sessions, eventually arrived at a point where he needed to put his personal needs first. Dr. M.'s private practice had become stable enough that he no longer wanted to be away from his family, working three evenings a week. He informed his Monday evening patients that, beginning in two months, his schedule would be changing, and they would need to find new appointment times. Since Josie needed evening sessions because of her employment situation, she was one of the patients Dr. M. asked to reschedule.

Josie found herself in a painful dilemma as a result of Dr. M.'s decision to alter his work schedule. She could not regulate her work hours in order to leave early one day a week on a regular basis, because she could not determine in advance how long a particular job would last. Consequently, although she changed her appointment time to 4:30 P.M., Dr. M.'s last appointment time of the day, Josie could not be certain that she could be at her appointment on time. Even greater than her distress at the uncertainty of her third session per week, Josie felt profoundly wounded by Dr. M.'s assertion of his separateness. The comforting and pleasurable illusion that Dr. M. was completely "there" for her had been shattered.

Josie's anguish over the loss of the relationship she had had with Dr. M., and of whom Dr. M. had represented in her psyche (an all-loving and all-giving mother), did not cause her to flee or to rupture the therapeutic relationship. Instead, Josie shifted into a mode of bitterness and rage, railing at Dr. M. for having led her down a "garden path" only to abandon and betray her. She wanted to terminate the therapy, but felt too attached to Dr. M. to leave him, fearing that she would fall apart if she did not have access to him.

The relationship became stuck in an excruciating impasse: Josie came to every session hoping to restore a positive alliance with Dr. M., but she was unable to move past her anger and pain. Weeks passed by and Josie remained immobilized in each session. She either sat sullen and angry, using silence to punish Dr. M., or else she screamed out loud her rage and pain. Dr. M. repeatedly acknowledged to Josie how painful it had been that he put his needs ahead of Josie's, but his recognition and acknowledgment of the loss did not help. Josie's depression worsened because she despised herself for feeling angry at Dr. M., the one person she had been able to feel loving feelings for and feel loved by. The perceived loss of her capacity to feel love was perhaps the worst part of the impasse for Josie. For Dr. M., bearing responsibility for having injured a patient in such a vulnerable state was equally distressing.

As in the example of Lori and Dr. R., Dr. M. had considerable insight into the nature of the impasse, but he was unable to find a way to use his awareness to facilitate a change. Eventually Dr. M. referred Josie for a special consultation on their impasse. We will return to Dr. M. and Josie in Chapter Thirteen to see how the intervention of consultation affected the therapeutic relationship. For now, the impasse provides us with an example of a therapeutic relationship that became stuck in a state of idealization and harmony and that urgently needed to move to an expanded relational modality that could include disappointment, separateness, and anger.

When Defenses of Patient and Therapist Intersect and Create a Stalemate: Martin and Dr. F.

Patients and therapists who have a good enough fit with each other can nevertheless find themselves stuck in an impasse when their personal vulnerabilities and defenses intersect in problematic ways around specific issues. These impasses are difficult to anticipate because they are based on invisible contributing factors that may be outside the conscious awareness of therapist and patient. In the following case of Martin and Dr. F., the patient's attempts to address concerns that aroused anxiety in the therapist were thwarted by the therapist's unconscious defenses against the anxiety. Impasses of this sort require of therapists a capacity to identify and work effectively with their blind spots in relation to particular patients. Freud's precondition that therapists be well analyzed applies to this type of impasse, particularly in light of the powerful tendency for therapists automatically and unconsciously to perceive the patient as resistant rather than consciously to face their invisible defenses. When therapists are able to risk looking at themselves in interaction with their patients and to disclose personal material to themselves and to consultants without fear of judgment or of being pathologized, impasses of this nature are more likely to resolve and open up new developmental pathways for both therapist and patient.

Dr. F. had been working with his patient, Martin, for nearly eight years. When the therapeutic relationship began, Martin, a thin, tall, bespectacled man in his late twenties, was a struggling student in graduate school working toward a Masters degree in business administration. Martin toiled academically but not financially: His grandmother had left a large estate in trust for him, and the income supported him.

Eight years after beginning therapy, Martin had completed his graduate program and obtained a lucrative management position in a growing company. He felt ready to end the therapy, except for one remaining area of concern to him. Although his outer life was in good order, Martin continued to be troubled by persistent anxiety and fear, either about the state of the world, the safety of his environment, or his own well-being.

Now Dr. F. found himself feeling increasingly irritated with Martin, had difficulty taking his worries seriously, and was beginning to lose a psychological perspective. He felt that Martin simply needed a thicker skin, so that his worries would "run off" like water from a duck's back. The more Dr. F. responded to Martin's concerns with the belief that he needed to change his attitude, the more anxious Martin became.

The most recent impasse between them arose when Martin expressed concern about his "abnormal" tendency to masturbate too often. Dr. F. responded by asking him how frequently he masturbated. Martin disclosed that he masturbated about twice a week and added that masturbating was not interfering with his sexual relationship with the woman with whom he lived. Dr. F. asserted that he did not view the masturbation as a problem. The problem, Dr. F. believed, resided in Martin's critical and worried attitude toward the masturbation. If Martin were less self-critical and allowed himself the sexual outlet of masturbation, his anxiety and worry would decrease.

While Dr. F. was convinced that his understanding of the psychological meaning of Martin's problem was accurate, he was worried about the intensity of his irritation with Martin. He caught himself snapping at his patient rather angrily and realized that he needed to investigate his reaction further. He began to wonder whether his irritation might be preventing Martin from setting a termination date and might actually be causing Martin's anxious preoccupation. Dr. F. brought his concerns into an ongoing consultation relationship.

Consultation relationships that encompass the personal issues and adaptive modes of the therapist as well as the patient have the best chance of being useful in situations of therapeutic impasse. Because Dr. F.'s consultation had included his personal vulnerabilities, his consultant was able to recall for him significant elements of Dr. F.'s personal history that had been revealed in the course of their long relationship. Dr. F., like Martin, had once been a struggling medical school student. But unlike Martin, he did not have a trust fund from his grandmother. Dr. F. had worked his way through college and had gone to medical school on a combination of scholarship and student loans that he had only recently finished paying off. Dr. F.'s mother had died of cancer when he was sixteen, and he had been raised by his father. Dr. F. had always tried to be a responsible, good son who did not cause his father undue concern.

The consultant commented that Dr. F., unlike Martin, had not been free to feel his fear and anxiety after his mother died. On the contrary, he had tried diligently to take care of his overwhelmed father by being responsible and coping with whatever difficulties presented themselves. He thought it a luxury to wish that his mother had not died or to yearn for her to be there to take care of him, or to wish for ample money to support his education. Dr. F. instead learned to push aside his fears and anxieties in order to continue coping efficiently and effectively with his life. His consultant gently speculated that Dr. F.'s irritation with Martin might well have something to do with his envy of Martin, who, having the financial support and the safety of the therapeutic relationship, enjoyed the luxury of expressing and feeling his anxieties and fears.

Dr. F. heard the comments and knew immediately that his consultant was correct. Dr. F. recognized that he had been pushing Martin's anxiety away because of his envy of Martin and because of his resistance to letting himself feel his own yearning for support. He felt relieved to understand that he and Martin managed their anxieties with opposite strategies. Where Martin would rely on fear to keep him in touch with reality, Dr. F. was prone to deny truly frightening aspects of his experience.

Dr. F. thought that the different defensive modalities between Martin and himself had initially been helpful. Martin had been able to "borrow" Dr. F.'s defense of denial and to be less fearful. But around the termination process, Martin's anxiety could not be set aside. In disavowing his anxiety and needs in the face of loss, Dr. F. became prone to envy Martin's freedom to allow all his feelings into consciousness. His resistance blocked his capacity for empathy with Martin's plight.

Dr. F. could have returned to the sessions with Martin and simply exercised a different level of awareness without speaking aloud his insight. Because Dr. F. and Martin were in a termination phase, in which the patient relinquishes idealizing projections onto the therapist and becomes more aware of the therapist's real strengths and limitations, Dr. F. chose to tell Martin that he felt he had been minimizing Martin's anxieties because of his own different way of managing them. Martin responded that he had known that Dr. F. was responding in a "skewed" manner to his concerns and that he appreciated the work that his therapist had done in untangling their interaction. The impasse dissolved in a single session, and Martin was then able to set a termination date.

As these three cases illustrate, therapist–patient dyads reach impasses for different reasons at different phases of the therapeutic venture. Sometimes, as in the case of Lori and Dr. R., a "third" factor that can give the stalemated dyad new momentum will emerge unexpectedly from the therapist or patient. In other cases, such as that of Josie and Martin, consultation can provide the fresh perspective that is unavailable to the therapist or patient. The freer patients and therapists feel to identify and name stalemates as ordinary and expectable phases of therapeutic relationships to which both participants contribute, the greater the opening may be for the intervention of a "third term" (such as an unexpected insight or a consultation) and for gleaning insight from the impasse.

CHAPTER THREE

❖ A Complicated Knot: ❖
The Case of Lynn and Dr. K.

Eventually, as session after session passed by, I began to feel stuck
with Dr. K. The sessions were pleasant and even intellectually
challenging, but nothing of any significance seemed to be happening. I talked about my concerns with Dr. K. and he understood my
feelings, but talking about them didn't change anything. Nothing I
tried made any difference. And then everything fell apart . . .
—Lynn

It's been three years now and I still feel like I failed Lynn. I didn't
realize how we had slipped off track and then it was too late. She's
a resourceful person and I know she'll be all right. I wonder what
happened after our termination.
—Dr. K.

The preceding chapter presented case vignettes in which the factors
contributing to the stalemate were clustered conceptually around a
single predominating factor—the patient's inability to use the therapist, a need for the therapeutic relationship to shift relational modes,
and the problematic intersection of the patient's and therapist's issues
and defenses. But therapeutic relationships commonly reach impasses
when these and other factors combine in a complicated knot. The
process of identifying and disentangling the factors can be a difficult
but rewarding—in the sense of consciousness-enhancing—task for the
patient and therapist. Patients whose therapeutic relationships rupture
in complex impasses, and who are not blocked by feelings of shame
and failure from exploring what transpired, are apt to find that the
process of gaining understanding and making meaning continues on
over time. Patients and therapists can continue to acquire new insight
at various junctures in their lifespan.

The case of Lynn and Dr. K. will be presented in greater detail
than the cases in Chapter Two in order to allow the complexity of the
impasse to emerge fully. The case also demonstrates that *therapists who*

are experienced and highly regarded have areas of unconsciousness that may lead to failures of empathy, misperceptions, and major errors with certain patients. Patients who are psychologically minded, motivated, and who function successfully in the world may be unaware of or disavow their therapists' limitations and their own profound impact on their therapists. We will see in the relationship of Lynn and Dr. K. how the factors that operated separately in the cases in Chapter Two combine to create a complicated impasse, almost as if several therapeutic relationships were operating simultaneously. Their story, a fictional account based upon an actual therapeutic relationship and consultation, is told in the present tense to convey both a sense of immediacy and the full impact of an experience of a complex therapeutic impasse in undiluted form. The details of the therapeutic relationship are presented without explanatory or theoretical comment in order not to detract from the experience of the relationship for both participants. The many tangled threads that resulted in the knot that patient and therapist tied round themselves will be partially disentangled in Chapter Four.

A Multidetermined Impasse: Lynn and Dr. K.

Lynn, an instructor in sociology at a community college, wife of a newspaper journalist, and mother of two young children, decides to seek psychotherapy when her youngest child is eight years old. In her mid-thirties, she looks forward to therapy to help her with a vague sense of dissatisfaction with her life, a sense of something missing. With her family and work life relatively stable, Lynn feels ready and eager, albeit with some anxiety, to embark on a journey of psychological exploration.

Lynn chooses Dr. K., an experienced and respected Freudian psychiatrist, with care. In addition to knowing that he had excellent training, Lynn is acquainted with one of his former patients. The former patient describes Dr. K. as a kind, responsible man and believes that Dr. K. helped him. Lynn thinks about Dr. K. for several months before she picks up the telephone to call him. By the time she finally makes an appointment with him, she feels as if she knows him.

Dr. K. is a man in his late forties at the time Lynn first meets with him. He has a well-established psychotherapy practice and is known and respected professionally. An introverted man, he takes pride in being restrained and compassionate. Unlike many of his colleagues, he maintains a reasonable fee range that enables patients of different economic backgrounds to avail themselves of his help. His vitality is most evident in his solitary intellectual pursuits, particularly his longstanding love of Shakespeare. When he talks about Shakespearean plays, his face lights up and he comes alive.

When Dr. K. greets Lynn for the first time, he sees a well-groomed, pleasant-looking, quiet woman with light brown hair and penetrating eyes. Lynn sees a masculine mirror image of herself: a neatly dressed, quiet man who averts his gaze when she looks directly at him and who seems rather subdued. Dr. K. ushers Lynn into a small office that is sparsely furnished with a modern leather analytic couch and two beige upholstered swivel chairs. Lynn sits in the patient's chair and takes a deep breath.

Surprised that tears begin to well up, Lynn begins the session by explaining to Dr. K. that she wants to bring all her anxieties and fears into the relationship with him. She is competent and successful as a mother and a teacher. Other people see her as an effective person, a good manager, reliable and dependable. But she wants to allow the hidden sides of herself to surface in the therapeutic relationship: her emotions, fears, and anxieties, the aspects of herself that others in her life rarely see. She knows that she could have more intimate relationships with her husband, children, and friends if she allowed these hidden sides to be more visible to others.

Dr. K. remains silent and attentive for the entire session. When the time draws to an end, he offers her a regular weekly appointment time. Lynn pushes aside a wish that Dr. K. would offer some preliminary thoughts about her, but she assumes that he chooses to be silent rather than to speak prematurely. She tries to engage him by asking him if he thinks she should meet with him twice a week instead of once.

Dr. K. hesitates and then replies that he has some feeling that twice a week might be better, but he is not certain. Lynn feels a certain relief that he is not pushing her into a more intensive therapeutic relationship right away. She begins to perceive Dr. K. as the helpful therapist that she wants and needs him to be.

For more than a year, Lynn conscientiously keeps her weekly appointments and enjoys the freedom to use them to talk about whatever is on her mind. Sometimes she talks about work-related issues, and sometimes she brings up the dilemmas that arise with family members, including her husband and children, her mother (her father died four years ago), and younger, learning-disabled sister. She carries a small spiral notebook in her purse to record any significant interpretations that Dr. K. offers, along with the occasional dreams she remembers. The simple fact of having a place to come fifty minutes a week in which she can pay attention to herself dissipates the sense of something lacking that plagued her before she began therapy and helps her feel energized and alive.

Dr. K. continues to remain essentially silent during the sessions, allowing Lynn to occupy the time and space as she chooses. Because Lynn presents herself in such an organized, articulate manner, he sees no reason to intervene. Lynn often pauses somewhat hopefully as she talks in order to give Dr. K. every opportunity to offer a comment. She falls into a pattern of resuming her monologue when he remains silent. He generally offers a summarizing statement near the end of the session reflecting back to her the themes she has raised. Because Lynn enjoys the attention and the experience of sharing her thoughts and feelings, the pattern of relationship that becomes firmly established is comfortable and pleasant. Lynn, accustomed to accommodating, does not know how to access or articulate other needs and feelings in a manner that will elicit responses from others.

When Lynn brings her dreams to her sessions, assuming that Dr. K. will be interested in them, she quickly senses that Dr. K. is awkward and ill at ease. He asks for her associations but rarely comments on the dreams beyond reflecting back to her their general themes. In one session, Lynn asks Dr. K. if he likes to work with dreams, and she appreciates his honesty when he tells her quite openly that he does not see himself as particularly skilled in understanding them.

Dr. K. looks forward to the sessions with Lynn. He is interested in her and enjoys her vitality as she shares stories about her family and work, figuring out solutions to the inevitable problems that arise. He comes to admire her intelligence, her thoughtfulness, and perhaps, above all, her empathy. She has an ability to intuit what others need and to supply it without their asking. He has been on the receiving end of her empathy. He recalls how on one occasion he came down with a bad cold but felt self-conscious about calling attention to himself. He appreciated the way Lynn expressed concern but refrained from engaging him with direct questions, as if she did not want to be a problem for him when he did not feel well. On the rare occasions when she asks him a direct question, he finds that he enjoys answering her. Unlike other patients in his practice and other women he has known, Lynn's temperament is even and she makes virtually no emotional demands on him. He can relax and enjoy her positive feeling for him, her appreciation of his attentiveness, and he knows that she enjoys his admiration of her. But he is also aware that Lynn has no rough edges. She has a seamless presence that lends him no ready opening to engage with her.

Lynn comes to depend more and more upon Dr. K.'s unflagging reliability and consistent presence. She feels safe and secure with him and both recognizes and appreciates that his needs do not impinge upon her. But at the same time, she becomes aware of the vague but growing sense of dissatisfaction, the same sense of lack that brought her to therapy initially. Although the relationship is pleasant and pleasurable, it also lacks "juice," her word for emotional energy and intensity. Dr. K. does not interact with her, and his silence leaves her wondering what he is thinking, what he perceives her problems might be, and how the therapy might help her.

Lynn is not sure what to do about her sense of lack and tries to focus on appreciating Dr. K.'s unwavering, reliable presence rather than on criticizing or making demands on him. She does not realize that she is afraid to risk even feeling critical of him, let alone expressing criticism. She is unaware of her fear of being perceived as an ungrateful, bad person, or worse, of provoking him into a furious rage at her, patterns that were established early on in her relationships in her family and to which she adapted by finding ways to avoid conflict. Consciously Lynn interprets Dr. K.'s silence as related to a choice to keep his needs from impinging upon her. She decides that he knows how responsible she is for the well-being of others both at home and at work. Instead of asking for more from him, she decides that Dr. K. is deliberately choosing to give her the freedom to talk about whatever she wants without being encumbered by his opinions.

The therapeutic relationship settles into a harmonious state that Lynn is invested in maintaining. Unaware of her paralysis around criticism—she fears that her anger will annihilate him or drive him crazy—Lynn continues to feel only the vague sense of lack. Two discordant notes eventually interrupt the static harmony of the relationship with Dr. K. Each time, Lynn mentions the discordant elements in the next session, but Dr. K. does not ask her to talk more about them or to explore their significance. Dr. K. is unaware of their importance, and without active encouragement from him, Lynn quickly pushes the incidents aside. The opportunities to access the roots of the stasis in the relationship consequently pass by.

The first discordant note sounds when Dr. K. telephones her at home one evening during the dinner hour. Until the telephone call, neither of them had initiated any contact outside of the regular appointments. Without preamble, Dr. K. asks her for the name of a medical specialist that her husband had been seeing. At first Lynn is taken aback by the unexpected call and does not know what Dr. K. is talking about. But then she remembers that she had praised the specialist during a recent therapy session. Surprised at Dr. K.'s request and at his calling her at home instead of waiting until their next scheduled appointment, she hesitates and then provides the information he asks for. Before she quite knows what has happened, Dr. K. has said goodbye and hung up the phone.

Lynn is left holding the silent telephone receiver, wondering why Dr. K. wants the information and for whom. Another patient? Himself? Is there another person who, like her younger sister with a learning disability, needs attention more than she does? Feeling herself sliding into potentially problematic territory, she stops her alarming thoughts and feelings by telling herself that she should be pleased that Dr. K. regards her as a competent person and not merely as another "neurotic" patient. She should be pleased that she can help him.

Neither Lynn nor Dr. K. refer to the telephone call in the next session. Lynn knows that therapists rarely call patients for personal reasons outside a session, and she expects that he will mention the telephone call in their next meeting. She is unaware that a yearning for someone to understand her and intuit her basic needs without her asking for anything has been reawakened in the therapeutic relationship, structured as it is to provide her with the undivided attention of an adult whom she admires. She has a nagging and disturbing feeling that Dr. K. is overlooking the connection between his telephone call and a familiar pattern in her family of origin—that attention is once again being deflected away from her toward someone else whose needs are perceived as more pressing. But she does not want to question Dr. K. or to feel that, by calling upon her for a need of his own, he has been inattentive to her. Not wanting to face her disquieting critical feelings, not knowing she does not want to face them, caught in her yearning for him to know her needs without her having to ask for anything, Lynn resumes her familiar role with him.

Dr. K. in fact does hesitate briefly before calling and asking Lynn for the name of the medical specialist. But a good friend needs the referral, and wanting to be helpful, Dr. K. decides to ask Lynn for the name even though she is his patient. He has some feeling that he is taking advantage of her, but he ignores his feeling in the same way that Lynn ignores her sense of lack. After he makes the call, he puts it out of his mind. By the time the next session rolls around, he has literally forgotten about his request.

Several months after the telephone incident, Lynn increases the frequency of her sessions to twice a week. The therapy has begun to seem so bland and unproductive that Lynn can no longer ignore her sense of lack. Dr. K. does not have a strong sense of why she feels the lack, but he takes her feeling seriously. When Lynn suggests that meeting more frequently might enliven the relationship and bring more issues to the surface, Dr. K. is immediately responsive and offers her a second weekly appointment time.

As soon as Lynn increases the frequency of sessions, her feelings about Dr. K. and about being a therapy patient intensify. She begins to feel a renewal of hopeful energy. Perhaps the long period of testing Dr. K.'s constancy has come to an end and the real work of psychotherapy is about to begin.

Lynn uses the additional session to begin a serious, prolonged exploration of the ways she shaped herself to fit into her family of origin. She confronts her need to repress and disavow critical and negative feelings toward her parents and toward her younger sister, Alice, by literally recording conversations with family members and reading them aloud to Dr. K. so that she can see what feelings she might be avoiding. She begins to respond in new ways to family members, always with Dr. K.'s encouragement and support. She spends time exploring her relationship to her father and mourning his loss. But she does not recognize the similarities in how she relates to Dr. K., and he does not focus her attention on their relationship or on her feelings about him.

Dr. K. consistently helps her face the darker side of herself and her family—the way her mother continues to worry about and hover over Lynn's younger sister, Alice, who struggled with a severe learning disability in childhood. He points out how her mother treats Lynn as if she is invisible, the way she expects Lynn to be successful and happy and never lets her talk about her troubles. He is comfortable with conflict and criticism when directed toward others, rather than toward him, and Lynn is afraid of being overtly critical. Appreciative of his unwavering support, Lynn begins to look forward to seeing Dr. K. and often holds conversations with him in her mind between the sessions, imagining his responses to her.

The second discordant note sounds in the midst of this phase of the therapy. Late one afternoon, once again during the busiest part of her day, the telephone rings. Dr. K.'s voice is as startling to Lynn on this occasion as it had been months before when he asked for the name of the medical specialist. He tells her that something has come up, that he will have to cancel her appointment the next morning. Could she come in the late afternoon instead?

A small voice inside Lynn that she has never heard before wants to cry out: Don't you know how important my regular appointment times are to me? Don't take away my time for something more important! Shocked at the unexpected intrusion from within, surprised at how important the reliability of her sessions has become, Lynn is temporarily immobilized.

Dr. K. repeats his request. Would 5:30 P.M. work for her? Confused, Lynn reaches for her appointment book and sees what she already knows: The late afternoon is always free because she reserves it to be home with her children. Her classes at the community college are routinely scheduled for weekday mornings or early afternoons. Even though she regards the loss of the time at home as a sacrifice, her unexpected need for contact with Dr. K. takes precedence. Yes, she tells him, silencing the unexpected inner cries, she can come at 5:30 in the afternoon and she is happy to be able to help him out.

The next morning, once her class is over, Lynn feels disoriented with the gap in her schedule. She tries to fill it productively, but ends up wandering aimlessly around her favorite bookstore, not registering any of the titles in her mind. By 5:30 P.M., sitting in Dr. K.'s waiting room at the unfamiliar time of day, she is tired and yearns to be at home.

When the session begins, Lynn complains that this is not the best time of day for her. Dr. K. waits silently for her to continue, unable to appreciate the significance of even a small complaint, unable to see through her composed, competent exterior to her distressed state. Lynn waits, too, hoping he will notice that she is complaining uncharacteristically and will acknowledge that the change in time has been a loss for her. Caught in her wish for his empathy for her unspoken needs, Lynn is silent.

Lynn realizes that Dr. K. is preoccupied or worried and does not want to cause him further distress. As his silence becomes prolonged, Lynn tries to ignore her discomfort by groping unsuccessfully for something else to talk about. The ensuing session is disjointed, uncomfortable, and feels like a waste of time, but Lynn does not know what to do with her disgruntled feelings. Whatever muted version of her feelings that she tries to put into words seems to dissipate into a vacuum because Dr. K. is unusually unresponsive. Lynn struggles to set aside her feelings. After all, she thinks, he has made an effort to meet with her instead of canceling the session.

Dr. K. is unfortunately struggling with a therapist's worst fear: the suicide of a patient. An extremely depressed patient, a man he had been working with for less than a year, ended his life by running carbon monoxide into his car. A funeral service had been planned for the morning of Lynn's appointment, and Dr. K. felt he should attend it.

Dr. K. had no warning that the patient was planning to act on suicidal impulses. Although the patient was depressed, he had not conveyed to Dr. K. how serious the depression was. Nonetheless, Dr. K. feels responsible and continues to agonize over what he might have overlooked. Dr. K. dreads encountering the patient's family at the funeral service. He imagines that the family blames him for the suicide and fears that they are enraged with him because he did not foresee the risk of suicide.

Conscientious, not wanting to fail other patients at a time when he feels vulnerable because he may have failed the patient who ended his life, Dr. K. reschedules rather than cancels his morning appointments. The funeral is an ordeal, even though his fears of being blamed do not come to pass. The combination of the funeral and doing a full day's work afterward takes its toll. Depleted of energy, Dr. K. barely manages to sit through his afternoon sessions.

A few days later, Lynn inadvertently discovers the cause for the change in her appointment time at a lunchtime gathering of women friends. One of the women happens to know the family of Dr. K.'s patient and talks about the suicide and funeral service. A shock ripples through Lynn as she realizes in an intuitive flash that Dr. K. changed her appointment time so he could attend the service. In a further intuitive flash, Lynn guesses that Dr. K. was the therapist of the man who had killed himself.

Trusting her intuitive knowledge, Lynn finds herself impaled on the crossroads of two conflicting sets of feelings: compassion for Dr. K. and anger on behalf of the patient who had not been helped. The anger is the more dangerous but more compelling feeling. Why had Dr. K. been unable to reach his despairing patient? Why had Dr. K. been unable to hold onto his patient until the patient found a reason to live? What would happen to her if she were to descend to that level of hopelessness and loss of meaning? But these questions are far too daring and cruel for her to ask, particularly when Dr. K. is understandably upset.

But Lynn wants to hear the truth from Dr. K. even if she withholds her upsetting questions. At her next appointment, she asks him directly, with unusual determination, if he was the therapist of the man who killed himself and if he had changed her appointment time so he could attend the funeral service.

Dr. K. explains that he cannot answer Lynn because of the confidentiality of patient–therapist relationships. But his face turns grey and somber, and because Lynn believes that he would otherwise have reassured her that he was not the therapist in question, she is certain that Dr. K. is the therapist involved.

Dr. K. neither asks Lynn what her feelings would be if he were the therapist of the man who had killed himself nor maintains his silent stance. Instead, recognizing that Lynn is aware that he was the therapist involved and that maintaining confidentiality is impossible, he confides to her how hard it had been for him to attend the funeral service, how he imagined the others who were there would hold him responsible for his patient's death, how he had envisioned being openly criticized by the mourners.

His shame and guilt affect Lynn powerfully, overriding her concerns for herself and her feelings about his disclosure of his feelings. She responds protectively that she wishes she could have been present to shield him from their criticism. She sees tears in his eyes as he thanks her for her understanding and concern, and she, too, is moved to tears to have touched him so intimately.

Dr. K. is acutely vulnerable when he discloses his feelings to Lynn. When Lynn catches him off guard and asks him a direct question, an unusual behavior on her part, he finds himself divulging his feelings and then feeling overwhelmed with gratitude for her caring and compassionate response.

The moment of shared intimacy around Dr. K.'s guilt, shame, and humiliation is pivotal for Lynn and permanently alters the course of the therapeutic relationship. She is afraid to let herself wonder what would happen to her if she allowed herself to expose her deepest despair to Dr. K. After all, she sometimes has thoughts of suicide, feelings that life is unbearable. What if Dr. K. could not help her and were to let her die? Neither she nor Dr. K. can face directly and openly the consequences for her of having received her therapist's private feelings of shame, humiliation, and failure. Both veer away from the dangerous territory of distressing feelings and conflict. Their personal issues mesh harmoniously and keep them from engaging in ways that might help Lynn alter an entrenched and constraining relational mode of disavowing her needs and accommodating to others. Dr. K. puts the interaction out of his mind. Lynn thinks about it but pushes aside her distressing feelings rather than endanger the positive alliance that is not only pleasurable but that has been important to the psychological work she has been doing in relation to her family of origin.

Trying to locate safer ground without knowing that she is searching for it, Lynn expresses a longing for more experiences of genuine, intimate contact with Dr. K. In an unusual moment of rebellion against accepted psychoanalytic tenets, trusting Lynn's statement about what she needs, and drawn toward her empathy for him because, like Lynn, he yearns for moments of intimate connection, Dr. K. responds to her longings by beginning to disclose details about his personal life. Partly on his own, partly in response to Lynn's questions, he eventually tells her about his family, his children, and his interest in Shakespeare.

Encouraged by Dr. K.'s new willingness to talk to her about himself, Lynn avidly begins reading Shakespeare. She listens with interest to his comments about the plays and admires his intelligence and knowledge. Dr. K. and Lynn spend many gratifying and pleasant sessions discussing Shakespeare as well as theoretical ideas about therapy. Dr. K. begins bringing in copies of articles on psychotherapy or on Shakespeare that he thinks Lynn might like and gives them to her as gifts. Lynn also lends books to Dr. K. On one occasion she repeatedly asks him to return a book, and he eventually reports that he has misplaced it. She also begins reading books and journal articles about psychotherapy that she finds in the school library and brings them to Dr. K. for discussion. She does not notice that the articles she brings to Dr. K. are often an ironic commentary upon the therapeutic relationship with him. One article Lynn comes across is entitled "The Patient as Therapist to His Analyst" by Harold Searles.[1] Lynn tells Dr. K. that the article makes her think about the ways she tried to be the healer in her family in relation to her parents and sister. She does not notice that she has fallen into the role of healer with Dr. K., working to bring energy and vitality to the relationship.

As time goes on and the sessions pass by, Lynn begins to feel mired in the positive relationship. The sense of lack that haunted her when she had only one therapy session per week returns with even greater intensity. The sessions are enjoyable and stimulating intellectually, but what is she learning about herself? She misses the progress they had made when they worked on her relationships to her family.

Lynn begins to talk with Dr. K. about her feelings. He understands her concerns, but talking about the impasse does not bring about a change. Without direct guidance from Dr. K. and assuming that the problem resides either in her or in the structure of the relationship, Lynn takes the initiative in trying to bring about a shift. The possibility that the therapeutic relationship might be caught in a mutually-created impasse never occurs to her.

Taking full responsibility for having created the lack as well as for fixing it, Lynn experiments with changing the structure of the therapeutic relationship. She brings up the possibility of increasing her sessions to four times a week. Lynn asks Dr. K. if he is willing to participate equally with her in the therapeutic relationship. She does not want to be the only one who puts energy into it and who takes the risk of exploring new psychological terrain, making changes while Dr. K. offers comments but remains personally untouched. Dr. K., challenged by the prospect of working with Lynn four times a week, assures her that the idea of being an equal participant sounds exciting to him, an adventure. When the frequency of sessions does not alter the relational mode, Lynn changes her position on the analytic couch so she cannot see Dr. K., hoping that she will feel less protective of him if she cannot see him.

Dr. K. can see how hard Lynn is trying and feels pained that the efforts she makes are not bringing about results. He has some sense of not understanding Lynn, of not being able to empathize with her, but he does not know what to do about it.

Eventually life itself intervenes to bring about a shift in Lynn's state. Lynn, her husband, and her children join Lynn's mother, her sister, and her sister's husband for Thanksgiving. Lynn and her sister, Alice, leave in the car to do some errands. A car driven by a drunk driver crosses the center line of the road they are on, and a collision ensues. Lynn, who is in the driver's seat with an air bag, survives with bruises, but her sister is seriously hurt. Alice has a concussion, fractured pelvis, broken legs, and deep facial cuts.

Lynn and her family remain with her mother and brother-in-law for several extra days, long enough to see that Alice is healing properly in the hospital, but then they return home and carry on with their ordinary lives. Over the next six months, Alice recovers from her injuries but is left with permanent difficulty in walking and with chronic pain. Lynn, who had coped effectively with the accident at the time, finds herself unable to recover psychologically from the trauma.

Having always been able to manage stressful situations and to keep her feelings under control, Lynn is not prepared for the intensity of grief and guilt that flood her after the accident. Why is she always the "lucky" one? Why does Alice always have the worst of things? Lynn was not even required to sacrifice any aspect of her ordinary life because the burden of care fell to her mother and to Alice's husband. Her anguish over the accident and the consequences spill out defiantly from underneath her rational defenses, retreating only temporarily as if to gather strength in order to burst forth once again.

For the first time in the four years since they had begun meeting, Lynn goes to her sessions with Dr. K. in a state of genuine need. The despair she sometimes feels comes into sharp focus around the traumatic car accident and erupts in the therapy. "I'm never going to be able to live with my guilt. I feel terrible about Alice's situation and I feel angry at her for always coming first. I can't stand it. What am I going to do?"

Dr. K. is taken aback by the drastic change in his patient. At first he feels disbelief, as if Lynn is merely acting upset rather than actually feeling distraught. He finds himself saying, "Come on, Lynn!" with impatience when, in one session, she seems to drift away, as if she is playing a game with him. When he realizes that she is not playing a game, he is immobilized by a feeling of helplessness and panic. Are these the same feelings that she is struggling with? He experiences an urgent need to help her feel better and offers whatever he can find.

When Lynn complains of exhaustion because she cannot get back to sleep at night when she awakens, Dr. K. is pleased to be able to prescribe medication. When she says she feels too upset to come to her sessions, he tries to soothe her by suggesting that she wait until she feels better. He tells her he will not charge her for the cancellations.

Instead of feeling grateful and appreciative, Lynn finds herself feeling worse in response to each of Dr. K.'s efforts to help her feel better. She believes that by giving her medicine or accepting her cancellations he is backing away from her distress. She quickly finds herself struggling with critical feelings toward Dr. K. and troubling questions about him, in addition to the feelings of guilt, grief, and anger in relation to her sister. She loathes having critical thoughts about Dr. K., who is clearly trying hard to be helpful, but her doubts and criticisms will not go away.

Lynn begins to imagine that Dr. K. is afraid of the intensity of her feelings and wants her either to mute her feelings or to go away. She finds herself leaving every session feeling worse than when she arrived. Eventually she comes to dread the appointments altogether. She knows that she will leave his office shouldering not only the same grief, guilt, and self-hatred with which she came in, but also the additional weight of her disillusionment and disappointment in Dr. K. for his inability to offer her the help she needs.

Unable to find what she needs in the sessions with Dr. K., Lynn tries to work with her feelings of guilt and loss on her own. She finds a support group for family members of accident victims through a local hospital and also hooks up with a fellow teacher at the college who lived through a similar experience and is glad to take the time to talk with her.

On more secure psychological footing, Lynn makes an effort to restore her therapeutic relationship with Dr. K. to its positive ground. But she finds that she cannot return to her former role. Her profound disappointment in Dr. K. has brought about a shift in her perception of him. Instead of seeing him solely as the "good" therapist she wants him to be, Lynn faces the possibility that he is no longer a good therapist for her. He was helpful for a long time in allowing her to look at herself in relation to her family of origin, but he is not able to take the next step of examining the ways she interacts with him.

Lynn finally decides that the relationship has progressed as far as it can. Although she finds it difficult to think of terminating the relationship—she is still deeply attached to Dr. K., and her daily routine is organized around her four sessions per week—continuing to attend and pay for therapy that offers her little in return no longer makes sense. She tells Dr. K. her perceptions.

Dr. K. is saddened by the change in Lynn's attitude toward him. He values the relationship with her. He is aware that he has somehow failed her, but facing his inadequacy and failure evokes memories of the devastating time when his patient committed suicide. The memories arouse more guilt than he can tolerate. The combination of his guilt and hurt in relation to Lynn impels him to detach from the relationship by withdrawing psychological and emotional energy from it. The withdrawal is not made with conscious planning or effort but seems to happen of its own accord, as most defensive responses do.

Lynn senses Dr. K.'s withdrawal but does not know how to respond to it. She asks him where he has gone, tells him that she feels he has disappeared, but, unaware of his defensiveness, he denies that he is psychologically absent. After numerous attempts to reach him fail, Lynn decides to act. She announces that she wants to begin reducing the number of weekly sessions over the next few weeks and then to stop altogether.

To her surprise, Dr. K., who has never taken a strong position on any issue that arose over the years they had been meeting and who has never been assertive, announces emphatically that he thinks Lynn should not give up any of her weekly sessions. Lynn finds herself consumed by anger: Why is Dr. K. taking such a strong stand now, when it's too late? He let her cancel her sessions without any concern when she was in the worst of her pain over Alice's injuries. Anger arising from her disappointment in him, critical feelings that she had managed to suppress, disavow, and ignore over the years begin to surge forth, gathering momentum until Lynn can no longer restrain them.

Dr. K. surprises himself as well as Lynn by his insistence that she continue as his patient. The surge of energy that went through him when Lynn tried to set a termination date was unexpected. But he feels good about his stance, and the renewal of his energy fuels a determination on his part to keep encouraging her to express her angry feelings. But wanting to be helpful by such encouragement and actually withstanding the anger without defensively warding it off are not the same. His defenses operate automatically, keeping him from appreciating the extent to which Lynn's anger itself is a defense that protects her more vulnerable, wounded self.

Lynn spends a sleepless night as anger interferes with sleep. Unable to tolerate her agitation until her next appointment, she telephones Dr. K. in the morning.

When Dr. K. picks up Lynn's message from his answering service, he feels a mixture of resentment and panic. What is he in for now? He has done his best to listen to her criticisms, but he is at the limit of his tolerance for what he now feels are unjustified attacks. He calls Lynn back with a sense of dread.

When Lynn tells him that she is too angry to tolerate waiting until her next appointment and that she has been up all night, he immediately recommends a new sleeping medication that will not have a hangover effect. But Lynn does not want medication. She wants Dr. K. to tell her that he understands she is angry, that her anger at not having her needs met is long overdue, that feeling and expressing her anger and needs represent progress on her part, and that he expects her to bring all her feelings to her next session. She tells Dr. K. what she needs from him, but once again he appears to be immobilized and frightened. She hangs up the telephone in despair, angry at herself for trying to elicit responses from Dr. K. that he cannot provide.

Dr. K. is left with his worst fears confirmed—Lynn's anger is spiraling out of control. Perhaps if she got some sleep she would feel better. But when he recommended the sleeping medication she rejected that too. Nothing he offered felt right to her, and she could not see or appreciate the effort he was making to do what she asked. Not knowing what to say to her, not wanting to lash out in anger, he had controlled himself and said nothing.

Lynn goes to her next session the following Monday able for the first time to feel and give words to all of her feelings. She feels a new sense of personal power and strength, as if she had been mute all her life and had suddenly been given her voice. But Dr. K. cannot see the change in Lynn and responds to her in such a peculiar manner that she begins to feel alarmed.

For the first time in the six years they had been meeting regularly, Dr. K. withholds the monthly statement that he always gives her on the first day of the month. She asks whether he is afraid to give it to her because she is angry at him and he fears she might complain that he had not earned it. He explains that he is experimenting to see if the same sequence of behavior that occurred the preceding Monday will occur this Monday. If he gives her the bill, the sequence he is looking for will be influenced by a change in his behavior from last week to this week.

Dr. K.'s reasoning makes no sense to Lynn, and she not only points out the problems in his reasoning but adds that she is a therapy patient, not a subject in a behavioral research study. A heated disagreement ensues over what sequence of behavior had in fact transpired the previous week. Dr. K. argues with Lynn, another unusual behavior on his part. He tells her that he is sure he is right, that he wishes he had tape recorded the previous Monday session so he could prove to her that he is right.

Lynn, able to recognize and express her feelings, asks him what is more important to him: proving that he is right or understanding her experience? She leaves the session feeling a mixture of relief and anxiety. She is relieved at having been able to recognize and express her authentic feelings. But she is disturbed by Dr. K.'s responses to her and his inability to see any value—or psychological function—in her anger. She is worried that she might defeat Dr. K., knowing that defeating him will mean a larger loss for her.

Dr. K. feels desperate after the session. He has been trying hard to tolerate her anger, but whatever he does makes things worse. He feels like she is driving him crazy, and he wants her to go away. Knowing that he is beginning to feel out of control, Dr. K. decides to get emergency consultation before the next session.

When Lynn comes to her session the next day, she has barely sat down in the patient's chair when Dr. K. begins to talk. Usually he waits for her to begin the sessions, so his initiating a topic for discussion is another unusual occurrence. Dr. K. begins with an interpretation, another surprise, because he rarely offers interpretations.

He tells Lynn that he believes that he missed an opportunity in their session the day before. He had felt that *she* was not empathizing with *his* experience in their session, and the feeling of not being understood by her had been terrible for him. His feeling of not being understood must have been analogous to what she had experienced as a child. He believes that he missed an opportunity to understand her early childhood experience through the vehicle of his inner response to her during their session.

Dr. K.'s interpretation to Lynn is psychologically accurate, but Lynn cannot assimilate it. Hanging on to her anger as protection, she feels that his focus on her early experience, a focus once wished for and not received, is inappropriate now. Lynn believes she is reacting to his real failures in the present. His sudden and unexpected shift of focus to her past seems to her to be yet another avoidance of her feelings. From her point of view, the fact that she has at long last stopped trying to empathize with his experience and is finally demanding that he pay attention to her reality is a personal triumph, not a fatal flaw. Transformed from the compliant, caretaking patient that she had been, Lynn readily lets Dr. K. know her feelings.

Unable to appreciate the positive aspects of the change in Lynn and not knowing how to help her shift to a more receptive state in relation to him, Dr. K. is deflated. He had hoped that the interpretation would restore an empathic connection and bring back Lynn's capacity to reflect upon her anger. Her indignation stops him in his tracks and leaves him without a clear sense of what to do next.

After a number of confusing exchanges with Dr. K. that alarm Lynn because his responses no longer make sense, Lynn finally tells Dr.

K. that she sees no point in continuing the therapy. She says that ninety-five percent of her believes that she should terminate the relationship even though five percent still feels hopeful that something might change.

Dr. K. asks her how it will feel to give up the last five percent of her hope. Lynn tells him that if he really wants her to continue in therapy with him, as he said, he ought to be asking her how they could augment the five percent of her hope. He counters that she once again has misunderstood his question, that he is not intending to side with the part of her that wants to leave. He adds in a distinctly bitter tone of voice that no one else would interpret his question the way she has. Feeling accused and attacked, Lynn stands up and tells him that she thinks she had better end the therapy right away. The therapy has become destructive to her. She leaves his office and later that afternoon contacts his answering service to cancel all future appointments—a bitter triumph.

The final contact that Lynn and Dr. K. have with each other takes place over the telephone the following week. He calls her and tells her that he has met with a new consultant who is willing to work with him. He says that he now has new information that he thinks will help them.

Lynn is caught in conflict. She wants desperately to restore the therapeutic relationship to prevent terminating in a disastrous breach and she is tempted to hear Dr. K.'s new information. But her past efforts to make the therapy work have ended in disappointment, and in recent sessions both she and Dr. K. have been alarmingly out of control and destructive. Her wish to avoid an abrupt and disappointing termination of their therapeutic relationship prevails. The idea that Dr. K. has new and useful information lures her back into the relationship she thought she had finally been able to end.

Lynn tells Dr. K. her dilemma: She does not want to remain his patient only to be disappointed again, but she also does not want to miss anything that might help her. Dr. K. asks her if she wants him to tell her his information right then, over the telephone. She tells him that not knowing what the information is, she has no way to decide what would be best. He is the therapist and he should decide what to do.

Dr. K. hesitates for a moment, uncertain what to do. Somewhat impulsively, eager to save the relationship, he tells her what he has learned. His consultant has suggested that Lynn is reenacting a painful time from her childhood. When her mother was distraught over repeated problems with Alice in the first six years of Lynn's life, Lynn feared that her needs had driven her mother crazy. Now Lynn is trying to drive Dr. K. crazy, and she needs him to be able to withstand her attempts.

The interpretation catches Lynn off guard. Delivered over the telephone after a week of no contact and with no scheduled sessions, attributed to an unknown and new consultant, the interpretation comes hurtling across the telephone wires at Lynn. Normally articulate, she finds herself stuttering and stammering, literally gasping for breath. Finally she manages to communicate that his interpretation feels like an attack, that he is acting irresponsibly in telling it to her at all and certainly in telling it to her over the telephone, that he is blaming her for the problems in the therapy. His facts about her early experience are not even accurate. Her mother was depressed, not crazy.

Not realizing that she is retaliating for what has felt like an attack, Lynn goes on to tell Dr. K. that she wonders if he failed the patient who killed himself the way that he is now failing her. Bitterly, she says she would like to ask the man's wife.

Dr. K. answers her calmly, as if she has made a genuine and quite reasonable request. He tells her that he will be happy to arrange a meeting with his patient's wife, implying that the wife would not only be willing to meet with an unknown, angry patient, but that she will take Dr. K.'s side. More than the content of his words, Dr. K.'s calm, quiet voice in uttering them has a chilling effect. Lynn realizes that Dr. K. is out of control and that she needs to extricate herself from an impossible situation. Not knowing what else to do, she simply hangs up the telephone.

As Lynn gradually collects herself, she comes to understand what has transpired on her side of the telephone interchange with Dr. K. Her understanding calms her down, and she is able to place another call to Dr. K.

When Dr. K. answers, his voice is subdued. Lynn explains that she was upset in the prior call because she cannot stand being called crazy or to be accused of driving others crazy. She asks him why he chose that particular interpretation to share with her out of all that he and his consultant must have discussed. Could it be, she asks, that he feels she really is driving him crazy and that he cannot stand it?

A subdued Dr. K. tells her he thinks she is correct. He recalls her request that he be an equal participant in the relationship when they began to meet four times a week. Even though he felt challenged at the time, some part of him had not wanted to be equally involved in the therapy with her. He adds that he realizes that he has an internal block against empathizing with her. He asks Lynn if she will consider returning to therapy because he believes that his consultation will help him work more effectively with her.

Although Lynn is impressed by his honesty and tempted by his offer, she is held back by her conviction that the relationship is too dangerous. She believes that she now represents a pathway for his continuing psychological growth and development, but that he cannot provide that same pathway for her. Her sense of her destructive power in relationships is tragically reaffirmed.

Lynn and Dr. K. end their six years of work together at the safe distance provided by the telephone. Dr. K. never sends Lynn a bill for her last four sessions, an omission that she takes to mean that he is assuming some responsibility for the abrupt and painful end of their therapeutic relationship.

The task of mourning the end of the relationship and the loss of contact with Dr. K., a therapist to whom she was deeply attached despite his limitations, and the challenge of understanding what happened to bring about the stalemate and rupture remain hers alone. Lynn ultimately has to relinquish the illusion of Dr. K. as an expert therapist who has "worked through" his personal issues and can therefore help her. She has to consciously face Dr. K.'s vulnerabilities and the extent to which he unconsciously fell into them. In doing so, she is forced to confront her own: How she learned to shape herself around the needs of others for fear of annihilating them with her anger or of being annihilated by them. How she learned to preserve the psychological stability of others even if she had to sacrifice her own feelings, needs, wishes, and thoughts. She has to face her need to disavow his vulnerabilities and her own, as well as come to understand both the personal and cultural context of her need not to see them.

Beyond a conceptual understanding of how and why the therapeutic relationship of Lynn and Dr. K. reached an impasse and ended in a rupture are the tantalizing questions their experience raises. Can we distinguish avoidable failures of therapists from defeats brought about by the powerful defenses of patients that become engaged around vulnerabilities? If Dr. K. had been able to empathize more effectively with Lynn, would she have needed to protect herself from him with her rage? When therapeutic relationships do rupture, how can we sort out the positive aspects of the rupture from the destructive ones? Lynn defeated Dr. K. with her anger, a victory that was also a loss, but she survived without destroying either herself or him. For Lynn, who lived with a terror of destroying her parents and sister were she to have unleashed the full force of her rage, was the survival itself a developmental gain?

In working with impasses, wounding, and ruptures in therapy, we profit most if we can both work toward answers and at the same time hold onto the challenging questions.

CHAPTER FOUR

❖ *Untangling the Knot* ❖

Into the isolated, physically immobile life of the analyst comes a succession of intelligent, mostly personable younger people who bring with them the breath of many different lives. They share with him their deepest feelings, as well as feeding into him considerable instinctual stimulation by the stories they tell, by their appearance, their voices and their smell. On the whole, analysts manage this situation well, but considerable instinctual inhibition is involved.

—John Klauber[1]

I believe that patients, even very disturbed, withdrawn, or narcissistic patients, are always accommodating to the interpersonal reality of the analyst's character and of the analytic relationship. Patients tune in, consciously and unconsciously, to the analyst's attitudes and feelings toward them, but inasmuch as they believe that these observations touch on sensitive aspects of the analyst's character, patients are likely to communicate these observations only indirectly through allusions to others, as displacements, or through descriptions of these characteristics as aspects of themselves, as identifications . . .

—Lewis Aron[2]

The psychoanalytic situation provides many opportunities for people to observe their analysts closely. These observations are inevitably woven into the fabric of patients' transference experience. Because the observations can be uncomfortable for the analyst, there is a constant temptation to ignore or deny the plausibility of the patients' perceptions. . . . Thus, countertransferential self-protectiveness is a constant, inescapable threat to our work, and our theory itself may provide a shelter from some of the harshest storms. Continuing awareness of this threat is necessary if we are to sustain the respectful and affirmative presence that Schafer (1983) has so aptly termed the "analytic attitude."

—Jay R. Greenberg[3]

Underemphasized Aspects of the Therapeutic Relationship

The process of disentangling the impasse of Lynn and Dr. K. illustrates how the determinants of impasses that are initially obscured by the complexity of the therapeutic relationship can be sorted out and understood. However, because we are operating in the realm of subjective meaning, the factors that operated together to bring about their impasse and derail the therapy are not objective, fixed truths. Rather, the factors that will be discussed are intended to serve as flexible models of subjective meaning. *The various contributing factors together create a conceptual understanding, a composite, that can only approach the true complexity of the relationship.*

The example of Lynn and Dr. K. illustrates potentially problematic aspects of therapeutic relationships that tend to be underemphasized because they occur automatically and are consequently difficult to render visible. As the quotation from John Klauber suggests, *therapists are vulnerable to experiencing intense feelings toward their patients*—a factor that can contribute to therapeutic impasses. Lynn worked to forge a special bond with Dr. K., in part because of a reactivated yearning for an unattainable bond with her father. Her efforts were expressed in her empathy and concern for him and in adopting his interests (Shakespeare and psychotherapy) as her own. Her efforts met an acute and equally unconscious need in Dr. K. for a soul mate, a kindred spirit, a kind of intellectual companion. Dr. K. came to rely upon her for the intimacy she could provide and unknowingly abandoned his stance as her therapist. If he had not done so, he might have been able to reflect on both his needs in relation to her and her yearnings and wishes in relation to him. Like Dr. K., therapists are at risk of relying unconsciously on certain patients to meet personal needs. Like Lynn, many patients yearn to experience a special intimacy with their therapists.

Patients' automatic efforts to protect their therapists by disavowing perceptions of the therapists' vulnerabilities constitute another potential source of impasses. As the quotation from Lewis Aron indicates, patients accommodate to the interpersonal reality of their therapist, accurately sensing their therapist's feelings and attitudes toward them. *But when they intuit that these feelings and attitudes are related to areas of vulnerability in the therapist, they often hold themselves back from talking explicitly about what they perceive.* Lynn sensed but disavowed her perception of Dr. K.'s need to be enlivened by her interest in him, to receive her compassion in the face of his shame and guilt, and to avoid intense affects and conflict in the relationship. Lynn repeatedly held herself back from putting Dr. K. on the spot by not sharing her responses, evidenced in her reluctance to raise her concerns both about his telephone call outside the session for a referral and about his guilt over his suicidal patient. Fearful of the destructive power of her critical, angry feelings, Lynn created him, albeit unconsciously, into the helpful therapist she needed him to be. She had protected herself in her family of origin by disavowing her feelings of anger in order to protect herself from feeling like a bad, unloving person and to provide herself with a loving family. Like Lynn and Dr. K., patients' tendency to disavow the perceived limitations of their therapists may mesh harmoniously with the therapists' need to preserve a particular sense of self. Like Lynn, who was unaware of her core sense of being bad and destructive, patients are often unable to "see through" their own defenses to the vulnerable core the defenses protect. Their defenses can effectively hide the vulnerable core from their therapists as well.

Therapists may unconsciously contribute to impasses, as Dr. K. did, by warding off expressions from patients that would disrupt their sense of self. As the quotation from Jay Greenberg indicates, *therapists are prone to deny or ignore their patients' accurate perceptions of them because of the discomfort the perceptions cause*, another common source of therapeutic impasses. For example, Dr. K. had difficulty asking himself how he might be contributing to the stalemate in the therapeutic relationship because of the psychological disequilibrium that such questions would have caused. If Dr. K. had asked himself, for example, why he was giving Lynn articles on Shakespeare and psychotherapy rather than asking her what her wish to share his interests might mean, he might have uncovered his unmet needs for a soul mate. He might then have confronted his reluctance to seek consultation or psychotherapy. Had he done so, a range of disavowed feelings about himself might have been consciously available to him rather than defended against in ways that limited and derailed the therapy.

Three Factors Contributing to the Stalemate Between Lynn and Dr. K.

In addition to the contribution of these general and underemphasized aspects of therapeutic relationships to the impasse of Lynn and Dr. K., there were (at least) three other specific contributing factors. These factors, like those discussed in Chapter Two and the preceding section, are not unique to Lynn and Dr. K. but rather represent common sources of impasses in therapeutic relationships.

First, Dr. K. did not make explicit connections between Lynn's early history and the kinds of interactions that occurred in therapy. Thinking through these links, regardless of whether or not he shared his ideas with Lynn, would have helped him adopt a reflective stance toward her. Without a mutually created conceptual narrative to provide a platform from which both Dr. K. and Lynn could look at and explore her mode of relating to him, Lynn could only continue attempting to influence their relationship through familiar relational modes. Dr. K., like a boat without a rudder in stormy seas, could only react to Lynn without conscious reflection and an orientation to guide him. A conceptual formulation was essential because of the function it would have served in protecting Lynn and Dr. K. from being lost together in their jointly created relational mode, not because it would have constituted a statement of objective truth about their therapeutic relationship.

Second, Lynn and Dr. K. related to each other without an awareness of the personal vulnerabilities and defensive adaptations that might otherwise have been provided by a reflective stance on their part, alone or in consultation. Naming the vulnerabilities and adaptive mechanisms that had become engaged in the therapy could have served the same function as a narrative frame for the relational dynamics: facilitating a reflective stance (without regarding the stance as objective truth). Dr. K. could not penetrate Lynn's seamless protective shield to see her fear of her anger. He did not recognize that his vulnerabilities were causing him to back away from Lynn when her personal sensitivities were activated. Lynn was unaware of her fear of her destructive potential and did not realize that Dr. K.'s distancing from her served a self-protective function for him. Like many patients, Lynn attributed Dr. K.'s distancing himself to her blameworthy and unlovable core. Dr. K.'s emotional and psychological withdrawal caused Lynn to react with panic and anxiety, which in turn led her to increase her efforts to connect to him. Ironically, Lynn's renewed efforts to reach Dr. K. and the anger that defended her wounded self only drove him further away from her. Without a recognition and understanding of their relational pattern that would have provided some distance from it, the stalemate between Lynn and Dr. K. could only worsen.

Third, Dr. K.'s failure to create with Lynn a narrative understanding of her personal history, and to identify and work psychologically with their mode of relating to each other, took place within a broad, culturally determined matrix that underlies therapeutic relationships between men and women. This matrix often operates invisibly, outside the conscious awareness of therapists and patients, yet its influence on the relational patterns that develop within it is profound. Therapists and patients can profit from working together to make visible and name the cultural field in which they operate.

An aspect of the cultural matrix that affected Lynn is connected to female socialization. Many women are socialized to relate to men in ways that support and affirm the man's sense of self. Women oriented toward men in this way are unable to receive support from men for the development of a strong sense of a female self.[4] Male therapists are best able to facilitate the unfolding of the unique female self of their patients when they remain conscious of their susceptibility to disavowing personal vulnerabilities and relying upon women to enhance their sense of self. With conscious awareness of the pitfall created by cultural conditioning, male therapists can make use of their empathic and relational skills in the service of enhancing a woman's sense of self.

The remainder of the chapter will consider the stalemate in the therapeutic relationship of Lynn and Dr. K. with respect to these three specific factors: the lack of attention to Lynn's personal history and the transference context of the relationship, the failure to attend to the intersecting personal vulnerabilities of both patient and therapist on the relationship, and the unconscious enactment of culturally influenced gender roles.

The Missing Transference Context

Lynn did not realize until the end of the therapeutic relationship that Dr. K. had not kept her personal history in mind. She had told him significant stories from her early life and assumed that he retained them as a backdrop against which he could better understand her responses to her current life and her modes of relating to him. The narrative structure that Dr. K. might have created with Lynn and kept in mind would have been based upon the following history.

Lynn is the elder of two daughters. Her father, an executive salesman for a large company, and her mother, a housewife, were preoccupied with caring for their younger daughter. Alice required extra attention as a result of a learning disability that was detected when she was in the first grade. Unlike Alice, Lynn functioned exceptionally well in school and required virtually no assistance.

Lynn's father, unlike Dr. K., was extraverted and outgoing, but, like Dr. K., he had always been a solid, reliable, stable presence and behaved in an overtly loving manner. He was not given to talking about his feelings nor did he engage in self-reflection, so Lynn had always felt distant from him and yearned to be closer.

Lynn also felt removed from her mother because she felt excluded from the bond that Alice and her mother shared. Her feelings of envy and deprivation often caused her to be angry and difficult with her mother. Consequently Lynn's relationship with her mother was emotionally intense, fraught with conflict that upset her father, and left Lynn feeling guilty and unhappy.

Lynn's relationship with Alice alternated between protective concern and angry envy. Alice adored Lynn and had an engaging, loving personality. Lynn was never able to remain angry at Alice for long, partly because of Alice's personality and partly because Lynn felt guilty that Alice's learning problem made her life so difficult.

Lynn had learned to mute her needs, thoughts, and feelings in relation to her mother and father in order to minimize conflict and to maximize the chances of maintaining a positive connection to them. She accurately perceived that they were stretched to their psychological limits in their effort to take care of Alice. If Lynn pressed them with her needs, she created conflict. Conflict caused family members to lose control of themselves with eruptions of anger that frightened her. As a child, she blamed herself for the family conflicts, becoming in her mind the "bad" child in the family. Her egocentric child's mind determined that if she were "good"—less hateful toward Alice, less greedy for attention, less demanding—the family would be able to sustain a loving equilibrium.

Cumulative experiences of blaming herself resulted in a split in Lynn's conscious sense of self. She experienced herself as "bad" when she spoke out, precipitated conflict, felt angry or complained, or could not control fluctuations in her mood. She experienced herself as "good" when she was compliant, attentive to the needs of others, and demonstrated competence in taking care of herself.

When Lynn entered into the therapeutic relationship with Dr. K., she was unaware of the adaptation she had made to her family and of the split that operated unconsciously in her experience of herself. She had only a vague awareness that aspects of herself other than the competent, undemanding, reliable, caretaking, "good" self were not allowed into consciousness. The vague awareness emerged in the request she made in the initial session with Dr. K. to be able to bring the less visible sides of herself into the relationship—the emotions, fears, and anxieties that she kept hidden inside, aspects that others in her life rarely saw.

The first phase of therapy was helpful to Lynn. She experienced Dr. K.'s silence as positive. He did not impose his needs on her, nor did he have strong ideas about her that might have replaced her own, as her mother's too often did. At first she dared show him only her "good" side by being a competent, responsible, capable patient. But she interpreted his unhesitating response to her requests for additional sessions as an invitation to her to include within the therapeutic relationship the sides of herself that she experienced as bad: her anger, criticality, strong opinions, fears, dependency needs. During this phase, Dr. K. proved helpful in facilitating a broadening of her perception of her parents and younger sister, supporting her in facing the previously disavowed limitations.

The two pivotal incidents, referred to by Lynn as "discordant notes," in which Dr. K. asserted his needs in the relationship, precipitated a reenactment of Lynn's role in her family and led to the second, stalemated phase of the therapy. Lynn automatically responded to Dr. K.'s needs without explicit acknowledgment between them that she was doing so. Her feelings about taking care of Dr. K. went underground, just as they had in her family: first, by supplying the name of her husband's medical specialist, disregarding her concern that he was relating to her only as a competent adult and not as a vulnerable patient; and second, by expressing care and concern for him when his patient committed suicide, suppressing her worries about the reliability of his careful focus on her.

The therapeutic relationship entered a phase of impasse. Lynn was aware that the therapy was stuck and made efforts to bring about a shift. Dr. K. responded willingly to her efforts. She tried to intensify the therapeutic relationship by increasing the frequency of the sessions to four times a week. But the range of what the relationship could include did not expand. Confused, Lynn assumed that the problem resided in the structure of the relationship or in her. The possibility that Dr. K. might be contributing to the impasse did not occur to Lynn, as is the case with many patients and therapists who tend to locate problems exclusively in themselves or in the therapist (where they may at times reside) rather than to consider the intersection of their vulnerabilities and defenses.

The crisis in Lynn's life precipitated by the automobile accident in which her younger sister was seriously injured catapulted Lynn and Dr. K. into the third and final phase of their relationship. Lynn's anguish was so intense that she could no longer maintain her role as the good patient, nor could she continue to assume responsibility for what was not taking place in the therapy. As her needs caused Lynn to exert more pressure on Dr. K., she was pushed into a conscious confrontation with Dr. K.'s limits and vulnerabilities that she had previously needed to disavow. At the same time that Lynn faced Dr. K.'s limits, she was also forced to confront her defensive adaptation to his limitations and her own wounded core. She came to recognize the personal price she had paid to protect her "bad" side from overpowering the "good," to maintain an equilibrium in her family, and to preserve both a positive connection to her parents and a view of them as nurturing and supportive. She also was able to appreciate the extent to which she had repeated this pattern in the therapeutic relationship with Dr. K.

The final rupture in the relationship was inevitable, once Lynn's heightened state of need disrupted the balance. The impasse and the relationship ended in a painful and problematic way. But Lynn eventually reached an enhanced conscious awareness of self and other. Lynn came to appreciate consciously her own defenses, including her anger, and those of Dr. K. In the process, she relinquished the relied-upon "good" self that had served her well, integrated aspects of herself that had been suppressed as "bad," and consequently accessed a more authentic and powerful voice.

Lynn might be regarded as an unusual patient because she arrived at her new understanding of herself largely on her own, outside the context of the therapeutic relationship. Traditional conceptions of therapy assume that patients arrive at a new awareness of themselves as a consequence of psychological work that takes place in the ongoing relationship. But insights and psychological change often occur outside the therapy, because of the relationship but not necessarily within it. Hence, patients work with experiences that were part of therapeutic relationships long after the relationships terminate. Termination refers to the ending of regular psychotherapy sessions, not to the end of the relationship, which the participants continue to carry psychologically. Because of the assumption that psychological growth primarily occurs *within* an ongoing therapeutic relationship, patients often assume that their insights are "given" to them by the therapist, who is viewed as able to see aspects of them that they cannot see.[5] As therapists move toward claiming the "patient" in themselves, patients may analogously be helped to honor the "therapist" in themselves and to take responsibility for and appreciate their efforts on their own behalf.

Lynn was also left with a psychological residue that she would eventually address in another therapeutic relationship: Because she believed that she had overpowered and defeated Dr. K., she feared that she risked unleashing a potentially destructive force if she dared to speak, truthfully and aloud, her feelings and perceptions.

The Missing Vulnerabilities of Dr. K.

Dr. K., like Lynn, operated in the therapeutic relationship from a limited conscious sense of self. His introversion and temperament functioned to keep Lynn at a distance and warded off intense affect states either in her or in himself. He unwittingly made it difficult for Lynn to experience a feeling of connection with him most of the time. Dr. K. resembled Lynn's father in this respect, a resemblance that initially enabled her to feel at home with his silence and to perceive him as solidly present and reliable.

But unlike Lynn's father, who was confident of himself in relation to other people and enjoyed a ready popularity, Dr. K. had struggled with a lifelong sense of social inadequacy and reticence around people. His role of therapist operated like a protective shield, enabling him to have the semblance of intimacy without putting emotional energy of his own into the relationship. Lynn's yearning to relate to and connect with her father in a personal way awakened and met an equal and long-buried yearning for connection in Dr. K. He fell into the gratifying experience of sharing his intellectual interests with Lynn, unaware that by doing so he was meeting his own needs and abandoning her as his patient.

When Lynn perceived the relationship as "stuck," the block resided in their inability to stand back from the therapeutic relationship and discern the gratifying collusion that had become established between them. Dr. K. could not identify the early (pre-Oedipal) transference level of the relationship—that Lynn was searching for a way to bond to him just as she had wished to bond with her mother. He could not see that his need for connection and intimacy had overridden his focus on his patient's need for him to mirror psychologically her issues. Unconsciously immobilized by the prospect of facing the feelings that would be unleashed, he was unable to seek ongoing consultation or personal therapy. Consequently Dr. K. had no way to address the impasse in the therapeutic relationship with Lynn or the personal issues that had been activated and contributed to the stalemate. Lynn could not help Dr. K. reach an awareness of the transference matrix of their relationship because she, too, was unaware of the relational modes that were operating automatically.

Dr. K's difficulty with intimacy and relatedness, manifest in his marked constriction in Lynn's presence, made it impossible for him to work directly and explicitly with her perceptions of him. His demeanor of kindness and compassion, in tandem with her well-developed capacity for disavowal, made it difficult for Lynn to have critical feelings in relation to him. Lynn's primary defensive adaptation—her tendency to disavow negative aspects of herself (her angry, needy, critical feelings), her parents, and everyone else in her life—operated unconsciously with Dr. K. and he failed to help her identify it. Like many patients, Lynn attributed problems in the relationship to herself and not to the problematic intersection of vulnerabilities and defensive adaptations within the relationship.

When he allowed Lynn to comfort him after the suicide of his patient, Dr. K. fell into a mode of relying on her to receive his feelings and allowed himself to enjoy her interest in him. He was enlivened by their discussions of psychotherapy issues and by her wish to share his interest in Shakespeare. He remained unaware of his collusion in allowing her to relate to him in the same way that she related to her father and to her family in general—responding to perceived urgency of others' needs and minimizing conflict to ward off a loss of connection.

The automobile accident that left Lynn's already handicapped younger sister with permanent disabilities evoked in Lynn intense emotions of rage, guilt, and grief. The trauma of the accident revived emotional and psychological states that Lynn had already lived through in childhood. The current situation elicited Lynn's childhood guilt at being free from the learning disability that plagued Alice, as well as Lynn's envy of and anger at Alice for the special attention Alice received from their parents. Lynn had developed strong ego defenses to manage these feelings, but the force of past and present distress escalated until her defenses were overwhelmed and the feelings they were holding back burst forth. Dr. K. was unable to provide a solid, strong, empathic container for her feelings until her defenses could be restored with an expanded awareness. The opportunity presented by the catastrophe was lost.

The intensity of Lynn's feelings in response to her life crisis frightened and overwhelmed Dr. K. Unaware of his fear that the feelings would be more than his cognitive defenses could organize, he retreated from her by withdrawing psychologically and tried to stop her feelings by offering medication and encouraging her to cancel sessions. Had he been able to name his vulnerability openly, perhaps by acknowledging his difficulty withstanding the onslaught of intense feeling, had he been able to affirm Lynn's need to be in the presence of someone who could welcome her feelings, the abrupt and painful termination of the relationship might have been averted. Lynn might have been freer to express disappointment, disillusionment, and feelings of abandonment or criticism rather than compelled to revert once again to blaming herself or being reinforced in her belief that no one would ever tolerate her "bad" side. Instead, she left the therapy feeling that she had defeated him, a victory that only reaffirmed her fear of her destructive potential.

Dr. K. contributed to the painful and disillusioning end of the therapeutic relationship by being unable both to acknowledge his vulnerabilities and limitations and to shift to a different relational mode in response to Lynn's intensified needs after the traumatic automobile accident. Stating honestly and openly that his capacities had been temporarily exceeded, seeking consultation sooner, encouraging her to express her feelings, making interpretive connections to ways she had been shaped in her family before it was too late and in a less shocking manner, might have helped them make use of the opportunity embedded in the trauma of the accident. Instead, Dr. K. sought consultation too late and introduced interpretations that might have been useful in a different context in the midst of self-preservative defensive responses. The result was an unfortunate amalgam that made the relationship seem dangerous to Lynn.

In reflecting back upon the therapy, Lynn believes that if Alice's tragic automobile accident had not intervened to disrupt the stalemate, she would have persisted interminably in her efforts to make the therapeutic relationship work. At some point she would have given up and decided to terminate therapy. She imagines she would have done so in a planned way, exiting the relationship politely and thanking Dr. K. for his help. Although the termination that took place was profoundly disappointing and painful, Lynn feels some sense of accomplishment in having ended with an expression of her authentic feelings of anger and disappointment, without destroying either Dr. K. or herself. She went on to make use of a subsequent therapeutic relationship to address her fear that her critical feelings could overpower and destroy others.

Dr. K., unfortunately, did not make use of the opportunity for growth that his patient, Lynn, presented him with. He did not seek psychotherapy or ongoing consultation. However, he maintained a successful psychotherapy practice that included patients who felt he helped them.

The Invisible Cultural Matrix

An additional component of the impasse in the therapeutic relationship between Lynn and Dr. K. was their unconscious enactment of culturally influenced gender roles.[6] Lynn occupied the position of the "good daughter"/"good mother" and enabled Dr. K. to take the corresponding role of the "good father"/"good son." Dr. K. and Lynn fell into an unconscious enactment of a culturally influenced dynamic of a good father/good daughter alliance. Male therapists and female patients are particularly vulnerable to this particular enactment. Because of the special susceptibility of opposite gender dyads and the invisibility of the cultural matrix, this particular contributing factor, although last in order, may be of greatest importance.

Because male therapists and female patients in our culture are particularly at risk of falling into these roles unconsciously, awareness of the potential to do so is particularly important. Just as shifts are occurring in the underlying paradigm of psychotherapy, so are they occurring in our cultural attitudes toward women and men that will necessarily affect therapeutic relationships.[7] For example, Lynn's anger at Dr. K. may have been fueled in part by a long-suppressed anger of women in Western culture at the domination of men. Feminist activists, female scholars in fields ranging from literature, history, philosophy, psychology, political science, and religion, are rethinking and reenvisioning the role of women. In the process, women are being freed from unconsciously serving as empty vessels for the projections of men.

Women are becoming increasingly aware of how they have been socialized to relate to men predominantly as respectful and compliant daughters, as attractive sexual objects, or as dutiful wives. Beginning with the second wave of feminism in the late 1960s, women have been encouraged to pay attention to their subjective experience as women and to articulate it in language. Women are beginning to talk about aspects of female experience that until now have been disavowed. For example, women in ethnic minority groups have been writing about their experiences. Novels that depict the lives and struggles of contemporary women have become best-sellers. As this trend continues, female patients will have an easier time expressing and trusting their sense of themselves, and therapists in turn will evolve a more differentiated understanding of female psychology.

Men are helping in this endeavor by focusing increased attention on the different but equally powerful limits placed on their sense of a masculine self by their role as men in a patriarchal culture. As the rising "men's movement" and the best-selling popularity of books like Robert Bly's recent book *Iron John* and Sam Keen's book *Fire in the Belly* indicate (regardless of the validity of their assertions), men are beginning to pay attention to their subjective experiences of being male. As male and female therapists become more conscious of what it means to be men and women in contemporary culture, they will be able to relate to their female (and male) patients from a different foundation.

We are only beginning to evolve a differentiated psychology of women and of men and to understand the implications for psychotherapy to which a differentiated understanding of men and women would lead. Groundbreaking work by the Stone Center women,[8] Carol Gilligan[9], and others[10] toward developing a psychological understanding of women has not yet been fully absorbed by mainstream psychology and psychoanalysis. Jungian psychology includes a rich understanding of the masculine and feminine duality (as well as the dimension of spirituality that is absent from other psychodynamic perspectives), but Jung, too, has also been excluded from mainstream psychoanalytic thought.

Jung provides us with a metaphor that describes the special susceptibility of male therapists to falling into a reliance upon their female patients to meet personal needs. In Jungian terms, Dr. K. related to Lynn as an *anima figure* rather than as a woman in her own right. By *anima figure*, Jung referred to an archetype in the collective unconscious that embodies the feminine for men:

> in the realm of his [the son's] psyche there is an imago not only of the mother but of the daughter, the sister, the beloved, the heavenly goddess, and the chthonic Baubo. Every mother and every beloved is forced to become the carrier and embodiment of this omnipresent and ageless image, which corresponds to the deepest reality in a man.[11]

Because the anima is an archetype, it remains part of the unconscious psyche, but the influence of the anima in shaping the ways that the actual women in a man's life are perceived can become conscious. Jung cautioned therapists to be aware of the anima, so that its influence on conscious experience could be sed productively:

> Though the effects of the anima and animus can be made conscious, they themselves are factors transcending consciousness and beyond the reach of perception and volition. Hence they remain autonomous despite the integration of their contents, and for this reason they should be borne constantly in mind. This is extremely important from the therapeutic standpoint, because constant observation pays the unconscious a tribute that more or less guarantees its co-operation.[12]

With the concept of the anima as an inner aspect of men that is readily projected upon women, Jung gives us a means of understanding conceptually the nature of the specific projections that female patients are called upon to carry for their male therapists. The importance of the therapist's involvement in ongoing personal psychological work is particularly evident here. Unless male therapists are well acquainted with the anima, the imago of the feminine in their psyche, they are vulnerable to projecting it onto their female patients who, because of their socialization in our culture to offer themselves in this way to men, are all too ready to receive it. A commitment to being a therapist thus represents a commitment to being a patient, not necessarily literally, but in the sense of continuing to seek a psychological understanding of one's self and self-in-relationship.

Looking at the therapeutic relationship of Lynn and Dr. K. through the special lens of women's role in relation to men in our patriarchal culture provides an expanded understanding of their impasse and rupture. Lynn, in working to understand what had happened in the relationship with Dr. K., was compelled to separate his actual failures from her unrealistic expectations of him. She came to see that her unrealistic expectations were clearly involved in supporting her continued disavowal of his failures, in causing her to idealize his capacities and to expect that he would always be reliably there for her. But she also came to see that his failures were not all the result of her unrealistic expectations. His responses after the crisis of the automobile accident undeniably communicated his need for her to feel better and to return to her former mode of being a gratifying patient (sharing his interests, never demanding much, attending to his needs with her empathic skills) or to go away so that she would not disrupt his equilibrium, communicated through his attempts to prescribe tranquilizing medication and his acceptance of cancellations.

Lynn recognized that the car accident in which her younger sister, Alice, was injured catapulted her into a psychological state that rendered her unable to function for Dr. K. as a gratifying patient, as a woman who met his unacknowledged needs for mirroring and positive affirmation. Lynn's unconscious messages were present but disavowed, as exemplified by her request that Dr. K. return a book that he had borrowed from her. Lynn reminded him several times to return the book, but he had misplaced it. Neither Lynn nor Dr. K. could reflect upon the psychological meaning of his inability to find her book or upon what "losing a part of her" might signify to her.

Looking back on the therapeutic relationship, and the ways in which Dr. K. failed her in reality, as well as ways she perceived him as having failed her because of her unrealistic expectations, proved to be invaluable for Lynn. She eventually recognized that without an abandonment of this magnitude by her male therapist, and consequently by the "father" on a psychological and archetypal level and by the patriarchy he represented on the historical-cultural level, she would not have been forced to confront how her sense of a female self had been shaped around deferring to men. As a consequence of her accommodation to Dr. K.'s needs, and of Dr. K.'s unconscious mode of relating to women as "good mothers," Lynn was visible to him only when she confined the facets of herself that she presented to him to the narrow channel of the nurturing feminine. Her only visible and acceptable aspect, both in the therapeutic relationship and with respect to her experience of herself, was that of the "good daughter"/"good mother."

Jungian analyst Marion Woodman describes this aspect of Lynn's disillusioning and disappointing therapy with a man. Woodman states that what appears to be a healing, positive relationship may be instead an unconscious reenacting of the father complex on the part of both the male therapist and female patient. The patient sees the positive father in her therapist, while the therapist feels fatherly pride in his daughter's achievement. Both parties remain unaware of the old patriarchal dominance residing in this situation, within which the female patient can only remain an "anima woman operating out of a male psychology."[13] What must happen to disrupt this collusive stalemate, and what could not happen for Lynn and Dr. K., is, in Woodman's words:

> a profound, revolutionary realignment of the relationship — a realignment that is as huge a challenge to the male ego as it is to the father complex that feeds that ego. The analyst who has been the best little boy in the world and has tried to be the most loving father in the world may have a very caring professional persona, but when it comes to real feeling, he may find himself at a total loss. A woman who is fighting for her own life is going to demand genuine feelings, and she has a right to an honest response.[14]

Painful as the termination of her therapeutic relationship was, it forced Lynn to see the extent to which she experienced herself as visible only when behaving like a "good mother." She further realized that she was able to take in positive affirmation of herself as a woman only when she operated in that familiar and gratifying channel of the nurturing feminine, whether in the role of patient, teacher, wife, friend, or mother. She saw that if she deviated from that stance, regardless of her role, she tended to experience herself as the embodiment of the "terrible mother," as wounding, abandoning, rejecting, and as having failed the other person in a way that inevitably resulted in injury and distress.

Lynn's sense of herself as simplistically divided into "good mother" versus "terrible mother" needed to yield to a more complex and differentiated notion of the feminine or of being a woman. In one sense, Lynn transformed the impasse and painful termination of her therapeutic relationship with Dr. K., as part of the psychological work she went on to do after the termination, into an *initiation into the realm of the feminine, into a more complex and differentiated sense of a feminine self.* Because psychotherapy occurs in a realm of subjective meanings, which are often different for therapist and patient, transformations of the meaning of experiences often occurs after the therapeutic relationship ends. Lynn's conception of the painful termination of the therapeutic relationship as an initiation can be understood as a change in the subjective meaning *to her* of the experience in psychotherapy with Dr. K. Jungian analyst Betty Meador describes the experience of an initiation or descent into the realm of the feminine:

> For a woman to grow into her fullness, she must find her way to the feminine aspects of the Self. Her ego will then reflect, express, and root in the divine feminine. That is to say, aspects of that complex energy we call the archetypal feminine will inform her ego orientation . . .
>
> On a larger scale, I am looking at a passage or a crossing over, as a woman shifts the support of her female self from the patriarchy to the archetypal feminine. *In this process she will let go of attitudes she has imposed on herself from the outer culture and foster those attitudes spawned by her instinct, as these begin to appear to her in dreams, imagination, and feeling* [emphasis added].[15]

Woodman also acknowledges the necessity for women to undergo an initiation into an experience of the feminine. Female patients with male therapists have the opportunity to experience such an initiation, if both participants in the therapeutic relationship bring to it an understanding of the cultural influences on their gender roles and therefore on their psyches. Woodman writes:

> The experience of psychological abandonment in women who are born and reared in a patriarchal culture is their initiation into mature womanhood. It is the experience that confers identity and takes them out of the father. Many women can accept their destiny in a patriarchal relationship, finding within its obvious limitations— socially, intellectually, spiritually—compensations that are important to them. Others accept that destiny and resist the limitations but are forced for financial, political, or social reasons to stay within its framework. Others go through the initiation. These women . . . are by inner necessity creators in the Keatsian sense of soul-makers. *They reject collective consciousness as an imposition from without, and they seek from within to construct an identity which almost inevitably brings them into collision with the very force they are struggling to integrate: the idealized image of the father* [emphasis added].[16]

When female patients come into full awareness that they have abandoned themselves in order to accommodate to their therapist's needs, either as a good daughter, good mother, or sexual object, they are likely to react with intense rage.[17] The rage is partly related to anger on their own behalf, a consequence of the recognition of the price they have paid to preserve an attachment to a man. But it is also a rage on behalf of all women who have suppressed and accepted a diminished sense of self. Women who come into awareness of this rage have forged a connection to what poet Susan Griffin refers to as "The Roaring Inside Her," a phrase from her book *Woman and Nature: The Roaring Inside Her*.[18]

The rage often erupts in an explosion that can seem to be of volcanic proportion, terrifying in intensity to the male therapist at whom it is directed. Male therapists who are unaware of its psychological under-pinnings, who view it exclusively as personal, and who place a high value on being "good sons" and "good fathers," typically react instinctively to protect themselves from it. Regardless of the specific defenses they employ—psychological withdrawal (Dr. K.), retaliatory anger expressed directly or indirectly in the form of hostile and pathologizing interpretations, or fragmentation and anxiety—the therapists leave their patients vulnerable to the experience of being misunderstood and left alone with their painful new realization. Even for those male therapists who appreciate the significance of the anger as part of their female patients' new and important awareness of self, withstanding the initial onslaught can be difficult. Male therapists, ordinarily human, are vulnerable to feeling guilty about and responsible for their patients.

As the influence of culture becomes better understood and articulated, therapists and patients will be more aware of the potential to enact without awareness culturally determined gender roles. As awareness of these roles and their impact on the psyches of men and women increases, the number of unfortunate impasses and terminations, such as that of Lynn and Dr. K., will be minimized.

*   *   *   *   *

As I have emphasized, the profession of psychotherapy is enlarging the paradigm in which an expert therapist applies a specific technique to a troubled patient to include the psychological impact of therapist and patient on each other. As this expansion progresses, impasses may have a better chance of being worked with constructively by both participants, whether or not the therapeutic relationship continues. Therapist and patient will be able to orient themselves toward an exploration of their mutual impact rather than holding a view of the patient as too troubled to be helped or the therapist as inadequate. An exploration of the mutual impact of therapist and patient may enable the relationship either to continue with expanded awareness on both sides, or to terminate with an understanding of the dynamics and a sense of resolution, rather than in a painful rupture with feelings of anger, blame, and inadequacy.

Because changes in the conception of psychotherapy filter slowly through the profession and reach the general public even more slowly, the burden currently rests too frequently with patients to confront on their own the ways in which their therapists' vulnerabilities and defenses have meshed problematically with their own. As therapists increasingly confront and work with their personal sensitivities in relation to their patients, *as therapists find new ways to incorporate these sensitivities into the therapeutic work*, and as we develop new models for consultation and intervention, the responsibility both for understanding impasses and painful terminations and for acknowledging the existence of unresolved areas that are part of all therapeutic relationships can be shared on a more equal basis between therapist and patient.

In the following chapter, the predicament that arises in therapeutic relationships when patients and therapists are wounded in areas of extreme personal sensitivity—the realm of primary vulnerability—will be addressed. These predicaments are not only particularly painful, but they also provide fertile ground for a catastrophic rupture in the therapeutic relationship.

CHAPTER FIVE

❖ *Wounding in Areas* ❖ *of Primary Vulnerability*

I have, in particular, wished to emphasize *the analyst's own part in the analytic process*, and the need for recognizing the effects upon the patient of the analyst's ways of working and interpreting. . . . Ignoring these effects can be as detrimental to the understanding of the patient as overlooking the real effects of early environmental failure. Not all of the analytic experience is to be understood in terms of inner reality or as projections by the patient. The analyst, as much as a parent, has a real impact upon the patient.

—Patrick Casement[1]

In retrospect, after Ann reminded me about the therapy, I wish I had been able to respond to her differently. I simply did not understand the vulnerable state she was in and I underestimated her reliance upon the therapy. Given who I am and the state I was in at the time, I don't think I could have acted differently. I don't know what would have helped us.

—Dr. L.

It never occurred to me to think about Dr. L. making a mistake, at least not for very long. Even if I had the thought that he did something wrong, I kept coming back to the feeling that I should have handled the situation differently, that there was something the matter with me for being so extremely hurt and upset. But every time I think about what happened at the end of the therapy, I get as upset as if it happened yesterday.

—Ann

When patients are wounded by therapists in areas of special sensitivity, a particularly painful predicament results that can jeopardize the viability of the therapeutic relationship. Patients and therapists, like participants in any intimate relationship, are at risk of being wounded by each other. But all wounds are not alike. I have used the concept of *a realm of primary vulnerability* to identify the kinds of wounds in the context of a therapeutic relationship that patients (or

89

therapists) often experience as intolerable. The concept of a realm of primary vulnerability, developed in Part II, provides a useful working model (rather than an objective truth or reality) because it gives us a means of understanding patients who feel that they have been damaged by a therapeutic relationship. My research and clinical experience indicate that *patients who are left feeling harmed by a therapeutic relationship that terminated abruptly in a painful impasse are in most cases patients who have been wounded in an area of primary vulnerability.* The wounding, instead of being contained and worked with in the relationship, has brought about a rupture and a particularly painful termination.

The extended case example of Ann and Dr. L. that follows, like the case of Lynn and Dr. K., is a fictionalized account based on an actual therapeutic relationship and consultation. Their story gives us access to the experience of a patient who is wounded in an area of primary vulnerability and to the experience of a therapist who is unaware that his primary vulnerabilities have become activated in the therapeutic relationship. The significant aspects of their relationship are presented in the present tense in order to convey the complexity and intensity of an experience of wounding in therapeutic relationships. The intention in presenting the case is neither to judge, diagnose, or blame either the patient or therapist, nor to contribute to the illusion that wounding can be avoided, but rather to acknowledge openly that situations of profound wounding arise in therapeutic relationships, to make them easier to talk about, and to evolve creative and flexible ways of providing essential psychological and relational support for therapeutic dyads grappling with them. Like Lynn's therapy with Dr. K. in Chapter Three, the relationship of Ann to Dr. L. will be referred to in subsequent chapters in order to illustrate a flexible, elastic use of theoretical concepts.

Wounding in Therapeutic Relationships: Ann and Dr. L.

Ann first seeks therapy when she is twenty-five years old. She has been married for three years to her husband, John, and works as a receptionist in a busy medical office. She and John are in the midst of trying to decide whether or not to have a child, and Ann believes that psychotherapy can help her resolve her ambivalence about becoming a mother.

Ann approaches her first hour with Dr. L., a therapist who has been recommended to her by one of the doctors she works for, with a mixture of hope and excitement. The popular Simon and Garfunkle song "Bridge over Troubled Water," which she listens to on the car radio as she drives to her appointment, seems to her to be a positive omen: "I will lay me down, like a bridge over troubled water, I will lay me down." Perhaps she will finally be able to let go of her sense of responsibility for managing everything and rely upon someone else. For as long as she can remember, she has always been competent, dependable, and responsible, regardless of the amount of personal stress she has to bear. Ann has no idea how resentful she is at the responsibility she has to carry nor how much she needs always to be in control.

Ann is the third of five children. While she was growing up, her parents both worked full time to support their large family, leaving Ann essentially on her own. She developed a fierce determination to be self-reliant, not to count on anyone other than herself. She is unaware of the vulnerable underbelly of her strong drive toward independence—a profound wish for a harmonious attachment to another human being who would be a reliable caretaker, for an indestructible attachment, a bond so solidly forged that it might bend but could never break.

Although Dr. L. has been trained as a psychoanalytically oriented therapist, he does not focus explicitly on Ann's early life experiences or on how her determination to be independent was shaped by growing up as a middle child in her large family. But he unwittingly encourages her to rely upon him by recommending in the first session that she meet with him twice a week and by his policy of charging for missed sessions, regardless of the reason, whether or not she cancels well in advance. Ann, who had expected to meet weekly, responds to his recommendation of twice a week with some anxiety, but she is pleased at his interest in her. Not wanting to pay for sessions she does not use, she makes certain never to miss an appointment.

Over the course of the first year of regular, biweekly therapy sessions, Ann's relationship with Dr. L. grows steadily stronger. He proves to be a person upon whom Ann can consistently rely for empathy and support. He helps her understand her reluctance to have a child for fear of being tied down, of having her freedom and independence encroached upon, and her need to reduce the responsibilities she carries. He supports her growing belief that she can have a child while preserving her feeling of freedom and independence, that she does not have to choose between being a mother and having a life of her own.

Ultimately Ann and John decide to have a child. When Ann becomes pregnant in a matter of months, Dr. L. shares her delight.

When her son is born, he accepts her decision to terminate without pressuring her to continue meeting with him. Ann is delighted that he allows her to terminate the therapy rather than telling her she is not ready to stop.

Two years later, Ann finds herself overwhelmed by the demands of a young child and her job. She feels as if she is drowning. The possibility of preserving the sense of independence and freedom that she had been able to hold onto during the time she was meeting with Dr. L. seems hopelessly lost. In a state of despair, Ann calls Dr. L. to see if he can meet with her again. Dr. L. responds warmly to Ann and offers her an appointment time.

For the next year and a half, Dr. L. once again meets with Ann twice a week. Ann is indebted to him for rescuing her. She feels grateful to him for the psychological work that she is able to accomplish. Her marriage had been foundering under the stress of parenting, and through his work with Ann, Dr. L. helps Ann and John restore a secure, loving relationship. He helps them make a decision to have a second child and assumes a supportive stance in relation to Ann's ensuing pregnancy.

The frequency of Ann's contact with Dr. L.—two individual sessions per week—in combination with her gratitude for the important role he has played in her life provide fertile ground for a strong attachment to him to develop. Ann conceals the depth of that attachment to and dependency upon Dr. L. both from him and from herself. The only overt sign of it is her unflagging attendance at all scheduled sessions.

Ann's attachment and dependency needs are apparent in her reactions to Dr. L. on several occasions, but neither she nor Dr. L. notices them. On one occasion, Dr. L. fails to appear in the waiting room to retrieve Ann at her scheduled appointment time. She waits for more than twenty minutes, and just as she is about to leave, he appears. The stress of the unusual situation creates a crack in her ordinary mode of relating to him and enables feelings of loss and fears of abandonment to break through her ordinarily unruffled surface.

Although Dr. L. explores her fantasies of what had caused him to be so late and ultimately explains that he had overslept, Ann's feelings of loss and abandonment and their unusual presence in the session escape further notice. The opportunity to explore her response to Dr. L.'s perceived abandonment and to identify her heightened experience of dependency needs and fear of loss as a means of access to an area of primary vulnerability pass by.

During the fourth month of her pregnancy, another significant incident occurs. Ann contracts a virulent flu and must miss several weeks of appointments. She leaves uncharacteristic messages canceling her sessions—her appointments are so important to her that she has never canceled because of illness. Ann is miserable. She is suffering physically because her pregnancy prevents her from taking medication to relieve her discomfort. She is suffering emotionally because she is worried about the potentially damaging effect of the virus on her unborn child and because she misses the support and sense of security that Dr. L. provides. Ann wishes, hopes, and even expects that Dr. L. will call to find out why she is missing so many appointments. But days pass by and he does not call.

When Ann finally recovers, she returns to her appointments and expresses her hurt that Dr. L. neglected to telephone her. Dr. L. immediately explains that he had been unusually busy and simply had not noticed how much time had elapsed. Once again neither of them recognizes that her hurt feelings are a manifestation of her attachment to and dependency upon Dr. L. as well as a response to feeling dropped from his conscious awareness. Once again an opportunity to label an area of primary vulnerability passes by.

As the final months of her pregnancy approach, Ann begins to feel increasingly anxious. She has been having bouts of uterine contractions that the doctor feels may put her at risk for a premature delivery. The doctor has recommended bed rest for the last month of the pregnancy to prevent an early delivery. The month of bed rest is unfortunately scheduled to begin just as Dr. L. plans to return from a one-month summer vacation. Consequently Ann will be without the sustaining bond to Dr. L. not only for an extended time, but also during a pivotal transition from pregnancy to motherhood.

Although Ann is aware of anxiety about the impending separation, she does not connect it to her fear of allowing herself to depend upon a caretaker for support. Nor is she aware of the special vulnerability of women in the last stages of pregnancy, the state of primary maternal preoccupation aptly described by psychoanalyst D. W. Winnicott.[2] But Ann knows that she is dreading the long separation from Dr. L. and that she will miss him. She has even numbered the days on her calendar until his return.

With only six precious sessions remaining before the long interruption, Dr. L. makes an unexpected announcement: He is raising his fee substantially beginning with his return from his vacation. Although a fee raise might appear to others to be a simple business transaction, in the context of Ann's vulnerable dependent state and the nature of her relationship to Dr. L., the change in fee, the timing, and the manner in which Dr. L. introduced it take on broader significance. The prospect of shifting her attention to his personal needs, represented by the fee increase, at a time when she is struggling with the imminent separation from him and the birth of her child (a significant separation from a former sense of herself), overwhelms her. She is angry with Dr. L. for picking such a difficult time in her life to change his fee, and worse, she is afraid to feel angry at him because she does not want the physical stress of bearing intense emotions to bring about the early labor and delivery she needs to avoid.

Ann pleads with Dr. L. to set aside the fee raise to talk about after the baby's birth and the vacation break. But Dr. L., in what seems to her to be an uncharacteristically rigid and cold manner, refuses to set the fee raise aside even temporarily. He insists that he is raising his fee for all his patients, that his action is not personal to her, that he waited a long time to raise her fee, and that therapists sometimes do ask their patients to take care of the therapists' needs.

Ann feels trapped. She cannot agree to pay a higher fee because if she agrees, she knows that she will feel enraged with him for choosing such a vulnerable time in her life to ask her for more money. She does not dare to allow herself to feel enraged. She fears that she will put her unborn baby at risk, not knowing that on a more elemental level she is afraid her rage could destroy Dr. L. and herself. But if she refuses to pay the higher fee, she fears that their important relationship will be in jeopardy. More than anything, Ann wishes that Dr. L. would reappear as the supportive, empathic person he had been when she first met with him as a patient, as if his support will magically protect her now just as it did during her first experience giving birth. Humiliated and ashamed of her need for him, she pleads with Dr. L. to change his mind, to put the fee increase aside temporarily. She thinks to herself how simple it would be for him to say, "I picked a terrible time to bring up a change. Let's wait and talk about it again after the break." But once again he refuses to set the issue aside or to acknowledge that his needs are impinging upon her at a difficult time. The opportunity for Ann to learn how to remain connected to others when she is angry or frightened passes by.

In the face of his lack of empathy for her reactions, his failure to recognize and appreciate how he is wounding her, and his inability to suggest a way out of their stalemate over the fee raise, Ann resorts to one of the most powerful forms of communication available to patients: She threatens to terminate. She hopes that by communicating her feelings in such a powerful form, Dr. L. will understand the impact of his action and move to restore their now-fragile connection. Her threat to disconnect from the relationship is in fact a drastic attempt on her part to preserve it.

But Dr. L. refuses to modify or postpone his plan to raise his fee or to acknowledge that he is adding a significant stress to an already stressful time. Ann, struggling to maintain composure and dignity in the face of her disbelief that he can allow their relationship to end in a rupture, falls back upon her familiar mode of being self-sufficient and independent. Without knowing, she relies once again on the defense of annihilating the other person with self-righteousness, unable to tolerate not being seen and having her needs acknowledged. She announces that she can no longer continue to be his patient.

After Ann leaves the session, she is confident that Dr. L. will find a way to reach out to her. Her conviction that their relationship will endure survives the discordant final therapy session. She expects a telephone call or message from him asking her to return to her sessions. But the telephone call she hopes for never comes. Ann does not contact Dr. L. to resume her appointments. The therapeutic relationship has ended in a rupture.

Early in the morning of the final week before his departure on his vacation, Dr. L. telephones and awakens Ann, who is still counting the days that remain until he leaves. For a brief moment she feels hope and relief wash over her. But then he explains that he is only returning a call that he thinks might have come from her; the name on his answering machine was not recognizable. Ann explains that she did not leave the message, and they say a polite goodbye. Immersed in feelings of abandonment and rejection the telephone call elicits, Ann does not consider the possibility that Dr. L.'s unexpected telephone call may signify that she is also close to the surface of his conscious mind.

The abrupt and unexpected severing of the attachment to Dr. L. leaves Ann bereft, in a state of acute grief and mourning that persists despite her efforts to control or at least mute her feelings in order to protect her unborn baby. Disoriented and lost without the regularity of the sessions upon which she had counted, she ruminates for hours about her decision to end the therapeutic relationship. She tries to dissipate her rage at Dr. L. during the night when she cannot sleep by writing innumerable letters to him that she never mails. The intensity of her anger and grief frightens Ann, who begins to feel that she has a psychological defect because she allowed Dr. L. to become so important to her. She berates herself for having let herself need and depend on him. She worries that she made a personally costly mistake by terminating. Perhaps she should not have been so upset by Dr. L.'s timing in bringing up the fee increase. But in spite of her recurring feelings of self-doubt, Ann cannot find any meaningful explanation of why Dr. L. changed so abruptly from being the person he once was to her, from offering his psychological support and understanding in an unflagging way. She has no way of knowing that the opportunity to learn to remain in relationship to another person through the vicissitudes of their fluctuating states of being has been missed.

Eventually Dr. L.'s vacation and Ann's month on total bed rest pass by and her healthy baby, a second son, is born. In the hospital, one of the first telephone calls she spontaneously makes is to Dr. L. Her attachment to him persists through the ruptured termination, despite the abrupt severing and loss of the ongoing relationship. Dr. L.'s response to her on the telephone is cordial, contributing to the outer appearance of a positive connection. But beneath the surface appearance, in Ann's private inner self, distress over the rupture in the relationship persists. She cannot make sense of their unresolvable deadlock over the fee, nor can she understand how a fee raise could have caused such an important relationship to end so abruptly and painfully. Unable to perceive her own defenses, she persists in wondering why Dr. L. was so stubborn and unyielding.

Ann has no way of knowing the circumstances of Dr. L.'s personal life. His marriage is ending in divorce despite attempts at couples' therapy. When Dr. L. overslept and missed Ann's appointment, he had been wakeful through the night after an argument with his wife. When Ann had the flu, he was preoccupied with the stress of his marital relationship. When she was pregnant with her second child, his envy of her intact nuclear family operated unconsciously in a destructive manner. Unaware of his feelings of envy, Dr. L. consciously believes himself to be devoted to Ann's welfare. He feels justified in raising his fee and regards her as the one who is preventing the therapeutic relationship from continuing by being unyielding and stubborn. He interprets her destructive impulses in leaving—"You're depriving yourself of a happy termination"—and is unable to appreciate either her vulnerability or her attachment to him. Certain that he is right, he can see only his own position. Certain that she cannot tolerate her anger without endangering herself and her baby, Ann sees only her position and experiences Dr. L. as permanently lost to her.

As months pass, Ann is able to put the therapeutic relationship out of her mind, but every time she does think of it, the feelings of hurt and anger surface as powerfully and immediately as if the rupture has just happened. She tries not to lose sight of the fact that Dr. L. was helpful to her in her joint decision with her husband to have children, but she believes that she made a mistake by letting herself depend upon him, and she remains convinced that she will never seek therapy again.

Some years after the birth of her son and the ending of her therapeutic relationship with Dr. L., Ann encounters him by chance at a local movie theater. He greets her warmly and takes her aside to chat for a moment. When she mentions that she still feels hurt by the painful termination of their therapeutic relationship, he is baffled. He has no memory that they engaged in a bitter struggle over his fee increase or that they ended in a painful rupture. He has no idea that his way of bringing up the fee raise and responding to her distressed feelings was wounding and that the wounding, occurring in an area of primary vulnerability for her, was profound. He does not understand that Ann not only dared to become attached to and rely upon him, but that she also risked openly exposing to him the full extent of her need for him. Dr. L.'s inability to recognize and appreciate the full psychological significance of Ann's attachment and of the exposure of her needs, not merely the fact of the fee raise, contributed to the traumatic wounding.

The Realm of Primary Vulnerability

The notion of a realm of primary vulnerability brings together a general area of concern that can be found in a number of different theoretical perspectives. Before considering the concept of a realm of primary vulnerability in relation to the existing theoretical frameworks that many psychotherapists currently rely upon, I would like to evoke an intuitive sense of its meaning by anchoring it in our ordinary experience as human beings. I have observed that each of us has areas of primary vulnerability that are activated by ordinary interactions with others. We trip into these vulnerabilities even in casual interactions with others because they were formed in the context of our earliest relationships and because we cannot completely control our impact on others or their responses to us.

An experience I had while going to a lunch meeting with a small group of therapists who were attending a psychotherapy conference, and who were interested in discussing my ideas about areas of primary vulnerability, provides an ironic example of how easy it is for any of us to fall into this realm. Although the behaviors of the therapists involved may seem to be merely reactions to the immediate situation, their responses were influenced by underlying areas of sensitivity.

The group consisted of one man and nine women. At the end of the morning conference session, we gathered to decide where to go for our lunch meeting. After a prolonged consideration of our options—we had come to the conference from an assortment of locations across the country and did not know our way around very well—we finally agreed upon a seafood restaurant, a specialty of the area we were in, and managed to arrange ourselves to go in three cars.

Those of us in the car that I was riding in had difficulty finding the restaurant, but we finally managed to locate it. One of the two other cars was already there after also having gotten lost. We assumed that the third car had given up hope of finding us. The remaining group of therapists consisted of four women and one man. By this time the five of us were extremely hungry. Moreover, I was worried about having enough to say about the realm of primary vulnerability to justify the trouble that everyone had gone to.

The man ordered one of the more expensive items on the menu, a lobster stew, while the women ordered seafood salads. After the waitress brought the food, we noticed that the man was staring at his stew with distaste. Like him, the rest of us saw an unappealing bowl of thin, milky broth with puddles of greasy butter on top and a mere two lumps of lobster meat. This was not the thick stew, full of vegetables and fish, that the man had envisioned. Although he did not want to eat it, he was also sensitive to the fact that the rest of us were hungry. He did not want to create a fuss or a further delay by sending the dish back to the kitchen. We could say that in these circumstances, taking care of his personal needs would contribute to added stress that might threaten the equilibrium of his self-state.

The women at the table had similar perceptions of the unappetizing lobster stew and encouraged the man, against his resistance, to send it back. One of the women, who was clearly more comfortable being assertive than the rest of us, called the waitress over and explained the problem. She said quite firmly to the timid young waitress, "This doesn't look like a stew, it looks awful, and you have no business charging so much money for these two little lumps of lobster meat!"

The waitress hesitated, uncertain and uncomfortable about responding to the complaint (we might say that interpersonal conflict and her fears of antagonizing her manager and losing her job activated areas of vulnerability). "I don't think I can take it back just because you don't like it, but I'll check," she said.

The waitress left our table and consulted the manager while, the women sat politely, despite our hunger, with uneaten salads sitting in front of us. The lobster stew, which had been pushed to the center of the table, was cooling rapidly.

After a seemingly endless wait, the manager, an attractively dressed woman, came to the table and firmly told us that there was nothing wrong with the stew, that the waitress could bring something else, but the man would have to pay for whatever he ordered as a substitute and for the stew. The assertive woman, speaking for the now-silent man, insisted that the restaurant take back the unappetizing and expensive dish and added that the man should not have to pay for it.

Clearly stifling angry feelings, the restaurant manager went off to get the cook. In a matter of seconds the cook, a young woman with reddened cheeks who was visibly upset, arrived at our table. By now other customers in the restaurant were unabashedly staring at our group. I was helplessly pondering the irony of the conflict: Here were five experienced psychotherapists, attending a conference focused on relationships and interested in psychological vulnerabilities, who were apparently unable to resolve an impasse over food.

When confronted with the complaints about the problematic lobster stew by the four women and the man, who by now undoubtedly wished he had never voiced a complaint, the cook flew into a rage, as if she were being personally attacked or treated abusively. "I've been making this stew according to the same recipe for ten years," she declared, nearly shouting at us. "There's nothing wrong with it and I won't take it back! I serve good food here!"

"There must be some way out of this impasse," I muttered weakly, but events were now moving faster than any voice of reason could hold back. "I don't think he should have to pay for this!" one of the women announced, stubbornly holding her ground.

After a silent moment, the cook ended the stalemate. "I am going to take back all your food and ask you to leave the premises." With that pronouncement she whisked away as many of our uneaten dishes as she could carry and walked off.

We left the table with as much dignity as we could muster and regrouped at a hamburger stand down the road where we abandoned any lingering concerns about cholesterol and fat and rapidly consumed extra-large cheeseburgers and french fries. Our hunger assuaged, I took charge: "Let me tell you about the realm of primary vulnerability . . . !"

The incident at the restaurant had in fact given us a real-life experience of being catapulted into the *edges* of our individual realms of primary vulnerability. In therapy, patients and therapists are catapulted into the *center* of their areas of vulnerability because social conventions and the constraints of civility are more likely to be overridden. The man's anxiety about causing trouble by attending to his needs, the assertiveness of the woman who fought for his rights, my heightened sense of responsibility for the well-being of the group and anxiety about conflict, the resistance of the other women to backing down once a stance had been taken, the distress of the cook in the face of the rejection and criticism of her food, are all manifestations of areas of primary vulnerability. We differ from one another only in the extent and content of our personal vulnerabilities and in how successful we are in creating inner and outer structures that either keep us from descending into them, or that enable us to descend into them and bear the anguish of doing so.

Primary Vulnerability: A Working Model

I believe that the realm of primary vulnerability encompasses a central human psychological concern and sensitivity: *the preservation of the cohesiveness and connectedness of the self.* By self, I am referring to our conscious sense of self, our ego, or who we know ourselves to be.[3] By cohesiveness, I refer to an enduring inner relatedness of parts of the self. Much as we like to think of ourselves as unitary entities, we have different facets, or self-states, to which an observing-self often bears witness. How well our different facets or self-states are related to one another at a given moment determines how cohesive our sense of self is for that time. By connectedness of self, I refer to the maintenance and preservation of the bonds comprising our significant outer world relationships. Each of us, simply by being human, has a primary concern with sustaining an *inner* relatedness to different facets of ourselves as well as with maintaining connections to significant others in our *outer* relationships.

A concrete and dramatic illustration of the realm of primary vulnerability is provided by a story recounted by Heinz Kohut, about a group of astronauts on a mission in space several years ago.[4] Believing their spacecraft was malfunctioning, scientists managing the mission gave the astronauts a choice in the event that the problem with the spacecraft could not be corrected. The astronauts faced certain death, but they had the option of circling endlessly in outer space or of returning to earth and burning up in reentry. The astronauts unanimously and without hesitation chose to return to earth. The dread of the disconnection of self from whatever place is invested with the meaning of a home base is a universal, primordial fear.

Another example of the realm of primary vulnerability can be found in the philosophy behind the establishment of a California hospice for dying infants and children.[5] The hospice was created to enable terminally ill children to be cared for by parents and nurses around the clock so that there was no possibility that they would die alone and unattended in a sterile hospital room. In our culture, the image of anyone dying alone, particularly a helpless, dependent child, evokes the pain of being isolated from all human contact and connection and mobilizes our most fervent protective instincts. Tibetans, for example, believe that it is important for individuals who are dying to have someone else present to reassure them, to prevent panic as physical and psychological changes occur, and to enable the dying individual to focus on the significant event that is unfolding. Labor coaches who assist pregnant women during childbirth serve an analogous function. Disconnection from significant others jeopardizes our sense of internal cohesion. Each of us, by virtue of being human, lives with anxiety related to the realm of primary vulnerability.

Primary Vulnerability: Freud, Sullivan, and Jung

Having given anxiety related to primary vulnerabilities a central role in the wounding that jeopardizes therapeutic relationships, we can reexamine basic theoretical perspectives to determine what role, if any, such fundamental anxiety plays. Freud's views of anxiety, although they changed as his thinking evolved, were focused on the intrapsychic origins. Implicit in his view of anxiety is its power to disrupt the cohesiveness of an individual's sense of self. Freud's theory of the mind and of psychological functioning was predicated on a model of the mind as a unified, encapsulated entity. Freud was concerned with internal or intrapsychic conflict in a unitary mind among the agencies of the ego, id, and superego. He was also concerned with the boundaries between the conscious, preconscious, and unconscious contents of the mind. According to Freud, individuals rely on defense mechanisms such as repression, reaction formation, or denial to manage anxiety that arises from the arousal of forbidden impulses. He also conceived of anxiety as a warning signal of danger that surfaces in relation to specific internal fears, such as castration anxiety. Anxiety generated by forbidden impulses or because of conflict between ego, id, and superego would clearly threaten an individual's sense of internal cohesiveness and, indirectly, relationships with significant others.

Sullivan and other interpersonal theorists, in contrast to Freud, emphasize the social or interpersonal origin of anxiety that might disrupt an individual's cohesive sense of self. Anxiety arises at first within the mother–infant relationship and recurs later in life as a response to threats to an individual's sense of security. Individuals learn to avoid situations and behaviors that give rise to anxiety and are prone to regression in the face of intolerable anxiety. Sullivan and the interpersonal theorists thus focus on the individual's vulnerability to disruptions in bonds to significant others, which we can assume would then threaten the internal cohesiveness of a sense of self.

Jung extended the scope of Freud's original conception of the unconscious mind from that of a unitary container for repressed and forgotten experiences to a container that also includes a universal layer, one that connects all human beings.[6] Jung conceived of the universal layer of the unconscious mind as the collective unconscious. Believing it to be separate from the personal unconscious, he asserted that it exists in all human beings, linking us to one another psychologically through a common inherited psychic substrate. Jung's concept of an archetype gives us a means of understanding conceptually the universality of a realm of primary vulnerability.

Archetypes, as Jung explains them, are the building blocks that make up the collective unconscious. They provide the *forms* within which we represent significant portions of our experience. Examples of archetypal forms include the Mother, the Father, Hero and Heroine, Wise Old Man, and the Wicked Witch. Jung inferred the existence of archetypes in the collective unconscious because his patients reported images of archetypal figures from their dreams with whom they could not have had actual contact. He believed that these dream images could be understood as manifestations of archetypes that had surfaced from the collective unconscious layer of the psyche. Archetypes also account for the recurrence of similar themes and characters in myths and fairy tales across different cultures and historical time.

Because archetypes are unconscious, they cannot be known directly, nor can they be completely defined. Archetypes can only be experienced. They are hypothetical, *psychological* models, analogous to instincts, which are inherited *biological* patterns of behavior. Jung writes, "The archetype is essentially an unconscious content that is altered by becoming conscious and by being perceived, and it takes its colour from the individual consciousness in which it happens to appear."[7] Each of us fills in archetypal forms in a unique manner depending upon who we are and what we have experienced. The impact of culture would presumably occur at this juncture. For example, the mother archetype is particularly important early in life in Western culture. Babies, in Jung's view, do not enter the world as blank slates written on by experience but instead are born with an archetypal readiness to relate to a mother. As the baby grows in relation to her, all the unique, individual feelings, perceptions, experiences, and behaviors related to the mother–baby relationship shape the baby's *mother complex*.

A complex is Jung's term for a collection of associated ideas and images that are linked together by common image or affect. Jung, unlike Freud, did not believe in a unitary mind or psyche. Complexes operate like "splinter psyches" that take us over when they are activated.[8] Complexes are not inherently pathological but rather are the building blocks of a healthy psyche. But they can contribute to psychological difficulties when the experiences that comprise them are problematic. For example, an individual who has experienced good-enough mothering and satisfactory relationships with a mother will have a mother complex that does not create unmanageable problems. An individual who has had predominantly unsatisfactory relationship experiences with a mother can develop a mother complex that does create problems. Jung, minimizing the impact of culture, believed that we are born with a mother archetype by virtue of being human. The mother archetype forms the core of the mother complex, a complex that exists in each of us but that derives its particular nature from our unique personal experiences.

The Realm of Primary Vulnerability

The realm of primary vulnerability may be thought of in Jung's terms as an archetypal form that provides the core of the complex of primary vulnerability that takes its unique and individual shape from the interaction of our experiences in life and our innate temperamental or constitutional characteristics. The specific, personal way in which each of us fills in the archetypal realm of primary vulnerability will differ by virtue of our highly individual natures and our unique life experiences. Examples of individual manifestations of the archetypal realm of primary vulnerability that affect most of us to different degrees include fear of disintegration, issues of trust, fear of betrayal, separation, fears of failure or success, and anxiety around abandonment, rejection, and neglect.

Because having areas of primary vulnerability is inherent in being human, manifestations of sensitivities arising from them are evident in every adult. What we currently label as pathological are not the vulnerabilities themselves but rather the unproductive, self-defeating modes of managing, adapting to, and responding to them. Our primary vulnerabilities take on personally specific form and shape as our sense of self develops. We develop adaptive mechanisms and defenses that function to protect our vulnerable areas much as we apply bandages to protect wounds in our skin.

The area of primary vulnerability may remain unarticulated in words and operate invisibly to influence our mode of being in the world and of relating to others. We intuit its existence and infer its contents in the same way that astronomers postulate the existence of black holes in outer space in order to account for observable phenomena. Although we protect ourselves from falling into our vulnerable areas with the best adaptive mechanisms we can create, and even if we do whatever we can to heal ourselves, the underlying vulnerability remains.

Certain specific contents of our areas of primary vulnerability originate within the fabric of human relationships early in development, before the emergence of language and the cognitive skills necessary for us to think of ourselves as a coherent entity, as an "I." The first manifestations of primary vulnerabilities arise within the context of our early relationship to caretakers, who in the beginning of life occupy a powerful position in relation to dependent infants. Although a single traumatic event may give rise to a particular vulnerability (such as an early prolonged separation from a mother, illness or death of a parent, traumatic physical or sexual abuse), more often vulnerabilities are formed as a consequence of the repeated ordinary interactions that occur between infant and caretakers in the context of daily life.[9] The areas of vulnerability can be reinforced or modified by ensuing experiences in relationships, at first within the family and then with peers in school, teachers, and the community at large as life goes on.

The ordinary interactions that contribute to specific primary vulnerabilities in the beginning are influenced not only by the psychological makeup of parent and child but by their temperament and constitution. Specific vulnerabilities result from the complex interaction of the circumstances of our environment and our temperament, the physical and psychological "fit" between our infant self and our caretakers, and the responses of our caretakers to our changing needs as we grow and develop. Areas of sensitivity or vulnerability are inevitable and develop even with the best of circumstances, even with adequate parenting and even in the most harmonious of childhoods. As our lives continue, the areas of vulnerability become self-reinforcing, operating like filters in new relationships. Therapeutic relationships offer us the opportunity to "see" the invisible filters that shape our sense of ourselves and our relationships.

How we manage and express the anxiety arising from the universally human concern with the preservation of our sense of self and of significant bonds to others give rise to lifespan issues that we work on in different ways and for different reasons as we progress through our lives. The realm of primary vulnerability is apt to be accessed in the course of a long-term therapeutic relationship, just as it is likely to be accessed within other intimate relationships.

The example of Ann and Dr. L., to which we will return in the following four chapters, gives us an opportunity to notice that in therapeutic relationships the primary vulnerabilities of *both* therapist and patient are likely to be activated or avoided. Patient and therapist have a rare and unique opportunity to make visible (without the implication that the therapist automatically discloses personal areas of vulnerability to the patient) the vulnerabilities that operate for each of them like filters, influencing not only interactions in relationships, but the sense of self and other.

When primary vulnerabilities remain invisible and unnamed, patients are in jeopardy of being rewounded as adults in ways that echo earlier experiences and of missing an opportunity to review and reshape their fundamental sense of self. When areas of primary vulnerability of patients and therapists intersect in problematic ways, irreconcilable mismatches may result. When they remain invisible, unnamed, and avoided, stalemates may arise that immobilize therapeutic relationships. These situations are in need of our deliberate attention and exploration so that they no longer remain among the silenced dilemmas of psychotherapy.

Most theoretical perspectives that guide our understanding of psychotherapy focus only upon the vulnerabilities of patients in different conceptual languages. Therapists are presumed to have worked through their personal issues as part of their training and prior psychotherapy. The profession has not recognized explicitly that personal vulnerabilities in each of us endure and recur throughout life, that problematic interactions with therapists in therapeutic relationships can stem from areas of primary vulnerability in the therapist, not only from the primary vulnerabilities of the patient. *We have yet to formulate conceptual models that allow for the primacy of the intersection and interaction of the vulnerabilities of both therapist and patient as an integral part of the relationship. These intense and difficult phases in therapeutic relationships can profitably be addressed; they need not be perceived only as failure experiences that bring about a problematic derailing of the relationship.*

Because primary vulnerabilities often operate like invisible filters that shape the responses of therapists to their patients, and because these vulnerabilities may be activated in patients in ways that create both dangers and opportunities, the chapters in Part II will focus extensively upon our conceptual grasp of them and upon their origins early in life. A broad conceptual canvas for primary vulnerabilities may increase the possibility of working with them constructively when they are activated or avoided by either the patient or therapist in therapeutic relationships.

PART II

❖ **Primary Vulnerability,** ❖
**Relational Modes, and
Ruptured Attachments**

CHAPTER SIX

❖ Related Views ❖ of Primary Vulnerability

I intentionally did not say "the most intensive anxiety" [in referring to disintegration anxiety as the *deepest* anxiety man can experience] because the degree of anxiety that an individual actually feels is influenced by many factors. But I would not hesitate to state unequivocally that disintegration anxiety is not only man's deepest but also, *potentially*, his most severe anxiety.

—HEINZ KOHUT[1]

In my view the origin of the basic fault may be traced back to a considerable discrepancy in the early formative phases of the individual between his bio-psychological needs and the material and psychological care, attention, and affection available during the relevant times. This creates a state of deficiency whose consequences and after-effects appear to be only partly reversible. . . . As may be seen from my description, I put the emphasis on the lack of "fit" between the child and *the people* who represent his environment. Incidentally, we started with a similar lack of "fit"—between the analyst's otherwise correct technique and a particular patient's needs; this is very likely to be an important cause of difficulties, and even failures, experienced by analysts in their practice.

—MICHAEL BALINT[2]

At the stage which is being discussed it is necessary not to think of the baby as a person who gets hungry, and whose instinctual drives may be met or frustrated, but to think of the baby as an immature being who is all the time *on the brink of unthinkable anxiety*. Unthinkable anxiety is kept away by this vitally important function of the mother at this stage, her capacity to put herself in the baby's place and to know what the baby needs in the general management of the body, and therefore of the person.

—D. W. WINNICOTT[3]

In Part I, three categories of dilemmas that put therapeutic relationships at risk were discussed: mismatches, impasses, and wounding. The concept of a realm of primary vulnerability as a useful working model for areas of special sensitivity that are present in each of us was introduced as a means of understanding the virtually insupportable wounding that some therapy patients experience. When therapists respond to wounded patients through the filter of their own areas of primary vulnerability, a secondary level of wounding can occur that endangers the therapeutic relationship. If the relationship ends in a rupture, patients may feel harmed by the therapy, and therapists may suffer doubt and despair about the value of their profession. The chapters in Part II develop a working model of the realm of primary vulnerability in relation to other theoretical perspectives (Chapter Six), the maternal–infant matrix (Chapter Seven), relational modes that are established early in life with early caretakers and that recur in therapeutic relationships (Chapter Eight), and theories of and research on infant development (Chapter Nine).

The preceding chapter elucidated the concept of primary vulnerability and provided a case example in which a patient named Ann was wounded in this realm by Dr. L., her therapist. Dr. L., responding to Ann from his own area of primary vulnerability centering on feelings of envy and deprivation, unwittingly created an additional layer of wounding that I refer to as the *secondary level of wounding* (a concept that will be discussed in more detail in Chapter Ten). The therapeutic relationship ended abruptly in a rupture.

This chapter will discuss concepts analogous to the realm of primary vulnerability that have been put forth by three well-known and highly regarded theorists from different theoretical perspectives: Heinz Kohut, who founded Self psychology; Michael Balint, a member of the British Object Relations theorists who flourished in the 1950s; and D. W. Winnicott, a British pediatrician who became a psychoanalyst and, like Michael Balint, was a member of the British Independent School. The fact that representatives of different theoretical perspectives have concerned themselves with the notion of a realm of primary vulnerability attests to its significance in human psychological functioning. How primary vulnerabilities are activated in therapeutic relationships in both patient and therapist and how they can be worked with constructively are questions of central importance for the profession.

Kohut and Disintegration Anxiety

Heinz Kohut established the domain of psychoanalysis currently referred to as Self psychology. He introduced the concept of a selfobject, which refers to our experience of another person specifically with respect to the *functions* that person serves in preserving our sense of self.[4] Kohut asserted that each of us needs others to serve as selfobjects throughout our life, but that the nature of our selfobjects develops from lesser to greater maturity. Archaic selfobjects are those that exist in the early stages of development, in contrast to the maturely chosen selfobjects that optimally characterize adult life. When an adult experiences the self-cohering effect of a maturely chosen selfobject, the archaic selfobject experiences of the preceding stages of development also resonate unconsciously. Kohut provides the example of an adult who is uplifted by admiration for a cultural ideal, a mature selfobject. The experience of being uplifted revives in the adult the former uplifting experience of being picked up by a "strong and admired mother and having been allowed to merge with her greatness, calmness, and security."[5] Mothers frequently serve a selfobject function when they soothe their children, helping them restore a coherent sense of self. Spouses serve multiple selfobject functions for each other that are essential to the maintenance of a cohesive sense of self.

Kohut put forth the concept of disintegration anxiety—the primordial anxiety about the dissolution of our sense of self that arises when we are catapulted into our areas of primary vulnerability. Kohut conceived of disintegration anxiety as the fear of an experience that is virtually indescribable in words: "the deepest anxiety a man can experience."[6] Kohut noted that none of the forms of anxiety that Freud described are equivalent to it.[7] Disintegration anxiety, which may be experienced as subjectively similar to the fear of death, is a fear of the loss of humanness or of a psychological death. The trigger or specific source of disintegration anxiety is the loss of the essential selfobject environment that makes psychological survival possible.[8] Kohut believed that disintegration anxiety arises from an exposure to an indifferent, nonhuman world. Even hatred confirms the hated person's humanness. It is *indifference*, not hatred, that leads to the experience of a loss of self.

To embody the concept of disintegration anxiety in a case example, Kohut recounts an episode that occurred with a patient named Mr. U. Mr. U. was facing the reality that in terminating his therapeutic relationship he would be relinquishing Kohut's emotional support. He would have to face the remainder of his life with whatever selfobject support he could find on his own.[9] Mr. U. had a dream that expressed the massive anxiety evoked by the idea of losing his therapist. In his dream Mr. U. found himself in an unreal "stainless steel world" from which there was no escape and within which there was no possibility of communication with others. He woke up from his dream with intense anxiety, namely, disintegration anxiety, that persisted for some time.

Disintegration anxiety, according to Kohut, refers specifically to the "threatened loss of the self-cohesion-maintaining responses of the empathic selfobject."[10] We can conceptualize the intense anxiety that Ann experienced when Dr. L raised her fee as disintegration anxiety arising from the abrupt loss of the bond with Dr. L. Ann was abruptly deprived of the selfobject functions he provided. These functions were essential in helping her maintain a cohesive sense of self, particularly during the stressful final months of her pregnancy.

Some time in the course of a psychotherapy every therapist will inevitably fail to respond empathically to patients. In the best of circumstances, the failures will be manageable in degree. Kohut believed that no harm would ensue to patients if therapists responded appropriately to their patients by recognizing the specific nature and meaning of the empathic failure and interpreting it to the patients.[11] But we can infer from his assertion that psychological harm may befall a patient if the therapist's empathic failure is beyond a tolerable level, that is, if the therapist cannot respond effectively to a patient who has been tripped into an area of primary vulnerability. Patients like Ann, who have an experience of disintegration anxiety resulting from their therapists' unanticipated and massive empathic failures, are likely to feel that they have been harmed rather than helped by the therapeutic relationship.

From a developmental perspective, in Kohut's view, a healthy and cohesive sense of self is established when parents provide a matrix of idealizable and mirroring selfobjects for their children.[12] Patients who seek psychotherapy typically have experienced deficits early in development in the matrix of selfobjects available to them. These can be identified and worked through in the relationship to a therapist, where working through means experiencing the deficit in the context of the therapist's psychologically present and empathic adult ego. But these deficits may also be exposed and deepened when the therapist, knowingly or inadvertently, wounds the patient by failing to provide the necessary selfobject functions, failing to appreciate the extent of wounding, and allowing the psychotherapy to end in an impasse that cannot be resolved.

When we left Ann in the last chapter, she had returned to the determined, self-sufficient state that had been her adaptation to her family of origin. Her wish to be able to yield to a more intimate connection, expressed indirectly in her ambivalence about becoming a mother, was never explicitly acknowledged in the therapeutic relationship with Dr. L. Although she was able to decide to have children and was successful in establishing a nuclear family of her own, we do not know whether she feels that she is able to have as intimate a connection with her children and husband as she would like, nor do we know whether she continued psychological work on this aspect of her psyche in another therapeutic relationship.

Balint's Concept of Basic Fault

Michael Balint, an English psychoanalyst who was part of the British object relations group that included Fairbairn, Klein, Guntrip, and Winnicott, wrote extensively about a concept similar to that of primary vulnerability in his book, *The Basic Fault*, published in 1968.[13] For the purpose of conceptual clarity, I will discuss how his concept differs from and is similar to that of primary vulnerability.

Apart from certain clarifications and qualifications, Balint's book contains valuable insights and perceptions that are applicable to the concept of a realm of primary vulnerability. His insights are particularly relevant to impasses and ruptures arising from wounds that patients experience in the realm of their primary vulnerabilities.

Balint explicitly acknowledges that psychotherapy does not necessarily have a happy outcome. In the course of addressing the question of why some patients are more difficult than others, and why some therapies end in failure, Balint notes, "Processes initiated in the analytic situation must be conceived of as powerful or intensive enough to penetrate into deep layers of the mind and achieve fundamental changes."[14] Because of its special power in accessing the "deep layers of the mind," a therapeutic relationship has the potential to wound as well as to heal. Change is a neutral term—a patient may subjectively experience change as being for the better or for the worse. Consequently, as therapists, we must learn to negotiate the terrain we enter when the powerful forces to which Balint refers are activated. We must continually be aware that the meaning our patients attribute to the events that occur when such forces are activated may not be the meaning we hope for. As patients, we can be aware that powerful processes do become engaged in therapeutic relationships. Our fear when these processes are engaged need not prevent us from persisting through difficult times and putting them to constructive use.

Balint asserts that in the original two-person relationship between mother and infant, only the needs and wishes of the infant count. The caretaker, although experienced as immensely powerful, matters to the infant only in terms of its needs and otherwise does not exist. For the infant, Balint posits, there are objects that are safe and gratifying, those that are hazards to be avoided, or there are no objects. As the infant progresses developmentally into babyhood and early childhood, the capacity to perceive the caretaker as a more complex human being increases dramatically. In psychotherapy, however, the chronologically early state of infancy is activated when, as Balint puts it, patients regress to the level of the basic fault. Patients will then relate to therapists as if they are either safe and gratifying, as if they are dangerous hazards, or as if they are not there at all.

Balint accurately describes the experience of a patient in the realm of the basic fault or primary vulnerability when he writes that these patients are exquisitely sensitive to their therapists' mood. If the therapist is not in tune with the patient, the patient, dependent and in need of harmony in order to preserve the coherence and connection of self, reacts with anxiety, aggression, or despair. Adult language can be useless or misleading at this level, because words do not always have an agreed-upon, conventional meaning. At the level of the basic fault, every gesture of the therapist, let alone her words, matters enormously. The therapist is either loved or feared by the patient/infant. The patient named Lori, who was unable to make use of Dr. R. until a shift occurred in the relationship (see Chapter Two), may be said to have reached the level of her basic fault in her therapy.

Balint accurately notes that our theoretical knowledge and technical methods for dealing with the basic fault are less developed than the therapeutic methods we have developed for other issues. We are still grappling with understanding and responding in helpful ways to patients who reach the level of the basic fault. Balint puts the problems that exist for both therapist and patient in the form of questions: How can we help the patient receive help in this regressed state? How can the therapist bridge the gulf that exists between them and reach the patient? To what extent must the patient help bridge this gulf? What are the hazards faced by the therapist in dealing with phenomena associated with the basic fault? These questions still have no clearly defined answers. Perhaps no absolute answers exist, and we will be able to enumerate only general guidelines because each patient–therapist pair is as unique as each mother–infant pair. Unique relationships, like flexible sculptures, can be molded into distinctive and changing forms as the relationship develops, with the result that no definitive methods exist for dealing with the basic fault in every relationship.

Balint does offer some general responses to his questions, based upon his clinical experience. According to Balint, the therapist has the job of translating primitive behavior into conventional adult language. The therapist's task is to interpret and inform, regardless of which theoretical language is used. The therapist must be careful not to insist upon a given interpretation out of an irresistible urge to organize the patient's complaints and make sense out of them. She must also be careful to avoid fixing blame on either herself or her patient if the interpretations offered fail to stop those complaints. To therapists, who are each ordinarily human, these recommendations also constitute an ideal that cannot always be attained—hence, the urgent necessity for understanding the structure of therapeutic impasses and ruptured therapeutic relationships.

In a regressed state at the level of the basic fault, the patient wants perfect harmony, a meshing of her needs with what the therapist has to offer. But the needs of an adult are far more complicated than those of an infant, and no therapist can meet an adult's needs perfectly any more than a mother and father can meet perfectly the needs of their infant. Nonetheless, a patient in a regressed state experiences any disconnection from the therapist as an excruciating failure. On the other side of the relationship, the therapist who tries to be perfectly attuned is destined to fail. Balint believed that the therapist must recognize and resist the wish to respond to the patient with omnipotent behavior; namely, by analyzing, interpreting, organizing, or changing the environment. Otherwise, there is the danger of creating a delusional transference in which the patient becomes trapped in a state of dependency and need in relationship to the therapist. What the therapist should strive to do is to be a need-recognizing and, where appropriate, a need-satisfying and certainly need-understanding object. The therapist then should try to communicate the recognition of need to the patient. Only those demands that are necessary to secure the existence of the relationship should be met.

Balint asserts that the therapist can bridge the gulf to the patient and prevent a regression from becoming malignant by understanding what the patient needs and conveying the understanding to the patient, not through interpretations, but by creating an atmosphere of respect and tolerance. The therapist must accept all complaints and resentments as real and valid, even if the therapist has a different view, in order to allow time for the patient's resentments to shift to regret. Balint believes that interpretations will only impede this process. The therapist may need to tolerate long periods of violent (verbal) aggressiveness, followed by mourning and regret, not only about the therapist's present failures but about the original caretakers' failures and losses. Although the mourning process may last an exasperating length of time from the therapist's point of view, *it must be witnessed in full*. The mourning must occur in the framework of a two-person relationship.[15] Only then can the patient reassess her position and reexamine the possibility of accepting the often-indifferent universe. The goal of negotiating the treacherous territory of the basic fault is to bring about a new relationship between the patient and some part of her world that has been barred by the gulf created by the basic fault.

Balint understood the significance of the early infant–caretaker relationship in shaping areas of primary vulnerability that are evident in adult psychotherapy patients. He recognized and respected the power of reevoking in the therapeutic relationship the dynamics that once occurred early on in the coming-into-being of an infant. He recognized that adult patients can be retraumatized if the original failures are repeated, or they can be transformed in positive ways (in the sense of modifying entrenched beliefs about the self and other) if the original failures are recognized and mourned. Balint also draws our attention to the importance of the therapist tolerating intense affect states, recognizing the pain inherent in experiencing unmet needs, being a stand-in object for rage toward previous caretakers, and bearing witness to the process of mourning. These are responses that require the therapist's endurance rather than the active overcoming of obstacles. Balint in fact recommends that therapists resist the temptation to respond with action to overcome the patient's problems by making logical, rational interpretations in order to control the patient's feelings.

My use of the concept of primary vulnerability differs somewhat from Balint's conception of basic fault, which Balint used to describe an area accessed in therapy by patients who are regressed. He did not consider the basic fault to be inherent in being human but instead linked it specifically to deficiencies in caretaking that result in the psychological problems of adult therapy patients. In contrast, I am asserting that areas of primary vulnerabilities exist in each of us, regardless of the adequacy of our caretaking. Because Balint believes that a deficit in environmental provisions early in life brings about the basic fault, the term "fault" with its connotations of defectiveness is perhaps appropriate.

Even if Balint had intended his conception of the basic fault to refer to an area that exists in each of us, rather than only in individuals whose caretaking was deficient, I prefer to use the term "primary vulnerability" because "fault" has connotations of damage, defect, or flaw. The term "vulnerability" refers not to a defect but to an area of sensitivity, an area that is insufficiently protected, related to the Latin root for "wound."[16] If we are to shift our paradigm of psychotherapy to include the human vulnerabilities of therapists as well as patients, we are better served by a word that does not link the notion of damage exclusively to patients.[17] If we broaden the domain of psychotherapy from one that focuses on "objectively" defined psychopathology in patients, to one that includes the subjective experience of patients and therapists, the nonpathological terminology of primary vulnerability is more appropriate.

Balint refers to the basic fault as a level (rather than a position, conflict, complex, or situation) that belongs to a two-person relationship. The term "level" might be applicable to the concept of primary vulnerability to the extent that we speak of our "deepest" vulnerabilities or our "earliest" problems. However, my representational image of vulnerability, unlike Balint's, is more accurately described by such adjectives as "central" or "core" vulnerabilities. I envision the realm of primary vulnerability to be circular rather than linear, more like the core grain of sand inside an oyster, around which layers of pearl accrue, than like the first level of a multilevel structure.

Balint used the concept of basic fault in tandem with the concept of regression in psychoanalysis: Patients in analysis regress to the level of their basic fault and optimally work their way out of it once and for all. Because I believe that anxieties related to areas of primary vulnerability remain with us throughout our lives, although our understanding of and response to them change as we evolve, the term "regression" seems less descriptively accurate than the images of "falling into" or "reaching the heart of." Rather than regressing or reverting "back" into a realm of primary vulnerability associated with childhood, situations arise during the course of psychotherapy that cause us to "fall into" or "pierce the core of" the timeless experience of a basic human anxiety arising from the fear of losing the coherence and connection of our sense of self.

Balint believes that a state of perfect harmony existed before the trauma occurred that established the basic fault. I believe, however, that it is more accurate to say that a state of perfect harmony is simply not part of human life, even in the beginning and in the best of situations, although each of us has moments or extended times of contentment and happiness throughout our lifetimes. Every human being, and certainly every infant, is vulnerable to states of internal discomfort and to times when needs are either unmet or met imperfectly. The Garden of Eden that recurs in myth is a longed for-but unattainable ideal.

Balint views the original cause of the basic fault as the failure of the caretaking person to meet the biological and psychological needs of the infant. The failure creates a state of deficiency or deprivation, the consequences of which are only partly reversible. I am asserting that areas of primary vulnerability exist in each of us as part of being human and cannot be attributed solely to the deficiencies of the caretaker, although these contribute. Put another way, no ordinary person, no matter how devoted and psychologically aware, will avoid having areas of unconsciousness, sensitivity, and limitations. But there are specific threats to the experience of cohesiveness and continuity of self that do arise in the context of each mother–infant relationship. Rather than arising only from a failure or deficiency, problems reside in the ordinary, repetitive, mutually influencing interactions between infant and caretaker, in other words, *within the relationship that begins at birth between the mother and the actual baby and that begins at conception in the mother's psyche.*

Areas of primary vulnerability arise in part from the temperamental and constitutional qualities that infants bring with them into the world. Even the best mothering and fathering cannot circumvent the development of a specific vulnerability. For example, Erin, a first-born baby, suffered from that painful state of uncertain origin called three-month colic. Inconsolable and clearly in pain, she would cry for hours at a time. Her father walked and rocked her, and her mother let her nurse on demand. Erin responded by clinging to her parents with a fierce urgency, as if to a port in a storm. As her family watched her grow and develop into a young adult, they noticed in her traces of a basic vulnerability, a sense of the world as a dangerous place, of herself as inadequate to withstand its demands, and of a strong need to be attached to caretakers. We can speculate that her vulnerability may have originated in the experiences of her first weeks of life, during which her physical predisposition to colic contributed to a state of distress. Her distress became associated with her parents' diligent efforts to remove its causes and continually to soothe her. Ginny, another first-born child, evidenced a different form of specific vulnerability in which her temperament, evident from birth, interacted problematically with her parents' devoted efforts to be good-enough parents, attentions that were perhaps experienced as intrusive. From birth, Ginny maintained clear boundaries and a need for autonomy that functioned like an invisible shield around her, perhaps protecting a soft-hearted center. She displayed little need for holding or cuddling beyond that necessary during feeding. As she grew up, Ginny continued to ward off overt expressions of affection from her parents. Rick, the youngest child in a family of four children, was born with a happy outlook that continued throughout his childhood to keep him skipping safely over small moats of fear. His fears ranged from anxiety over natural catastrophes to imaginary kidnappers.

We can speculate how Ann's therapy with Dr. L. might have progressed if he had recognized the state of primary vulnerability that was activated when he raised her fee. The stress of her second pregnancy, the anxiety over separation from him, and her fear of an early delivery catapulted Ann into a state of dependency and need that in ordinary circumstances she sought to avoid at all costs. If Dr. L. had been able to understand Ann's fears in the context of her primary vulnerabilities, he might have been able to work in a constructive way with the wounding experience of the fee raise, creating an opportunity for connection rather than a devastating rupture.

We can further speculate that Dr. L.'s capacity for empathy was obscured by feelings elicited by Ann related to *his* areas of primary vulnerability. Dr. L. was dealing with significant loss in his personal life—the dissolution of his nuclear family—at a time when Ann was in the process of creating one. His deprivation and envy threatened his sense of a cohesive self. He managed his anxiety by channeling it into a need for higher pay, which was too pressing and strong to be contained or postponed until after his vacation and the birth of Ann's child. We can speculate that being in Ann's presence and sensing her potential to have what he was losing evoked more emotional pain than Dr. L. could tolerate. Unable to face his vulnerability consciously, he acted unconsciously by insisting on a fee raise and bringing about a termination. Dr. L.'s unconscious response brought about a *secondary level of wounding* that exacerbated the impasse with Ann and ultimately brought about a rupture in the therapeutic relationship.

The case of Ann and Dr. L. brings us to another speculation: *When a patient is wounded in an area of primary vulnerability and the therapist is unable to empathize with or help the patient understand the wounding, the therapist may herself have been catapulted into an area of personal primary vulnerability.* When the therapist is vulnerable, she has the urgent task of restoring a coherent sense of a competent professional self and consequently may lack adequate psychic energy to empathize with the patient. The therapist's efforts to restore a cohesive sense of self may lead to a *secondary level of wounding* that further injures the patient and places the therapeutic relationship in jeopardy. When the underlying matrix of vulnerability remains unacknowledged by the therapist and patient, wounding interactions are apt to continue unabated. The patient may be forced to terminate the relationship abruptly and feel harmed by the experience.

D. W. Winnicott and Primary Agonies

D. W. Winnicott, in a 1962 article, referred to what he called the "unthinkable anxieties" of infancy. These anxieties are clearly in the same conceptual domain as Kohut's disintegration anxiety. Winnicott considered unthinkable anxieties to be primordial, the "stuff" of psychotic anxiety.[18] The anxieties include going to pieces, falling forever, having no relationship to the body, and having no orientation.

In his final article "Fear of Breakdown," which was published posthumously in 1971, Winnicott refined his conception of unthinkable anxieties. Because he felt that "anxiety" was too weak a word, he referred instead to "primary agonies" that each of us must defend against.[19] He believed that an adult's fear of an impending breakdown is actually a fear of returning to a state of primary agony that she has already lived through as an infant, before the development of the cognitive capacities necessary to remember it.

We can look at the patient Ann through the lens of Winnicott's conception of primary agonies and the fear of a breakdown and create a narrative understanding of her early experience. We might speculate that as an infant of a mother who was occupied with two older children as well as with going to work, Ann was left alone at times when she experienced distress. Without the soothing and containing functions of her mother or another caretaker, Ann might well have had the experience of a newly forming and relatively fragile sense of self fragmenting under anxiety and stress. As an adult, Ann did not dare to allow another person to soothe, hold, and contain her because the danger of fragmentation, if the other person neglected or abandoned her, was too great to risk. When she did feel safe enough with Dr. L. to trust him, he failed her and then was unavailable to "hold" her (remain psychologically connected and available) through the experience of anxiety and fragmentation that ensued. Had Dr. L. insisted that Ann remain in relationship to him, especially in view of the injury that his fee raise brought about, Ann would have had an important opportunity. She might have lived through a "breakdown" experience—the injury of Dr. L.'s fee raise, the experience of his utter abandonment, her rage and disappointment—with full adult consciousness and without the loss of the important attachment/connection to him. In Winnicott's words, she would have reexperienced a fragmentation that first occurred in relation to her parents when she was not enough of a person (not cognitively developed enough) to live through it. As an adult in a therapeutic relationship, the fragmentation would take place when there was a "person" (ego) there to experience it. Instead, Ann lived through the breakdown once again, reenacting a traumatic disconnection from an important attachment figure. Ann's subjective sense of having been damaged by the relationship with Dr. L. was partially accurate, because the likelihood that she will risk another therapeutic relationship after the rupture with Dr. L. is diminished. The residue of his abandonment remains with her.

The experience of primary agony to which Winnicott refers need not be viewed as pathological, unless it comprises all there is of an individual's experience, nor does the concept of a "breakdown" necessarily have to mean a total inability to function in the world. Most adults are vulnerable to episodes of primary agony that may be fleeting or that endure for hours, days, or weeks. These states repeat a condition that was suffered when the adult was very young, in the presymbolic phase of development prior to language. What we refer to as "moods" are often the reexperiencing of such states. For example, any of us can experience states where all meaning and enduring value are lost, whether of a specific project, a career, self-worth, parenting capacity, or ability to love. These states can be precipitated by an experience of a loss of coherence of self, perhaps related to a failure or physical illness. These states can also be related to disconnection from others, perhaps because of an argument with a friend or losing someone who moves away. Disconnections from self and others can trip any of us into areas of primary vulnerability.

Winnicott, like other British object relations theorists and Kohut, believed that mothers (and other significant caretakers, including the father) provide their infants with a psychological buffer from the experience of primary agonies. If we consider the multiple functions that maternal caretakers continually provide for their babies early in development, Winnicott's assertion is true beyond question. Babies are consequently exquisitely vulnerable to developing psychological sensitivities early in life in the context of the maternal–infant relationship. We can turn to the British object relations theorists for an understanding of the significance of the maternal–infant matrix in the development of primary vulnerabilities. These theorists also contribute to an understanding of the nature of the anxieties that arise early in development and that are related to primary vulnerabilities.

CHAPTER SEVEN

❖ *Origins of Primary* ❖ *Vulnerabilities in Infancy*

Even as we grew up, my mother could not help imposing herself between her children and whatever it was they might take it in mind to reach out for in the world. For she would get it for them, if it was good enough for them—she would have to be very sure—and give it to them, at whatever cost to herself: valiance was in her very fibre. She stood always prepared in herself to challenge the world in our place.

—EUDORA WELTY[1]

The idea that mother is or should be all-giving and perfect . . . expresses the mentality of omnipotence, the inability to experience the mother as an independently existing subject . . . What determines whether hatred becomes the destruction that dispels idealization or, instead, goes inside where it requires idealization as a defense, is, finally, *what happens in real life*. The child can only perceive the mother as a subject in her own right if the mother *is* one.

—JESSICA BENJAMIN[2]

Primary Vulnerability: The Mother–Infant Matrix

The mothering person's care, regardless of whether mothers are idealized, or perceived realistically as Eudora Welty's epigraph suggests, initially serves as a buffer between the infant and intolerable distress, what Winnicott called the "unthinkable anxieties"[3] of infancy. Maternal care includes not only physical but psychological care, of which the mother's (and father's or other caretaker's) empathy for an infant's needs is an essential component. Infants begin life in what Winnicott calls a state of absolute dependence,[4] a state that renders them utterly vulnerable to the human environment in which they find themselves. Infants rely on maternal care to protect their psyches from overstimulation and neglect in the same way that we rely on our skin

122

as a protection for our physical body. In a state of absolute dependence, infants are unable to provide in any way for their own basic needs, although they are able from the beginning of life to elicit actively the caretaking responses they require. But their ability to evoke needed responses is contingent on reliable responses from the human caretaking environment. We now understand that psychological needs are as important as physical needs, as the research on failure-to-thrive infants and anaclitic depression affirms.[5] Including along with the needs for attunement, empathy, and love, other needs such as curiosity, the need for stimulation, and the need to feel effective and competent. Psychological needs include the need for attunement, empathy, love, stimulation, and the need to feel effective and competent. A therapeutic relationship, by re-creating in form the exclusive dyad of mothers and infants, encourages patients to experience, often unconsciously, yearnings that cannot always be adequately met for therapists to protect them from impingements, to provide essential care, and to be empathically attuned to them. Therapists, like mothers, are in danger of being increasingly idealized as the conditions under which they function become more difficult.

The seeds of the unrealistic expectations placed upon women in our culture as the primary providers of maternal care (and that women place upon themselves in nurturing others) may well begin with the initial vitally important functions that mothering persons necessarily serve for infants. As Jessica Benjamin's epigraph suggests, mothering persons tend to be idealized out of a yearning for perfect care or as a defense against hatred of them for their inevitable failure to provide perfect nurturing. Hatred arising from unmet needs for nurturing has the positive potential to enable mothering persons to be perceived realistically as ordinary human beings. The maternal concern that most of us feel for infants and babies (including for some individuals the strong feelings of distress elicited by the possibility of elective abortion), is rooted in our awareness of their absolute dependence and vulnerability to the caretaking environment. As adult human beings we share a common primary vulnerability: a fundamental fear of being helpless and alone with no one to notice us and to care for us. The seeds of the at-once unrealistic and yet necessary illusions of patients in relation to therapists originate in this domain.

Mothers can continue to serve the psychological function of buffering children from unmanageable anxiety throughout their lives, even though children develop their own mechanisms for managing anxiety and even though their relational networks expand to include fathers, siblings, peers, and teachers. For example, Rick, the boy referred to in Chapter Six, developed at age thirteen a terror of being abducted by aliens after he read Whitley Streiber's book *Communion*. When the book was made into a movie, Rick wanted his mother instead of a friend to go to the movie with him because he believed she could help him master his fear. Her presence served as a source of protection to him perhaps because of the psychological function and role she continued to occupy in his psyche, based on his actual relationship to her as an infant.

The concept of a realm of primary vulnerability in each of us, patient and therapist alike, acquiring its specific contents from the beginning of life in the context of the complex and cumulative interactions of infants with their mothering persons, takes us directly back to the mother–infant matrix (broadening the definition of mothers to include male mothers as well as biological and adoptive female mothers).[6]

Psychotherapists and theorists like Klein, Balint, and Winnicott began to pay close attention to experiences in infancy that shape the predominant psychological concerns of adult patients. Echoes of the mother–infant (and father–infant) bond reverberate at a nonverbal level in the therapist–patient relationship. These "echoes" need to be identified and named so that they do not overwhelm the patient and therapist and lead to the dangerous outcomes that Balint describes. For example, we can conceive of Ann's yearning for Dr. L. to provide her with absolute, consistent, unwavering support as a revived need for a reliable maternal and paternal presence as well as her current need for an attachment figure as an adult. Because Dr. L. addressed the fee raise only in a literal way, insisted upon being paid, and did not consider its psychological meaning on multiple levels, the opportunity to raise to consciousness echoes of the mother–infant relationship was missed. Even if Dr. L. had been aware of the echoes but had not communicated them explicitly in words to Ann, his response to her feelings about the intrusion of the fee raise into the harmonious relationship might have been less destructive.

Therapists have been evolving a language for mother–infant experience that is derived from and applicable to adult therapy patients. Winnicott was one of the first therapists and theorists to focus attention not only on the phase of infancy but on the mother–infant unit. As mentioned earlier, the mother, according to Winnicott, serves to buffer the infant from unthinkable anxieties in the realm of primary vulnerability. Winnicott, who initially worked as a pediatrician, had a special gift for understanding mother–infant relationships. He is well known for his recognition that "there is no such thing as an infant."[7] Babies cannot exist without their mothers and therefore cannot be considered as psychological entities separate from their mothers. In the first phase of life, the totality of an infant's experience occurs in the context of its relationship to the mothering person. Today most infants are cared for by more than one person, each one a significant attachment figure. Winnicott's conception of "mother" may be broadened to include all "mothering persons" without altering his conception that babies develop a sense of self within a relational context. In ensuing discussions of Winnicott and mothers, we can expand the conception of mother to reflect the extended network of caretakers that raise infants.

Winnicott suggests that an infant develops two kinds of relationships simultaneously with the mothering person. The infant relates both to an "environment mother," who optimally provides a reliable holding environment, and to the mother as a separate object, or the "object mother."[8] As the baby matures, these two aspects of the mother come together. A "capacity for concern develops" in the infant when it begins to realize that its behavior affects the mother as a separate person.

The concept of an environment mother and an object mother has relevance to the patient's relationship to the therapist. For example, Ann had been relying upon Dr. L. in the transference level of the relationship as an environment mother (or parent). When his separate needs unexpectedly intruded via the raise in his fee at a vulnerable time for Ann, Ann and Dr. L. lacked access to the language of the maternal–infant relationship as a context for understanding both the distress that Ann was in and Dr. L.'s inflexible stance in response to her distress. Had Dr. L. been conscious of and able to name explicitly the abrupt shift in the maternal transference level of the relationship (from functioning as an environment mother to becoming an object mother), a fruitful exploration of the meaning of the painful turn in the therapeutic relationship instead of a devastating rupture might have been possible.

Thomas Ogden sharpens Winnicott's (1960) notion that "there is no such thing as an infant" and his concept of a mother–infant unit by introducing the term "matrix," derived from the Latin word for "womb."[9] Ogden writes:

> it was not until Winnicott that psychoanalysis developed a conception of the mother as the infant's psychological matrix. From a Winnicottian perspective, the infant's psychological contents can be understood only in relation to the psychological matrix within which those contents exist. That matrix is at first provided by the mother. . . . Because the internal holding environment of the infant, his own psychological matrix, takes time to develop, the infant's mental contents initially exist within the matrix of the maternal mental and physical activity.[10]

The quality of the maternal "mental and physical activity" to which Ogden refers will necessarily differ from mother to mother (once again expanding the concept to include significant caretakers), depending on a complex amalgam of her physical constitution, her personal experiences as an infant and as a mother, her attitudes toward mothering, her feelings about herself as a mother and toward her baby, her perception of her relationship to her mother, father, husband, and siblings, and finally, on the unique nature of her infant. The cultural level of the ideals and forms of mothering that women have been taught by "professionals," as well as the economic and social factors that influence their lives, provide an essential context for these complicated personal ingredients.[11]

Understanding the nature of the psychological matrix within which an adult therapy patient's sense of self took shape helps the patient and therapist understand the patient's areas of primary vulnerability. Ann's relatively unavailable mother and Ann's adaptive response to maternal unavailability of suppressing dependency and attachment needs in favor of self-sufficiency created fertile soil for the impasse that erupted with Dr. L. Analogously, although Ann could not have known, Dr. L.'s experiences as a younger brother whose older brother was adored created fertile soil for his feelings of envy and deprivation.

Christopher Bollas, an American psychoanalyst who is a current member of the British Psychoanalytical Society and who follows in the tradition of Klein, Bion, and Winnicott, gives us additional language for articulating early experience and the mother–infant relationship. He also demonstrates how preverbal experience can recur and be worked with productively in the relationship of a patient to a therapist who is knowledgeable about as well as comfortable and skillful in working with the primitive, presymbolic (before language) realm of experience. Bollas describes the relationship of mothers to infants in the following terms: "the mother is less significant and identifiable as an object than as a process that is identified with cumulative internal and external transformations."[12]

Bollas, refining Winnicott's notion of the "environment mother," refers to the mother as a "transformational object." He means that the mother is an object that the infant comes to identify through the mother's association with caretaking processes that alter (transform) the infant's state of being. For example, a mother who repeatedly soothes an irritable infant becomes to that infant a transformational object associated with the alteration of a state of being from agitated to calm. The infant's experience of the mother is not carried in words or language but rather exists on a presymbolic level. The infant's experience of the mother exists outside of language as an "unthought known," literally something that is known by the individual but not yet articulated in language, that can be recovered (or put in language) in the process of psychoanalysis.

As an infant grows and develops, the relationship to the mother "changes from the mother as the other who alters the self to a person who has her own life and her own needs."[13] (Winnicott would say that the mother changes from being primarily an environment mother to being primarily an object mother, or that the mother has been destroyed as an object existing solely under the infant's omnipotent control and, if she survives and does not retaliate, becomes for the baby a subjective object or person with a separate center of initiative. Klein or Ogden would say that the child has reached the depressive position.) Traces, or the "shadow" of the early transformational object that the mother once was for the infant, remain visible in the behavior, thoughts, and feelings of the adult patient in relation to the therapist and in the corresponding feelings engendered in the therapist while being with the patient. Bollas provides the example of a patient named Peter who was helped not by the content of Bollas's interpretations but by the sound of his voice in uttering them:

> what he wanted was to hear my voice, which I gradually understood to be his need for a good sound. My interpretations were appreciated less for their content, and more for their function as structuring experiences. He rarely recalled the content of an interpretation. What he appreciated was the sense of relief brought to him through my voice.[14]

By paying close attention to the nonverbal experience and feeling-states elicited in them by patients, therapists can glean what the patient's earliest experiences of self and other—experiences that occurred before the achievement of language—were like.

To understand how the theoretical notion of the maternal–infant matrix can inform our understanding of therapeutic relationships, we return to the patient Ann and her experience with Dr. L. Although Ann's attachment to and dependency on Dr. L., particularly during the last stage of her second pregnancy, is visible and clear, the maternal–infant matrix that was activated in the transference may be less obvious. Ann had come to lean upon Dr. L. as a presence who, unlike her mother, soothed and calmed her, rendering the world safe and secure. His presence, registered by Ann through nonverbal (outside of language) aspects of his being, such as his calm, consistent demeanor and quiet tone of voice, became part of his identity as a transformational object. In Bollas's terms, Dr. L. was operating not only as a separate adult person but was functioning as a transformational object in the transference matrix of the relationship, buffering Ann from the anxieties of reality.

When Dr. L. unexpectedly raised his fee just before his vacation, he suddenly loomed large in Ann's subjective view as an adult person, separate from Ann, jolting her out of the safe cocoon of his secure maternal presence. She reacted to the sudden change in nonverbal aspects of his demeanor (e.g., the alteration from his calm, quiet voice to a harsh, impersonal tone) as much as to the content of what he said. The sudden absence of his presence as a familiar transformational object was more than Ann could tolerate. She could not withstand being catapulted into a state of primary vulnerability and then being left alone there as a consequence of the sudden change in him. Without his help in identifying and affirming the change that had occurred, Ann withdrew from the relationship altogether in order to restore a coherent sense of herself as a separate, adult person.

Dr. L., suffering from his personal primary vulnerabilities centered in feelings of envy, deprivation, and loss, was unable to continue to function as the maternal presence buffering Ann from the intrusion of anxieties from the outer or inner world. Unfortunately he was not sufficiently aware of his own state of vulnerability either to manage it on his own or to convey it to Ann so that she might have understood his behavior in conceptual terms. An acknowledgment of and way of thinking about what had occurred in the relationship would have allowed Ann to experience the loss of Dr. L. while in relationship to him instead of alone without him. *Moving through a painful experience in the context of an ongoing relationship with a therapist is worlds away from moving through it without the relational tie.* A consultant can serve this function for a patient when the therapist is unavailable, as the chapters in Part III demonstrate. Patients are able to tolerate profound shifts in the transference matrix of the therapeutic relationship as long as the therapist remains in relationship to them and can acknowledge the nature of the shifts. But Dr. L. was caught in his own vulnerabilities and in his needs for Ann to remain available to him. Allowing Ann to terminate as his patient enabled him to reduce his ongoing exposure to the sense of loss, deprivation, and envy that she elicited in him.

Had Dr. L. been able to remain in relationship to Ann and her experience, as well as to convey to her something about his vulnerable state and the way his anxieties were interacting with hers to produce an impasse, the therapeutic relationship might have been preserved. *However, the relationship would have been permanently altered, and the permanence of the alteration would need to be explicitly acknowledged.* Therapists may resist relinquishing the gratification inherent in functioning as a positive maternal caretaker and consequently may have difficulty acknowledging with the patient that a permanent change in the therapeutic relationship has occurred. Patients generally welcome their therapists' acknowledgment of a permanent change. Even when vulnerable facets of a patient's self are activated in the maternal–infant transference matrix of a therapeutic relationship, the adult part of the patient's self continues to exist and can be called on when necessary.

Anxiety and the Realm of Primary Vulnerability

Object relations theorists, including Klein and Ogden, in addition to alerting us to the significance of the maternal–infant matrix, have also provided us with a conceptual grasp of the central anxieties that arise early in development and that correspond to the phases of development they believe all infants move through. The anxieties they name are directly related to the areas of primary vulnerability that are inherent in human beings and that are likely to be accessed in therapeutic relationships.

Freud's conception of anxiety was different from that of the object relations theorists. His perspective on anxiety changed as his thinking evolved, moving from a view of anxiety as a danger signal to a view of anxiety arising as a consequence of the arousal of forbidden sexual and aggressive drives. In contrast, the object relations theorists (and interpersonal theorists) considered anxiety in the context of experiences occurring in relationships to important others (or objects). In general, Freud's theorizing was biologically oriented, based upon a theory of human instincts in which basic libidinal and aggressive drives emerge from the id and are managed at first by the ego and, later in development, with the help and influence of the superego.[15] The object relations theorists who followed the object-relationship line of Freud's theorizing made a shift from an instinctually based theory to one of psychological functioning based on object relationships, in which "object" refers both to other significant human beings (outer objects) and to internalized representations of other human beings (inner objects). Freud was also less preoccupied with infancy and the first months of life than the object relations theorists who followed him.

Although Klein, who branched off theoretically from Freud, does not refer to a concept analogous to that of primary vulnerability, she does concern herself with the different forms of anxiety that arise early in human relationships and that are implicitly related to the realm of primary vulnerability. She conceptualized two positions in the evolution of an infant's sense of self: the paranoid–schizoid and the depressive positions. She wrote about the overwhelming paranoid anxiety, related to a fear of annihilation by a bad object, that characterizes the paranoid–schizoid position. Klein believed that the fear of annihilation arises from the projection of the infant's innate death instinct, which is too dangerous to contain within, onto objects in the environment that are then perceived as ominously persecutory.[16] The major adaptive mechanism of this phase according to Klein, is splitting, in which good and bad are separated and located in different objects. The self is experienced as good or bad, and the other correspondingly carries the opposite. If we consider Ann and Dr. L. from the perspective of the paranoid–schizoid position, we might say that they each struggled to locate the bad in the other and the good in themselves. Ann was unable to maintain her perception of Dr. L. as bad and continually shifted or fought against shifting the bad feelings to herself after the termination. She consciously experienced Dr. L. as behaving toward her in a persecutory manner. Analogously, Dr. L. attributed the rupture in the relationship to Ann's inability to allow herself to have a "happy graduation" in terminating therapy and was unwilling to assume responsibility for having been a part of the problematic ending.

In the depressive position, which occurs later in development, the infant is able to perceive the mother as a whole object toward whom the infant experiences ambivalence, or both love and hate. The anxiety arising in this position is related to fear that one's destructive impulses have harmed the object.[17] For example, viewed from the perspective of the depressive position, the patient Ann might have left the relationship for fear that her rage at the change in Dr. L. might harm him. She was consciously aware of a fear that her rage at Dr. L. would harm her unborn child.

Ogden, in his recent book, *The Primitive Edge of Experience*, extends Klein's theory by exploring three modes of organizing experience that he believes each of us relies upon. The modes remain in a dialectical relationship one to another throughout human life[18] and are particularly apparent in therapeutic relationships. Ogden conceives of the paranoid–schizoid and depressive positions not only as sequential developmental phases, but also as positions that remain accessible throughout life. He expands Klein's original two positions, the paranoid–schizoid and depressive, into three positions by positing the existence of an even more primitive mode which he names the autistic-contiguous position.[19] Building on the work of Bion, Bick, Meltzer, and

Tustin, he defines the autistic-contiguous position and the specific nature of the anxiety arising within it as:

> a sensory-dominated, presymbolic area of experience in which the most primitive form of meaning is generated on the basis of the organization of sensory impressions, particularly at the skin surface. A unique form of anxiety arises in this psychological realm: terror over the prospect that the boundedness of one's sensory surface might be dissolved, with a resultant feeling of falling, leaking, dropping, into an endless and shapeless space.[20]

A therapist who understands conceptually the patient's experience of collapsing into the autistic–contiguous position as a consequence of a threat to the patient's sense of self, as wounding in the realm of primary vulnerability is, may be better able to tolerate sitting with a patient who is in a state of fragmentation. The therapist has access to a conceptual language that provides an anchor and helps the patient restore a stable sense of self.

Therapists are vulnerable to the impact of their patients and are also at risk of collapsing into the autistic–contiguous position, as well as into the paranoid–schizoid and depressive positions. Patients whose behavior and affect states are intense and extreme may endanger a therapist's sense of self, giving rise to primitive anxieties in the therapist. Therapists who feel in jeopardy of fragmenting, leaking, or dissolving will necessarily need to distance themselves from the patient by relying on available defensive measures. In the case of Lynn and Dr. K., we could say that Lynn's rage had the potential to evoke in Dr. K. the unique form of anxiety characteristic of the paranoid–schizoid position (a threat of annihilation by the bad object). His distancing himself from her, pathologizing her, and attempting to medicate (subdue and quiet) her may be understood as manifestations of his defensive efforts in the service of preserving his sense of self, although he regarded them as his efforts to help Lynn.

Amplifying the theoretical contributions of Klein and Winnicott, Ogden delineates the specific anxieties that are related to the two other positions and modes of organizing experience: the paranoid–schizoid position and the depressive position. In the paranoid–schizoid mode of organizing experience, as Klein postulated, intolerable anxiety arises from the dilemma of loving and hating the same object. The conflict is handled by splitting the good parts from the bad so that the two aspects are separated from each other. Ogden emphasizes that to a person who has collapsed into the paranoid–schizoid mode, thoughts and feelings are not experienced as separate *creations* of one's self, but as *facts* that exist. Individuals operating from this mode have little capacity to mediate between (reflect upon) themselves and their experience. In therapy, for example, for patients operating out of this position, therapists would not simply behave "like" one's parents; they would actually become the parents. For therapists operating from this position, a patient might become the parent. A female therapist, for example, found herself enraged with a male patient who would not accept her advice to try an adjunctive group therapy experience for help with an addiction problem. The patient, who was anxious about participating in a group, refused to try the group unless the therapist would provide research articles documenting the effectiveness of such groups. The therapist, oblivious to the patient's anxiety, confronted the patient with his tendency to be suspicious and manipulative. The patient felt attacked and misunderstood and was unable to make himself attend the subsequent session. Meanwhile, the therapist worked with a consultant and became aware that the patient's cold, mistrustful manner resembled the way the therapist's father related to her. The therapist had reacted to her patient as if he were her father.

In the depressive mode, which is less primitive and developmentally more complex than the other two modes, individuals have the capacity to experience others as whole beings, as both subjects and objects. Others are perceived as separate human beings who have a life of their own, and not only as objects that are under one's omnipotent, magical control. In this mode of organizing experience, a new anxiety arises: "that one's anger has driven away or harmed the person one loves."[21] Patients operating from the depressive position will have difficulty expressing angry and critical feelings toward their therapists, fearful that the expression of anger will alienate the therapist or cause the therapist to forget that the patient also has good feelings for them. Patients who are catapulted into states of intense rage, like patients wounded by therapists in an area of primary vulnerability, do cause therapists to forget that they are also attached in positive ways. *When therapists are unable to hold onto the importance of the attachment, they make their patients' worst fear become a reality: The patients' anger does drive away or harm the therapist and endangers the relationship.*

To summarize, the existence of a realm of primary vulnerability, more specifically a sensitivity to the potential dissolution of a cohesive sense of a connected self, is basic to all human beings. From an object relations perspective, there are different forms of anxiety arising from areas of primary vulnerability, although all forms of anxiety continue to exist in dialectical relationship to one another in each human being throughout the lifespan. The object relations theorists, particularly

Klein, Winnicott, and Ogden, have evolved a useful conceptual scheme that encompasses a developmental progression of anxiety. Ogden, whose work is the most recent, describes the three positions, each with a different form of anxiety related to a primary vulnerability: the autistic–contiguous position, where the vulnerability centers on disruption of sensory cohesion and boundedness; the paranoid–schizoid position, where the vulnerability centers on the loss of space between one's experience and the capacity to reflect upon it (a loss of the separation between self and object); and the depressive position, where the vulnerability centers on the disruption of whole-object relations.

The metaphors of the three positions give us a means of differentiating specific forms of anxiety arising from areas of primary vulnerability into specific categories that can be linked in turn to phases of early development. Although the basic sensitivity that gives rise to the experience of vulnerability resides in each of us, how our human environment responds to us determines whether we are pushed further into a vulnerable state, or whether we are "contained" sufficiently by a relational network so that we can move through the vulnerable state with awareness.

We can return once more to Ann and Dr. L. in order to embed the object relations concepts in an actual case and speculate that both Ann and Dr. L. were catapulted into the paranoid–schizoid position by the stress of Ann's pregnancy. In understanding impasses in therapeutic relationships, typically only the dynamics of the patient are focused on. *But impasses, particularly those in which wounding has occurred in the patient's realm of primary vulnerability, often involve the vulnerabilities of both patient and therapist.* Understanding the interaction of the vulnerabilities of both patient and therapist is critically important if the wounding is to be worked through rather than allowed to disrupt the relationship altogether.

Dr. L. and Ann became to each other the abandoning parent, the "bad" object from whom they needed to flee. The rage and aggressive impulses that Ann felt toward Dr. L. for shifting attention to his needs were too dangerous for her to "keep" inside herself, particularly in view of her baby's presence inside her body. In psychological terms, Ann located the aggression and rage in Dr. L. and perceived him to be attacking her with his fee raise. Correspondingly, Dr. L. could not tolerate his envy inside himself and acted to "spoil" the source of his envy: Ann's pleasure in her pregnancy and growing family. As Ann, the patient, and Dr. L., the therapist, collapsed into the paranoid–schizoid position, the holding environment of the therapy shifted from being the soothing, safe, secure container that it had been and became a danger-ous place, filled with envy and rage, for both individuals.

When both patient and therapist are caught in a realm of primary vulnerability and when anxieties powerful enough to elicit primitive defensive responses are generated, neither patient nor therapist can function as the therapist in the situation. We might speculate about what might have happened to Ann and Dr. L. if they had been willing to utilize a consultant. A consultant could have met with each sepa-rately to provide the empathic channel they both needed. Ann might have been helped to identify her need for Dr. L. to function as a maternal environment mother, buffering her from the anxieties generated by her pregnancy. Dr. L. might have been helped to see Ann's need for him to function in the maternal–infant matrix of the therapeutic relationship as a positive object. A consultant might have helped Dr. L. consciously acknowledge his envy of Ann, his personal feelings of loss, and his needs in relation to Ann so that they would not have been unconciously discharged in the relationship. The theraputic relationship might not have been jeopardized or a ruptured termination might have been averted.

Except in situations of glaring abuse or neglect, the factors that influence and characterize each mother–infant pair are often subtle and complicated, difficult to isolate and identify, as they are in therapeutic dyads. Nonetheless, they are extremely important to name, not with an attitude of judgment or blame based on an idealization of motherhood or therapists, but with interest and curiosity about the intersection of mother–infant and therapist–patient vulnerabilities. Awareness of the extent to which they were buffered in infancy from primordial anxiety by their mother-person helps patients and therapists create a concep-tual frame for understanding the patients' (and mothering persons') primary vulnerabilities. With such a conceptual frame, patients (and therapists) learn to tolerate a broader range of self-states without fear of a permanent loss of cohesion and connection of self. Therapy with patients who seek an understanding of their early issues usually in-cludes the creation (and re-creation) of a narrative history that encom-passes the mother–infant relationship. The narrative history is created not only from memories, fantasies, and perceptions of early experiences conveyed by patients, but from the verbal and nonverbal relational experiences that patients and therapists live through with each other and reflect upon together.

In the following chapter we will take a closer look at concepts concerning mothers, infants, and the mother–infant relationship upon which psychodynamic theories of early development are based. Psy-chodynamic theorists have differed in how they view mothers, babies, and the nature of the dyad: whether mothers and babies begin in a state of merger with each other, whether babies arrive in the world with an inner life that exerts an influence on the caregiving environment, or whether they are blank slates that the caregiving environment fills in. These theoretical differences not only affect speculations as to how primary vulnerabilities arise early in development but also have implications for how these vulnerabilities are manifested in and worked with in therapeutic relationships.

CHAPTER EIGHT

Relational Modes:
❖ Mother/Infant and ❖
Therapist/Patient

From the observable and inferred beginnings of the infant's primitive cognitive-affective state, with unawareness of self-other differentiation, a major organization of intrapsychic and behavioral life develops around issues of separation and individuation, an organization that we recognize by terming the subsequent period the separation-individuation phase.

—MARGARET MAHLER, FRED PINE, ANNI BERGMAN[1]

Infants begin to experience a sense of emergent self from birth. They are predesigned to be aware of self-organizing processes. They never experience a period of total self/other undifferentiation. There is no confusion between self and other in the beginning or at any point during infancy. They are also predesigned to be selectively responsive to external social events and never experience an autistic-like phase.

—DANIEL STERN[2]

I once said: "There is no such thing as an infant," meaning, of course, that whenever one finds an infant one finds maternal care, and without maternal care there would be no infant.

—D. W. WINNICOTT[3]

No psychological theory has adequately articulated the mother's independent existence. Thus even the accounts of the mother-infant relationship which do consider parental responsiveness always revert to a view of the mother as the baby's vehicle for growth, an object of the baby's needs. The mother is the baby's first object of attachment, and later, the object of desire. She is provider, interlocutor, caregiver, contingent reinforcer, significant other, empathic understander, mirror. She is also a secure presence to walk away from, a setter of limits, an optimal frustrator, a shockingly real otherness. She is external reality—but she is rarely regarded as another subject with a purpose apart from her existence for her child. . . . Yet the real mother is not simply an object for her child's demands; she is, in fact, another subject whose independent center must be outside her child if she is to grant him the recognition he seeks.

—Jessica Benjamin[4]

The Origin of Areas of Primary Vulnerability

Areas of primary vulnerability originate in the context of human relationships early in development. These vulnerabilities inevitably develop in the context of our primary relational bonds, even in the best of circumstances and even with adequate or "good-enough" parenting. The specific nature of the vulnerabilities that arise in an infant depends in part on the kind of objects or *relational partners*[5] that mothers (or mothering persons) and infants are able to become for each other and how flexible and adaptive mother and baby are in shifting from one mode of relationship to another. The mother's and infant's capacities to use each other flexibly in the service of personal developmental needs and to preserve the relationship is determined by and influenced in an ongoing way by the defensive needs and wishes operating both in the moment and developmentally within mother and baby and by the context in which mother and baby are located. By context, I refer to the relational context of the father, family, and friends, the cultural context in the narrower and larger sense, and the historical or temporal context. When primary vulnerabilities emerge in therapeutic relationships, therapists and patients have an opportunity to identify and modify constraining relational modes and entrenched representations of self or the possibility of further reinforcing them.

Whether primary vulnerabilities and the adaptive mechanisms that babies develop in relation to them remain entrenched or are modified depends on ongoing life experiences. Human beings may be affected by experiences in significant relationships and as the life context changes. Because of *the special malleability of the sense of self that characterizes new mothers and babies,* the evolving mother–infant bond in tandem with the relationship to a father (or fathering person), is an especially important beginning phase in shaping an individual's sense of self and sense of self-in-relationship. Babies learn early in life what behaviors, responses, and representations of self will preserve both their important attachment bonds and a coherent sense of self.

Therapeutic relationships are protected from impingement by external influences, allowing the therapist to become central to patients, just as the mothering person once was. The relationship thus brings to the surface the patient's relational modes that originated to preserve vital attachment bonds and the patient's self-representations that evolved to shape a coherent sense of self. As the patient's relational modes and self-representations emerge in the therapeutic relationship, those of the therapist echo and resonate in response, as illustrated in the cases of Lynn and Dr. K. and Ann and Dr. L., even with the therapist's best effort to be conscious of them and to keep them from impinging destructively on the patient.

Implications of Psychotherapy Theories for the Conception of the Mother–Infant Relationship

As the epigraphs at the beginning of the chapter indicate, developmental psychologists and psychodynamic theorists have held widely divergent views of mothers, infants, and the mother–infant relationship. Most psychodynamic theories of early development have adopted a unidirectional conception of development and a unidimensional focus on babies and mothers. By unidirectional conception of development, I mean that the theories have focused on the development of the baby, who makes use of the mother (or the caregiving environment) as an object in the service of growth, rather than on the corresponding and interrelated development of the mother and infant and the mother–infant relationship. By unidimensional focus, I mean that theorists have attributed fixed characteristics to the mother and to the baby with respect to discrete variables rather than regarding both babies and mothers as occupying shifting positions on a continuum of interacting variables.[6] With the exception of the intersubjective and interpersonal theoretical perspectives, the same unidirectional and unidimensional focus has characterized theories of therapy.

External reality and the caregiving environment is an example of one discrete variable that some theorists have emphasized. Winnicott, Bowlby, and Mahler, for example, have viewed babies as particularly influenced by the reality of environmental care. By contrast, other theorists have placed primary emphasis on the capacities that infants are endowed with at birth. For example, Freud and Klein stress the importance of the internal reality of infants, their drives and unconscious fantasies.

Some theorists have emphasized the merged state of infant and mother that exists during infancy. Winnicott, Ogden, and Mahler assert that infants and mothers begin life as a merged unit, making it impossible to consider one without the other. Developmental psychologist Daniel Stern, whose work will be discussed in the next chapter, differs by asserting that infants and mothers have a separate and autonomous sense of self from the moment of birth.

Theories of therapy have been characterized by similar differences in assumptions. For example, Jung conceived of therapy as an alchemical container in which the psyches of patient and therapist intermingle. Balint conceptualized regressed states in therapy as characterized by a "harmonious, inter-penetrating mixup,"[7] or a state of psychological merger between patient and therapist. In contrast, Kleinians, British Object Relations theorists of the Independent School, Freudians, and Self psychologists, maintain a conception of the therapist functioning as a separate, autonomous person. *The emphasis in the conception of the maternal–infant relationship and the therapeutic relationship put forth in this chapter is on the elasticity or fluidity of both the relational modes and representations of self, other, and the relationship rather than on fixed attributes of either the mothering person and infant or the therapist and patient.*

If we *look through* the different theoretical perspectives concerning early development, we can identify different assumptions concerning the significant direction and dimensions of development involving the mother, baby, and mother–infant relationship. These assumptions, particularly as the theories have been applied over time, have come to be regarded not as assumptions or working conceptualizations, but as objective truths. When working conceptualizations assume the position of truth or reality, they begin to operate invisibly, causing the theories of which they are a part to lose their subjective status as ways of organizing information that are influenced by history, culture, and the psychological makeup of the theoretician. When the subjective and relative status of theories is obscured, the theories are liable to be used to shape our experience, rather than remaining flexible modes of representing experience that continues to be shaped by the very experiences they represent.

The current chapter identifies briefly the basic assumptions that underlie the prevailing major theories of early development and the implications of these theories for therapeutic relationships. The discussions are not intended to be comprehensive but rather to model a way of looking through the content of a theory to assess the assumptions that are often taken to be objective truths. The theories under consideration are those that most therapists draw on in thinking about the early history of patients and in identifying areas of primary vulnerability that were formed early in development. Two aspects of early experience that cut across theoretical perspective and operate outside of language will be identified and discussed: the modes of relating to each other that characterize mothers and infants and the representations of self, other, and relationship that mothering persons and infants form within these relational modes. These aspects of early experience—relational mode and representations of self, other, and self-in-relationship—will be considered with respect to their role in the formation of areas of primary vulnerability and their reverberation in therapeutic relationships.

Mother and Baby According to Freud

Freud's developmental theory emphasized the significance of the Oedipal phase and did not focus specifically upon infancy. He conceived of infants as dominated by biologically innate sexual and aggressive drives that are mediated by the ego and that gradually come under the control of the superego. According to Freud, development proceeds in relation to the parents who serve as the objects of the developing child's fantasies. Development thus proceeds on a unidirectional course, with Freud's theoretical focus centered exclusively on the development of the infant and not on the mutual growth of parents and infants in relation to one another. The impact of the developing child on the psyches of the parents (and the influence of the parents' psyches on the child) is not an essential part of the process. The impact of external reality and the cultural context is not significant, attested to by Freud's conception of the universality of the Oedipus Complex and his ultimate, though qualified, renunciation of his belief in the actual seduction of some of his female patients by their fathers and his emphasis on patients' fantasies.

This conception of mother–infant relationships is echoed in the prevailing view of therapist–patient relationships. Therapists operating with these basic assumptions regard themselves as fixed human beings with a neutral stance whose responses to patients occur primarily as encapsulated countertransference responses. They do not view themselves as human beings whose self-representations are in constant flux and who engage in relational modes that either shift fluidly or become entrenched.

Mother and Baby According to Klein

Klein followed Freud in emphasizing the salience of biologically based sexual and aggressive drives in infants, but differed from him in focusing on infant development in the earliest weeks and months of life. Looking through her theory to see the underlying conception of infants, we find that infants arrive in the world with a complex and tumultuous inner subjective life. Klein conceived of infants as filled with dangerous unconscious sexual and aggressive fantasies that they defensively project upon their mothers. For Klein as for Freud, development proceeds unidirectionally within the baby. The mother serves as an object or collection of part-objects to whom the baby reacts until it achieves the depressive position and can recognize the mother as a separate person. The literal external care provided by the mother, the father, and the larger culture in which the mother resides has less impact on the developing infant than the infant's fantasies, which are based on unconscious wishes and beliefs about the care provided. How the fantasies are managed defensively by the infant—for example, by splitting or by projective identification—influences how the infant continues to develop psychologically and ultimately influences the kind of therapeutic bond that the infant will form as an adult. The therapist's primary role, derived from Klein's view of mothers and infants, is to identify the fantasies and defense mechanisms that characterize the patient in relation to the therapist as therapy proceeds.

Mother and Baby According to Winnicott

Winnicott, who began his professional career as a pediatrician and who consequently consulted with many mother and baby dyads, placed great emphasis on the real nature of the facilitating environment mothers provided for their babies. Winnicott was also aware of the facilitating environment that fathers optimally provide for new mothers by protecting them from external impingement so they can immerse themselves in their babies. As the epigraph at the beginning of the chapter indicates, Winnicott conceived of a baby as part of a dyadic unit with the mother. The mother enables her baby to develop optimally by providing essential holding and mirroring functions, buffering her helpless and dependent infant from the impingement of the outer world. Good-enough mothers optimally support the baby's healthy sense of omnipotence by meeting their (good-enough) baby's needs adequately enough to allow the baby to maintain the illusion of having created what it needs. Up to this point in Winnicott's theory, the mother functions as an object the baby imagines to be under its omnipotent control. In the initial phases of therapy, therapists serve an analogous function for patients, providing a safe holding environment for the nascent True Self of the patient.

Unlike Freud, Winnicott does include in his theory a relational mode and a phase in therapy in which mother and baby come to be separate objects in relation to each other, individuals with separate lives rather than (subjective) objects under each other's omnipotent control. There is a necessary developmental phase in which, for the baby, the mother is "destroyed" as an *object* under the baby's omnipotent control. If the mother survives the baby's attack without collapsing or retaliating, she becomes a *separate person, an objective object*, to the baby. Like babies, patients in therapy must eventually place the therapist outside their omnipotent control, shifting from a perception of the therapist as an object that exists to provide what they need to a perception of the therapist as a separate person with a range of capacities, limits, and vulnerabilities.

Winnicott, although he did consider pathological mother–infant relationships in which babies are subjective objects for narcissistic mothers, did not conceive of the possibility of a mother being a separate (objective) object for the baby from the beginning of life. He viewed mothers primarily in terms of the adequacy of their functioning on behalf of their children, not in terms of their individual personhood. Mothers who could function effectively were "good enough." Presumably therapists who make mistakes with patients or who sometimes make use of patients to meet their personal needs can still be good enough. But the possibility that mothers and infants, or therapists and patients, fluidly shift relational modes moment to moment and have an ongoing mutual impact upon each other was not a central focus of his conceptual scheme.

Mother and Baby According to Bion

Wilfred Bion, a psychoanalyst who approached the contributions of Freud and Klein from a unique perspective, introduced the concept of the "container" and the "contained" to refer to the psychological function that mothers serve for infants.[8] Ogden's articulation of the concept of projective identification extended Bion's understanding of the container and the contained.[9] Mothers serve as psychological containers when they receive the projections of their infants, hold the projections internally and metabolize them, and then reintroduce them in altered, manageable form to the infant. The way in which mothers serve as containers for their infants, the "contained," occurs literally on a physiological level during pregnancy. The pregnant mother provides the unborn baby with nutrients and oxygen that are processed through her body. She receives the baby's waste products, processes and then expels them. Analogously, therapists serve as containers for their patients, processing the primitive thoughts and feelings that patients convey and elicit and returning them to their patients in modulated form.

Bion's model is unidirectional: The mother serves as a developmental object in the service of her baby's development. She either successfully contains and transforms her baby's projected impulses and thoughts, or she is unsuccessful in her function as a container. The mother is not regarded as a unique person in her own right who both influences and is influenced by the baby. Bion considers the mother–infant dyad in isolation, existing initially outside the context of the relationship with the father, extended family, culture, and place in history. The possibility of mother and infant fluidly shifting relational modes was not part of Bion's thinking, and would not be part of the attitude that a therapist operating with these assumptions would have toward a patient.

Mother and Baby According to Kohut

Kohut and the Self psychologists who have followed him focus exclusively on the psychological development of infants in relation to parents and not on the mutual impact of the participants in the relationships. Mothers provide functions for their babies that Kohut calls selfobject functions. Selfobject functions facilitate the evolution of the baby's healthy sense of self, and include, for example, soothing, feeding, mirroring, or admiring. Analogously, therapists serve needed selfobject functions for patients that the patient failed to experience earlier in their development in relation to parental caretakers.

Kohut's model has the potential to consider the *mutual relational impact* that babies and mothers have on each other, but the model has not been consistently applied in a mutual direction nor has the role of culture been included. The concept of selfobject functioning need not be limited to the functions that mothers or fathers serve for babies. Infants also serve selfobject functions that preserve and enhance a mother's or father's sense of self. For example, women in this culture who are mothers fit by definition into an acceptable category of female identity. Babies thus serve a selfobject function for their mothers simply by existing. Women who do not have biological children are vulnerable to judgments, to being pathologized or viewed as inadequate women.[10] Babies also serve specific selfobject functions for their mothers and fathers. For example, a happy baby might enliven a depressed mother, thus regulating her mood and self-state. A hearty male child might enhance the self-esteem and sense of masculinity of the father.

Kohut does include the role of the father in the child's develop-ment. In his view, the father provides specific selfobject functions for the developing child, who can also turn to the father when the mother is unavailable. Although the theory has the potential to examine the *mutual* influence of therapist and patient, it has been applied in a predominantly unidirectional manner. Echoes in therapeutic relation-ships consist of the patient's revived yearning for selfobject ties that were missing in early childhood, without explicitly including the possibility of a therapist's vulnerability to experiencing revived yearnings in relation to the patient.

Mother and Baby According to Mahler

Margaret Mahler, an American psychoanalyst, derived a theory of early development based primarily on her observational research studies of infants and mothers rather than on her clinical work. Her theoretical position is included here rather than with the infant research of developmental psychologists whose work is discussed in Chapter Nine because, unlike infant researchers, she investigated only one dimension of early behavior from birth to two years—the baby's separation from mother. To Mahler, babies undergo a biological birth from their mothers, but they are not born psychologically until later in their development when they have emerged from a primary state of psychological fusion with the mother.[11]

Mahler's theory of early development is unidirectional and unidimensional, focusing exclusively on the development of the baby rather than on the mutual impact of mother and baby on a wide range of dimensions that affect their evolving representations of self and other. The baby begins life as an enclosed, autistic entity, moves into an undifferentiated phase of union with the mother, and gradually becomes a separate, autonomous, independent person. The mother remains a constant.

We might speculate that therapists who accept Mahler's concep-tion of a developmental line of separation from fusion to autonomy would conceive of patients as progressing through the same sequence of separation phases in relation to their therapist. Their emphasis would be upon the patient's increasing capacity to separate, with a view of autonomy as a sign of psychological health. The coexistence of attachment and dependency needs with needs for independence and autonomy would not be considered to be part of psychologically healthy, adult functioning, nor would both sets of needs be considered part of the experience of therapists in relation to patients.

Mother and Baby According to Lacan

Jacques Lacan was a French psychoanalyst in the Freudian school whose reappraisal of Freudian theory has become a new vision of human development and the psyche. Lacan offers a theory of development that is radically and evocatively different from the theorists whose views have been considered thus far.[12] Lacan asserted that there is no innately predetermined self that evolves logically, as would be implied by Winnicott's notion of a True Self, Kohut's "nuclear self," or Jung's archetype of the Self as representing an image of wholeness. Lacan believed that the human passion or wish for certainty and for wholeness is not the same as certainty and wholeness itself. The human condition by definition is characterized by subjectivity, discontinuity, miscommunication, and ambivalence. In Lacan's view, the infant has no means of understanding its perceptions. Cognitive capacity, memory, and perception gradually mature through the mediation of human relationships and within language.

Lacan's theory of early development consists of two phases: the pre-mirror stage covering the first six months and the mirror stage that ranges from six to eighteen months of age. During the pre-mirror stage, the infant experiences its body as made up of fragmented parts and images. There is no original experience of unity. In fact, identity does not evolve from biological or developmental first causes, but rather is mediated by the mother and other relationships through images and language. Images and language exist before the birth of the baby and before genetic potentials unfold and influence each biological and developmental phase. The outside world is primary in structuring identity because of the utter helplessness and malleability of the infant. Through a process that Lacan called *primary identification,* the infant becomes aware of itself. The first object of identification is usually, but not necessarily, the mother. The father, who plays a critically important role in Lacan's view of development, confers the social order on the infant through language, rules, and symbols.

In the mirror stage, the baby achieves a sense of unity of self, literally by seeing itself in a mirror and recognizing itself as a coherent physical entity. The coherent outer form of the self that the baby sees in the mirror is at odds with the baby's inner sense of incoherence and lack of symmetry. This split between outer unity and inner discontinuity is the first alienation that human beings experience. The unity that the baby experiences in the mirror stage is artificial because it is imposed from without, determined by the cultural mediation of others rather than a consequence of innate and instinctual developmental sequences. The mirror stage thus serves as a metaphor for a vision of harmony of a subject who is essentially in discord.

Lacan, like Winnicott and Bion, conceived of the mother–infant unit as an essential element of the pre-mirror stage. The father eventually intervenes to disrupt the dyadic unit, thereby bringing about a separation from the mother that is traumatic to the baby because it signifies loss and difference. The mother symbolically continues to represent for the baby an unconscious source of primary identity, whereas the father, who is associated with the conscious sense of self, symbolically represents a secondary introjection identified with cultural values and ideals. Lacan's theory attributes specific functions to mothers and fathers in a way that discredits both mothers and fathers. Mothers can foster autonomy and independence in babies, and fathers can provide the source for a sense of primary identity.

Lacan, unlike the other theorists who have a unidimensional conception of mothers and infants (and fathers, to the extent that they are included) and a unidirectional developmental perspective, puts forth a more complicated view of the human psyche and of relationships. He conceives of each individual as both subject and object, not only in relation to herself but also in relation to others. The ego self, or *le moi*, is not a cohesive, unitary entity, but rather is both a reflection of the objectifications of others and a self that objectifies others. In contrast, *le je*, or the speaking subject, that appears, for example, in dreams, stands outside the objects and apprehends its own *moi* in fragments and in objects. Consequently, *le je* can restructure *le moi*.

Because of his complex view of human beings as both subject and object, formed by and formative of others, Lacan may be considered a theorist who paves the way for conceptualizing a multi-modal form of relationship between mother and infant that would have important analogues in the therapist–patient relationship. But Lacan's theoretical perspective has not had a unified impact on psychotherapists and has not been applied in a uniform manner, as might be anticipated in view of his emphasis on discontinuity, uncertainty, and ambivalence and on the multiple meanings attributable to language.

Mother and Baby According to an Intersubjective Perspective

Just as intersubjective or relational models of therapy are currently being articulated and are slowly changing the unidimensional and unidirectional focus of theories of therapy, intersubjective models of infant development and mother–infant relationships are also evolving. Jessica Benjamin, for example, discusses the importance of a dialectical relationship between the need to assert one's uniqueness and realize one's sense of agency and the equally essential need for *mutual recognition*. Mutual recognition includes experiences that infant researchers are currently investigating, such as emotional attunement and mutual regulation of affect states. Daniel Stern provides us with a conception of infant development that enables mother and infant to be subjects as well as objects in relation to each other. The Stone Center relational theory of psychological development stresses the importance of mutual empathy, engagement, and empowerment in relationships, and views self-development and differentiation as always occurring in the context of a network of relationships.

The Fluidity and Imbalance of Mother–Infant Relational Modes

We can envision how primary vulnerabilities come into being if we expand the unidirectional, unidimensional, and conflicting views of mother–infant relationships that have characterized the wide range of existing theories and adopt a multidirectional, multidimensional view of maternal–infant development. Instead of looking only at how mothers facilitate or impede the development of infants, as if mothers are constant relational partners while babies develop and change, or looking only at the developing capacities inherent in infants, we can view mother–infant relationships as comprised of a range of different and continually fluctuating relational modes. The concept of fluctuating relational modes is important and will be referred to again. *Therapist–patient dyads are analogously multidimensional and multidirectional*, even though we have conceived of them, like mother–infant relationships, as unidirectional and unidimensional and as operating outside of a historical-cultural context.

A multidimensional and multidirectional view of therapist–patient dyads paves the way for understanding the dilemmas that put the therapeutic relationship at risk. *Mismatches, impasses, and wounding in the realm of primary vulnerability occur when the patient's and therapist's relational modes vis a vis each other and their representations of self, other, and relationship intersect in problematic ways.* This statement, once made, seems obvious, yet it cannot be clearly recognized until we analyze what is missing from the theories on which we rely and until we look closely at what actually transpires in therapeutic relationships that are at risk.

I believe, as experience and infant research findings indicate, that mothers[13] and infants have a separate and unique subjective or inner experience of themselves and of the other from the beginning, *even though they function at times in the beginning of development as part of a shared and undifferentiated mother–infant matrix, and even though the infant's subjective experience, inferred rather than directly knowable, begins in a nascent state and becomes increasingly organized and differentiated as development progresses and perceptual and cognitive skills evolve.* Analogously, patients and therapists have a separate and unique experience of themselves and perceive the other to be separate and unique, even though at times they perceive each other to be having identical subjective experiences or are unable to discern at times which of them originates a particular thought or feeling.

However, I believe that the intersubjective relational mode that is possible between mothers/fathers and infants, as well as between patients and therapists, can never be fully mutual. There is an inherent imbalance in parent–infant relationships tilted toward the power of the parent arising from the inherent dependency, relative helplessness, and the less-developed cognitive-emotional capacities of the infant. Analogously, patient-therapist relationships are tilted toward the power of the therapist because of the structure of the relationship: Patients bring the most vulnerable facets of self to their therapists' strongest aspects, comprised of an accumulated body of knowledge and expertise.

Mothers (and fathers, although with less recognition and emphasis in theory) retain awesome psychological power over children even with the depotentiation of age or illness. Perhaps for this reason, our psychological theories of development have stressed the necessity of separation from the mother. Perhaps for this reason as well our language in describing the care provided by mothers has remained primarily a language of blame—mothers are deficient, destructive, or otherwise fail their children. A non-blaming language can be developed that includes the mother's negative impact on her children without stripping the mother of her separate subjective existence by including the vulnerabilities that underlie her problematic impact. For example, the statement that a mother constantly criticized and caused an enduring sense of worthlessness in her child leaves the mother objectified as blameworthy. The statement that the same mother had a primary vulnerability related to feeling worthless that she projected onto her child allows the mother to be a person in her own right with a problematic impact on her child rather than solely a defective or bad object in relation to her child.

Therapists, like mothers, maintain a position of analogous power in the eyes of their patients, even when patients, like children, perceive their therapist's limitations and vulnerabilities. But unlike mothers, therapists have tended to avoid becoming the objects of blame because the spotlight has remained focused on the pathology of patients (and their parents) while the vulnerabilities and limitations of therapists have remained in the shadows. Consequently patients suffer alone with feelings of self-blame, shame, and anger, and therapists suffer alone with feelings of guilt, remorse, and sorrow in relation to the hidden dilemmas of therapy. *With therapy, as with parenting, we need a language of intersecting strengths and vulnerabilities rather than a language of blame. We need a conception of dyadic relationships in which participants mutually affect one another as they shift relational modes and in which strong attachments form. We need to embed dyadic relationships in a broad context of relationships and culture rather than leave them isolated in a vacuum.*

If we align ourselves with the differing perspectives of the mother and the infant in turn, we see that mothers and infants continually make use of each other as relational partners in different ways just as therapists and patients do. They function, consciously or unconsciously, to advance each other along their separate individual developmental pathways and to preserve a coherent sense of self and an essential relational bond. Optimally, mothers and infants[14] and therapists and patients shift fluidly from one relational mode to another, sometimes visibly, sometimes subtly, sometimes with conscious awareness, and sometimes unconsciously. But when the needs and wishes of either mother or infant predominate and interfere with the fluidity and mutuality of the interaction, whether in macroscopic or microscopic ways, the mode of relating can become rigid and fixed rather than remain flexible and responsive to the continually changing developmental and immediate needs of both mother and baby. Analogously, in mismatches, impasses, and wounding that put therapeutic relationships at risk of a rupture, relational modes between therapist and patient tend to become rigid and fixed, losing the essential elasticity that characterizes therapeutic relationships that are working well.

Ideally the developmental needs of babies and patients predominate most of the time, but mothers and therapists are likely to have vulnerabilities that at times prevent them from functioning as developmental relational partners for babies and patients. For example, a mother who was shaped early in her experience to take care of *her* mother in order to ward off her mother's rages may be unable to tolerate the ordinary rageful crying of a frustrated infant. A therapist with the same primary vulnerability as this mother might fall into the same entrenched relational mode with patients who need to expand their understanding of how rage functions for them.

For the purpose of thinking about the complex and manifold modes of mother–infant and therapist–patient relating that are possible, I have organized them into three groups: developmental relational partners, coerced relational partners, and subjective (in the sense of having a separate subjectivity and center of initiative) relational partners. When a mother or infant (or an aspect of the mother or infant), or a patient or therapist, functions for the other in the service of furthering personal growth, she is serving as a *developmental* object, a term developed and used by psychoanalyst Calvin Settledge.[15] Bollas's conception of a *transformational object* represents one kind of developmental object that a mother can be for her infant and that recurs in the therapist–patient relationship. For example, when a mother sets aside personal needs for contact and facilitates the baby's development as an autonomous person by helping the baby separate and attend preschool, she is functioning as a developmental object or relational partner. When mothers consciously choose to function as developmental objects or relational partners, they feel the satisfaction that comes from furthering the development of another human being to whom they are attached. Therapists have analogous experiences of satisfaction in relation to patients for whom they function as developmental relational partners. For example, therapists are able to set aside feelings of envy of their patients when they can feel pride in having facilitated their patients' expansion or development.

Analogously, babies can function as developmental relational partners for their mothers in complex ways. For example, a mother who has difficulty leaving her baby can be helped by the baby to tolerate separation if the baby is able to insist on being separate and tolerates the separation well. Patients also function as developmental relational partners for therapists, although explicit recognition of this dimension of the therapeutic relationship is rarely made. That patients serve this function for therapists is evident in the case presentations that enable therapists to enhance their knowledge and experience of therapy and their professional status. Our understanding of the uncharted dilemmas of therapeutic relationships can be expanded through considering the nature of the relational mode that is operating as the dilemmas occur. For example, impasses often arise when the developmental needs of patients shift and the patient needs the therapist to function relationally in a different way but the therapist resists the shift[16].

When mother and infant, or therapist and patient, are made use of by the other to ward off an anxiety-arousing loss of equilibrium and to maintain the other's sense of self-coherence, they are serving as *coerced relational partners*. When mothers or infants are used as coerced relational partners, they function to protect the other from collapsing into the realm of primary vulnerability by preserving the coherence and connectedness of the other's sense of self. The mother, or infant, who is functioning as a coerced relational partner generally allows herself, consciously or unconsciously, to be used by the other in order to maintain an essential relational bond. By functioning as coerced relational partners for the other, mother and infant ward off an experience of fragmentation and preserve the coherence of their separate selves and the continuation of the attachment bond.

Our understanding of therapeutic relationships that are stalemated in impasses will be enhanced if we look for the relational modes that might be operating. For example, among the many relational modes that operated in her therapy with Dr. K., Lynn functioned as a coerced relational partner to him when she gratified his needs for a kindred spirit who shared his interest in Shakespeare. Lynn accepted her role as a coerced relational partner in order to preserve the relational bond. Dr. K. unknowingly served as a coerced relational partner for Lynn by remaining locked in place as a good father.

When mothers and infants, or therapists and patients, experience the other as having an inner subjective life that can be known and understood, they are *recognizing* (Jessica Benjamin's term) each other as *separate* individuals with a separate center of initiative and inner life.[17] The wish to know others and to be known, to share moments of intimate connection, and to impact the lives of others in positive ways, is perhaps a fundamental, deeply held, shared human yearning that is apparent from the beginning of life. We see it reflected in the pleasure and satisfaction on the faces of both babies and mothers when they share such moments. These special moments constitute, as Winnicott might have put it, "a good feed" for both mother and infant. Similarly, therapists and patients often experience rare and special moments of connection. The yearning to know others and to be known intimately— the wish for mutual recognition—can be reawakened, along with the resistances that accompany it, in a therapeutic relationship.

To complicate matters further in the service of developing conceptualizations closer to the reality of human experience, the same observable behavior can have different and multiple subjective meanings to the participants being observed. *In untangling the dynamics of therapeutic dilemmas, understanding the different subjective meaning that therapist and patient may attribute to the same interaction is of critical importance.* For example, Dr. K. believed he was helping (being a developmental relational partner to) his patient Lynn when he offered her medication to calm her anger. Lynn, however, experienced herself as a coerced object, compelled to stop feeling and expressing her anger in order to protect Dr. K.

When mother and baby, or therapist and patient, function in harmonious or complementary ways as needed relational partners for each other, the coherence and connectedness of their separate selves are preserved, a balance between separation and relatedness is maintained, and the individuals involved are protected from collapsing into a realm of primary vulnerability. But if a baby has repeated experiences of being unable to find in the mothering person a needed developmental, coerced, or subjective relational partner and/or is repeatedly required to function primarily as a relational partner for significant caretakers, areas of vulnerability can arise. For example, when a mother uses her baby as a coerced relational partner by repeatedly flying into a rage and withdrawing at any expression of separateness on the part of the baby, the baby may respond by remaining dependent rather than risk the loss of the mother as a needed attachment figure. The baby keeps the mother in place as a coerced relational partner by suppressing needs and remaining dependent, and the mother keeps the baby in place as a coerced relational partner who functions to preserve the mother's sense of self.

To foreshadow the ensuing discussion of therapeutic relationships, we can speculate about what might happen were this baby to become a therapy patient as an adult. We can surmise that the baby who is now grown will need to risk the imagined loss of the therapist by asserting her independent needs. If the therapist is relying on the patient as a coerced relational partner to be a "good" patient, uncomplaining and cooperative, the patient is in jeopardy of being retraumatized should she risk being difficult. If the therapist is able to recognize the subjective meaning and importance of the patient's behavior and consequently can function as a developmental relational partner for the patient, the therapist will tolerate and receive the patient's difficult behavior. The patient will then have a new experience of self and other.

A Multimodal View of
Therapeutic Relationships

Most conceptions of therapeutic relationships, like theories of early development, have taken a unidirectional view by focusing solely upon the psychological growth of the patient and a unidimensional view of patients and therapists. References are sometimes made to the personal development of the therapist as a consequence of the therapeutic relationship, but ordinarily as part of the final outcome of the work rather than with reference to aspects of the ongoing interactions. There are theorists who have appreciated the mutuality of therapeutic relationships: C. G. Jung, who asserted that both therapist and patient undergo transformation within the alchemical container of the therapeutic relationship; Ferenczi, who conceived of "mutual analysis";[18] the Stone Center theorists, who emphasize the fundamental importance of mutual empowerment, engagement, and empathy in relationships; and more recent psychoanalytic theorists, for example, those affiliated with the William Alanson White Institute in New York, with an intersubjective perspective.

The relational modes that have been described in relation to mothers and infants, and the view of human relationships that they imply, are applicable to all human relationships. Friends, lovers, colleagues, teachers shift fluidly among different relational modes, functioning at different times as developmental, coerced, and subjective relational partners for each other. Therapists and patients in therapeutic relationships also relate to each other in these different relational modes, even though we might wish to believe that psychotherapists serve only or primarily as developmental relational partners for their patients. The concept of patients using therapists as different kinds of relational partners is not new (these ideas are typically expressed in the language of object usage, in which therapists serve as different kinds of objects), but the concept has not been expanded to include both patient and therapist using each other as relational partners. Similarly, the variety of relational modes that occur between therapist and patient have not been a focus of attention, nor has a connection been made between entrenched modes of being made-use-of or of using others and areas of primary vulnerability.

The modes of making use of each other as relational partners that have been described with respect to the mother–infant dyad recur especially and particularly in therapeutic relationships because of the level of protected intimacy that is encouraged as part of the relationship. Therapeutic relationships have an unusual and unique complexity because, within them, the particular relational modes that were part of the patient's early experiences with attachment figures— the mother and the father—are revived in relation to the therapist. *More often than we have acknowledged, perhaps because of the current tendency to emphasize projective identification, relational modes that were part of the therapist's early experience can also be revived in relation to the patient.* At the same time, patient and therapist are establishing new patterns of relating to each other. *The challenge of sorting out revived relational modes from modes that are part of the present relationship is an essential part of the therapeutic endeavor.* To help in the process, we can examine mother–infant relational modes in order to develop a language that can be used to describe the relational patterns that emerge in a therapeutic relationship.

Just as mothers in our culture tend to be objectified in theories of early development, our psychological theories have objectified therapists. While mothers have been objectified in terms of their deficiencies and failures, therapists have been objectified as psychologically healthy, "good object" healers. If the therapist becomes a "bad object," we tend to assume that the therapist is a good object who is perceived by the patient as bad because of transference projections, that the patient is inducing a negative response in the therapist, or the patient's psychopathology is distorting her perception of the therapist. As a profession we have largely veered away from seeing therapists as problematic relational partners for patients because of their personal vulnerabilities, tending to view those times when therapists become personally involved either as avoidable mistakes or as personal countertransference responses that can be adequately resolved rather than as inevitable occurrences that are part of being human.

Perhaps the objectification of therapists as healers originated with the medical model, in which therapists are interchangeable service providers. Currently, even though we acknowledge the importance of the therapeutic relationship as a factor in successful therapy experiences and increasingly acknowledge the uniqueness of each therapeutic dyad, we have nonetheless retained an implicit conception of therapists as essentially fixed good objects. On a psychological level, the objectification functions to provide therapists with illusory protection from having their primary vulnerabilities activated and exposed in the therapeutic relationship. We have assumed that the patient's recognition of a therapist's vulnerabilities would be problematic for the patient rather than an instrumental and vital part of modifying entrenched and destructive relational modes.

Concepts such as analytic neutrality and nongratification function to provide a protective distance for therapists not only from their patients but also from their personal vulnerabilities and to convert therapists into *permanent good relational partners* for their patients. The protection is not only inadequate and illusory, but also harmful, because therapists cannot keep their personal vulnerabilities out of therapeutic relationships any more than they can be permanent, positive relational partners for their patients (or for anyone else). In this respect, therapists are also vulnerable when they embark on a new therapeutic relationship with a patient. They cannot know when a new patient comes through the door what personal areas of vulnerability will be activated in the relationship, any more than patients can know what kind of psychological journey they are committing themselves to. Anxiety, resistance, and defense are concepts that apply to both participants in a therapeutic relationship.

Our current challenge as a profession is to enable therapists to be predominantly developmental relational partners for patients, as well as at times and perhaps increasingly, without burdening their patients inappropriately, subjective relational partners for them.[19] We need to find ways to include within the theraputic relationship both the therapists' and patients' vulnerabilities, along with accompanying affect states (e.g., anger, grief, uncertainty, abandonment, loss, conflict, disagreement, envy, competition), without jeopardizing the attachment bond or diminishing the therapist's primary role as a developmental relational partner.

When the entrenched mode of relating between mothering person and infant recurs in a therapeutic relationship, the possibility exists, if the therapist is attuned to it, of noticing and naming it, and optimally of modifying it, albeit gradually and with a conscious effort on the part of both participants in the relationship. Examples of the problems that occur when the multidimensional levels of relational modes remain unconscious are provided by the extended case examples from preceding chapters. Dr. K. was unable to receive his patient Lynn's distressed feelings after her younger sister was injured in an automobile accident. He could not shift from relying upon Lynn as a gratifying (coerced) object who preserved his sense of self to serving as a developmental object for her. Had he been able to receive and transform her primitively expressed feelings, Lynn might have been able to have a significant experience in the therapeutic relationship that she missed as a child. Her parents, preoccupied with Alice, were unavailable to function as developmental relational partners for her by receiving her feelings.

In the case of Ann and Dr. L., Dr. L. shifted from functioning as a developmental object for Ann in helping her through the transformative experience of her second pregnancy and birth, as he had during her first pregnancy because his personal needs rendered him temporarily unavailable. He put pressure on Ann to function as a coerced object for him by receiving and digesting his envy (paying his increased fee). Ann, whose vulnerability as a pregnant woman about to give birth was intensified by her other vulnerabilities and defense modalities, could not relinquish her need for her therapist to continue functioning as a developmental object for her.[20] Unable to be made use of as a coerced relational partner for Dr. L., which might have been possible for her at a different time in her life and which might have enabled the therapeutic relationship to continue, Ann put pressure on Dr. L. not to force a change in the relational mode. Dr. L. resisted her pressure, putting his needs ahead of hers, and Ann found herself unable to remain in the relationship. Both Ann and Dr. L., like many patients and therapists in vulnerable states, had difficulty simultaneously holding in consciousness the human-caring and business-contractual dimensions of the relationship.

Unidirectional and unidimensional perspectives of mother–infant relationships and therapist–patient relationships are not only unrealistic as our conception of these relationships becomes increasingly differentiated, but they create serious problems, particularly when the perspectives lose their flexibility as modes of representing experience and become rigidified into authoritative truth. The patient Lynn and her therapist Dr. K. were ready candidates for the collusive therapeutic impasse they experienced because, like many women, Lynn was unconsciously accustomed to functioning as a coerced or developmental relational partner for others. She was unaccustomed to experiencing herself as a subjective relational partner in need of attention from a therapist whom she could use as either a developmental or coerced relational partner in the service of her psychological growth. Dr. K. relied upon Lynn to admire him, share his interests, and awaken his vitality.

Therapists have an additional challenge within the conception of flexible relational modes: remembering that even though they are literally addressing an adult person, they are at the same time talking on a psychological level to an infant, child, or adolescent.[21] For example, when Dr. L. raised his fee in a seemingly harsh manner at a particularly vulnerable time for Ann, he was simultaneously addressing a competent adult patient *and* a hurt and wounded child aspect of herself. By ignoring the hurt and wounded child and interacting only with the competent adult patient, Dr. L. unnecessarily intensified the wounding aspect of his behavior until the relationship ruptured, leaving Ann, the patient, in a state of acute distress. In working with areas of vulnerability, we do well to remember that there is a mother-in-the-baby and a baby-in-the-mother, just as there is a therapist-in-the-patient and a patient-in-the-therapist.

Psychotherapy becomes critically important both as a means of modifying unsatisfactory defensive adaptations to areas of specific vulnerabilities and as a means of understanding their origins. By carefully observing the ebb and flow of the ways that patient and therapist function as (separate) subjective relational partners, developmental relational partners, and coerced relational partners for each other, therapeutic relationships can serve as a medium both for psychological understanding and for change.

Contributions from Infant Research

Having examined the conception of the mother, infant, and mother–infant relationship through the filter of differing psychodynamic theories of early development, we are in a position to consider the findings of developmental psychologists from recent infant research studies. Developmental psychologists and specialists in infant research are arriving at an increasingly differentiated understanding of infants' capacities available to them at birth and of the gradual evolution of these capacities over time. Their findings, discussed in the next chapter, complement the delineation of mother–infant and patient–therapist relational modes by helping us understand how representations of self, other, self-in-relationship, and areas of primary vulnerability evolve from infancy on.

CHAPTER NINE

❖ *Support* ❖
from Infant Research

Anyone concerned with human nature is drawn by curiosity to wonder about the subjective life of young infants. How do infants experience themselves and others? Is there a self to begin with, or an other, or some amalgam of both? How do they bring together separate sounds, movements, touches, sights, and feelings to form a whole person? Or is the whole grasped immediately? How do infants experience the social events of "being with" an other? How is "being with" someone remembered, or forgotten, or represented mentally? What might the experience of relatedness be like as development proceeds? In sum, what kind of interpersonal world or worlds does the infant create?

—Daniel Stern[1]

My delusion was of total oneness, identity, and continuity with my mother, which I then transferred to Winnicott, with all the ambivalence belonging to it; for me he *was*, absolutely, my mother's womb. I had at some time to discover that in reality he was not; that he and I were not identical, or continuous; nor was he a part of myself that I projected. . . . He was very well aware of his countertransference and could use it positively, in reliable-enough "holding" and care of me and in direct relationship with me.

—Margaret Little, about her analysis with Winnicott[2]

Only recently have I realized that in fact, unwittingly, he [Winnicott] altered the whole nature of the problem by enabling me to reach right back to *an ultimate good mother, and to find her recreated in him in the transference.* . . .

He became a good breast mother to my infant self in my deep unconscious, at the point where my actual mother had lost her maternalism and could not stand me as a live baby any more. . . . Here at last I had a mother who could value her child, so that I could cope with what was to come.

—Harry Guntrip, about his analysis with Winnicott[3]

We see therefore that in infancy and in the management of infants there is a very subtle distinction between the mother's understanding of her infant's need based on empathy, and her change over to an understanding based on something in the infant or small child that indicates need. This is particularly difficult for mothers because of the fact that children vacillate between one state and the other; one minute they are merged with their mothers and require empathy, while the next they are separate from her, and then if she knows their needs in advance she is dangerous, a witch. It is a very strange thing that mothers who are quite uninstructed adapt to these changes in their developing infants satisfactorily and without any knowledge of the theory. This detail is reproduced in psycho-analytic work with borderline cases, and in all cases at certain moments of great importance when dependence in the transference is maximal.

—D. W. Winnicott[4]

The Development of an Infant's Sense of Self

During the past thirty years the field of infant research, investigating the capacities with which infants are endowed at birth, has expanded exponentially. The expansion is reflected in the burgeoning number of published studies and in the familiar photographs of tiny infants sucking pacifiers that are connected to revolving mobiles. These photographs no longer startle us; they appear not only in professional journals but in popular magazines for parents. Developmental psychologists, fascinated by the nature of the capacities and potentials that we now know exist from birth, are evolving elaborate schemes for investigating early capacities. They are able to identify and track both the developing capacities of infants to organize their experience and the domains of experience that become accessible to infants as they grow.

Whereas psychoanalysts evolve their conceptions of the infant and of mother–infant relationships from their work with adult patients, as the epigraphs from Little, Guntrip, and Winnicott demonstrate, developmental psychologists attempt to answer Stern's question in the epigraph from direct observational studies and research with mothers and infants. Developmental psychologists make inferences about how a sense of self develops based on their observations of children from infancy on. They shape their inferences into a theory of the development of the infant's sense of self, and that theory in turn shapes their observations. Therapists, working with adult patients' memories and stories, create with their patients a theory, often called a narrative or reconstructed history, of the development of the patient's sense of self. By considering the theory of the patient's early development against the background of a general theory provided by developmental psychologists, therapists can identify pivotal early experiences. Analogously, developmental psychologists can look to the concepts evolved by therapists for important variables that shape the development of a sense of self.[5]

Increasingly, developmental psychologists and therapists of adults are trying to communicate with each other, to exchange concepts, and to build bridges between the "observed infant" of developmental research and the "reconstructed infant" that comes into being in the offices of therapists. Constructing a bridge between developmental psychologists and therapists can help us articulate the complex interaction between interpersonal relationships (the infant and caretakers) and the unconscious beliefs and fantasies (the subjective reality) that the infant forms to make sense of these interpersonal experiences. Supported by such a bridge, therapists will be in a better position to help patients understand the evolution of their subjective sense of self in the context of early significant attachments, including the sense of self-in-relation to others. With an understanding of the origin of the ways they think about themselves, patients are in a better position to modify the conscious and unconscious beliefs that cause them difficulties and to find constructive ways of working with their areas of primary vulnerabilities.

The work of developmental psychologists provides support for the assertion that areas of primary vulnerability originate early in development, within the context of a primary relationship to a caretaker. Infants have an innate capacity that begins to operate at birth, if not before, to organize experience and to form categories of self and self-in-relationship that endure. The categories that serve to organize experience exist outside of conscious awareness and are not encoded in language. They then emerge nonverbally in the quality of the relationship that the adult patient establishes with her therapist. The emergence of these unconscious categories or beliefs provides an opportunity for the therapist and patient to name them. When they are accessible to conciousness, they can be modified if they are inhibiting psychological development and growth. But their emergence in the therapeutic relationship also provides dangerous and fertile ground for the rewounding of the patient in the vulnerable areas that are exposed.

The Work of Daniel Stern

Daniel Stern has organized the findings of a multitude of infant research studies into a general theory of the evolution of an infant's sense of self. He presents his ideas in the pathbreaking book, *The*

Interpersonal World of the Infant: A View from Psychoanalysis and Developmental Psychology. He also makes a beginning effort to explore the implications of his schema for psychoanalytic theory. His views conflict with some widely accepted psychoanalytic beliefs and support others. Because his work is seminal, and because his model offers the possibility of looking at mother–infant relationships from the multimodal relational point of view put forth in the preceding chapter, I will summarize it in some detail. I will indicate how Stern's categories of the development of a subjective sense of self correspond to the theories of therapy discussed in Chapter Eight.

Stern believes that infants do not begin life in a state of merger with the mother out of which they must differentiate themselves in order to form a sense of a separate, unique self. His assertion directly contrasts with the theories of Mahler, Winnicott, Bion, and Lacan. Instead of arriving as *tabulae rasae*, blank screens upon which the environment impacts, infants come into the world with capacities that actively impact their caretaking environment. These capacities include a *preverbal sense of self*—the sense of agency, physical cohesion, continuity in time, and intention. Capacities for self-reflection and language, which develop later, eventually come to work upon these preverbal experiences of self and both reveal their existence and transform them into new experiences. Organizational change within the infant and the interpretation of the change by the parents are mutually facilitative of the new integrations in an infant's sense of self. These new integrations come in quantum leaps that are noticeable at 2 to 3 months, 9 to 12 months, and 15 to 18 months, when observers sense a different qualitative presence in babies.

Infants have far more control over interactions and assert their autonomy and independence in more distinct ways at different ages than most theories of early development (specifically Erikson, Freud, and Mahler) have appreciated. For example, Stern has investigated visual gaze in mother–infant dyads with babies from three to six months of age.[6] He writes, "When watching the gazing patterns of mother and infant during this life period, one is watching two people with almost equal facility and control over the same social behavior."[7] The same interactional patterns are apparent later in life, with locomotive behavior substituting for visual gaze.

Irish author Christopher Nolan was severely handicapped as a result of a birth injury so that the only part of his body he could control was his eye movement. His autobiography offers a poignant description of the power of the gaze as a form of communication and interactional control or interpersonal influence. The following passage, evocative as well of the exquisite attunement and empathy of which his mother was capable, written later in life when he was finally able to communicate with the help of a computer, describes an interaction that occurred with his mother early in his life when he "spoke" to her with his eyes:

> He faced his mother. He gazed his hurt gaze, lip protruding, eyes busy in conversation. He ordered her to look out the window at the sunshine. He looked hard at her ear ordering her to listen to the birds singing. Then jumping on her knees he again asked her [with his gaze alone] to cock her ear and listen to the village children out at play in the school yard. Now he jeered himself. He showed her his arms, his legs, his useless body. Beckoning his tears he shook his head. Looking at his mother he blamed her, he damned her, he mouthed his cantankerous why, why, why me? Looking through his tears he saw her as she bent low in order to look into his eyes. "I never prayed for you to be born crippled," she said. ". . . . But. . . . you are loved by me and Dad. We love you just as you are."[8]

Within the matrix of maternal and familial love, attunement, and empathy, Christopher Nolan was able to evolve a sense of self strong enough to contain the emotional and physical pain and limitations of his severe disabilities.

Stern describes four aspects of a sense of self that define different domains of self-experience and social relatedness. According to Stern, these domains continue to grow and ultimately coexist throughout life: What some psychologists have regarded as the developmental tasks of infancy are actually lifespan issues. In Stern's conceptual frame, the first domain of self-experience, from birth to 2 months, is the *sense of an emergent self*—the experience of emerging organization. Infants in this domain of self-experience link separate experiences by means of the innate processes of amodal perception (recognizing invariants across modalities of vision, time, intensity and touch, such as identifying the visual image of an object that has been held but not seen); physiognomic perception (directly experiencing some aspects of people and things as categorical affects such as joy, anger, sadness); and vitality affects (dynamic terms such as fleeting, explosive, fading).

By emphasizing bodily experience as the raw material from which a sense of self begins to be organized, Stern indirectly affirms the significance of the autistic-contiguous phase that Ogden posits, in which repetitive physical movement serves the function of restoring a coherent sense of self. For example, an adult may find that repetitive physical activity, such as jogging, swimming, or using exercise machines, not only enhances physical well-being but provides a sense of psychological coherence as a physical being. Stern's emphasis on bodily experience also affirms the significance of a mothering person as a transformational object that Bollas addresses. For example, the sense of psychological well-being that exercise provides may have its origins in an infant's early repetitive physical experiences in the company of the mother, such as being rocked, walked, or patted.

Stern, unlike the psychotherapists who have sought to conceptualize infant development, does not explicitly recognize the significance of the primitive states that occur in infancy—the tantrums, crying fits, and rages associated with the primary agonies and anxieties to which Winnicott and Ogden allude.[9] Frances Tustin describes analogous primordial anxieties that have emerged in her work with autistic children and with the autistic core of adult patients. For example, Tustin describes fears of spilling away and dissolving or of leaking out of one's skin, that can beset autistic children.[10] Stern's theory is a highly rational one, oriented toward cognitive development in its emphasis on how infants organize their world conceptually. Unlike psychotherapists, Stern does not focus on the irrational states that infants experience. Consequently he does not fully consider how these states affect the organizational models that infants create to make sense of their experience and that then function outside awareness to shape the infants' ensuing experiences.

Stern asserts that the global subjective world of emerging organization that characterizes the phase of the emergent self is the fundamental domain of human subjectivity. He writes:

> It operates out of awareness as the experiential matrix from which thoughts and perceived forms and identifiable acts and verbalized feelings will later arise. . . . All learning and all creative acts begin in the domain of emergent relatedness. . . . The later senses of self to emerge are products of the organizing process.[11]

Most significant for therapists is the finding that infants have the innate capacity to organize experience and necessarily do so. *The task of therapists and their adult patients is to infer retrospectively, especially on the basis of clues arising in the transference, how the patient began as an infant to organize his or her world and how experiences throughout life shaped the organizational categories that became established in infancy.* Once these organizing principles are identified, they are available to be modified in constructive ways. For example, Erin, the colicky baby referred to in the preceding chapter, formed a perception of the world as unsafe. With awareness of the existence of this particular organizing principle operating automatically, Erin has the possibility of learning to discriminate degrees of safety in different contexts rather than remaining fearful much of the time.

Stern labels the second domain of the development of a sense of self the *sense of a core self*. The chronological time frame when this domain emerges and predominates ranges from 2 to 3 months through 7 months, but, like all the phases, the domain continues throughout the life cycle to evolve and to influence self representations. The core self is comprised of four self-invariants—aspects of the self that do not change across situations: self-agency (sense of volition), self-coherence, self-affectivity (feelings about one's self), and self-history (memory and continuity). These four self-invariants are necessary for adult psychological health. They are also aspects of the coherence of self that are essential: The individual who is unable to preserve them is in jeopardy of collapsing into the realm of primary vulnerability. Patients whose therapeutic relationships end abruptly in a rupture are likely to experience a discontinuity in their sense of self because the therapeutic relationship "holds" the patients' newly modified and changing sense of self until, during a planned termination phase, the patient can reclaim and hold the aspects of self that had formerly resided in the relationship.

Philip Cushman, in a provocative social-constructionist critique of Stern, asserts that Stern perpetuates a culturally influenced concept of the self as bounded, masterful, independent, cohesive, and preoccupied with relating to others.[12] Cushman believes that the invariants of self that Stern posits are not objective truths. The invariants are based in a historical context and correspond to the Western concept of the self. Stern derives his conception of these invariants from observable infant behavior. But Cushman believes that Stern makes too great a leap from simple observable behaviors to the more complex capacities of the self-invariants he posits. Consequently Stern attributes to infants capacities too advanced and complex to presume to be based on the relatively simple observable behaviors. However, even if we accept Cushman's criticisms as valid and recognize the importance of locating our theories in a historical context, adults who observe young children are able to identify the self-invariants or characteristics that Stern describes—a sense of volition, coherence, affectivity, and continuity. These qualities are essential and basic components of the capacity to function effectively in the Western world.

Stern asserts that the four self-invariants are integrated through the process of episodic memory, his term for a small but coherent chunk of lived experience that is indivisible. For example, babies form "Representations of Interactions that have been Generalized" (RIGs), which are analogous to an abstract concept of an interactive experience (e.g., a baby will form a RIG of breastfeeding experiences, which is an averaging of a number of separate and slightly variable discrete experiences). A significant part of this domain is the experience of being with a self-regulatory other such that self-feelings are changed, an experience that supports Bollas's concept of the mother as a transformational object. For example, a distressed baby who settles down in the presence of a calming mother has a positive experience of being with a self-regulatory other. A baby who is naturally quiet and is prodded into activity by a mother who needs a responsive baby has a negative experience of being with a self-regulatory other.[13]

We can assume that states we label "borderline" and "psychotic" include the temporary loss or nonexistence of the four self-invariants that Stern describes. Borderline and psychotic states thus can be thought of as a collapse into the realm of primary vulnerability where the invariants that stabilize a coherent sense of self are lost. Therapists who encounter borderline and psychotic states in their patients may find it useful to keep in mind the early relational origins of primary vulnerabilities. One example is provided by a patient whose first caretakers inhibited the expression of anger by withdrawing from her when, as an infant, she was angry. She became frantic with anxiety as a result of the disconnection from her caretakers. This relational pattern, established early in life, then emerged in her therapeutic relationship when as a patient, she reacted to her therapist's withdrawal by being catapulted into a state of acute panic. Rather than view the patient as borderline in a fixed, diagnostic sense, which could permanently and negatively alter the therapist's availability to her, the therapist has other options. The therapist might speculate that the disruption to the patient's cohesiveness of self caused by her rage brought about a relational disconnection that further augmented her anxiety. The therapist might then offer herself to the patient as a new and positive developmental object, by both reflecting an awareness of the sequence of events giving rise to the anxiety and by remaining psychologically and emotionally available in the therapeutic relationship. Patient and therapist together could then become aware of the potential for rage and/or the psychological withdrawal of a significant person to catapult the patient into the realm of primary vulnerability.

The specific self-representations that form the basis of the self-invariants Stern describes are not objective truths. They are subjective ideas or concepts that can function in helpful or problematic ways. If beliefs that are problematic are to be altered, an individual must relinquish familiar self-representations that have served her well so that new self- representations can take their place. For example, Dr. K.'s sense of self was organized around a conception of himself as a kind, caring man. This self-representation provided him with a sense of continuity, coherence, self-affectivity (good feeling about himself), and agency. Lynn's experience of Dr. K. as having abandoned her in a time of emotional distress imperiled a major component of his basic sense of self, threatening the coherence of his self-state. Had Dr. K. been more flexible, better able to tolerate a temporary experience of a loss of a coherent sense of self, he might have been available to tolerate the feelings that Lynn needed to be able to experience with him.

Stern labels the third domain, which predominates chronologically from 7-9 months to 15 months, *the sense of a subjective self*. In this domain, Stern believes that the baby discovers that inner subjective experiences can be shared without language. The baby makes the discovery of the subjective world of the mother through experiencing with her states that include joint attention, shared intentions, and shared affect states. Affective attunement of baby and mother–person, an experience that sets the stage for the later and more complex phenomenon of empathy, occurs in this domain. Affective attunement between an observed mother and infant pair manifests in the cross-modal matching of behavior (e.g., mother's sound "matches" the baby's physical movements) where the behavior being matched reflects the baby's feeling state. Such attunements occur automatically and out of awareness, unlike empathy, which involves the mediation of cognitive processes.

As a consequence of experiencing affect attunement, babies learn that internal feeling states are sharable forms of human experience. This awareness is the beginning of the experience of psychic intimacy. Stern's contention that babies learn about the existence of inner, subjective states that their mothers (or other carepersons) share supports Winnicott's notion that babies eventually relate to their mothering persons not only as "environment mothers" but also as "object mothers." His contention also supports Klein's conception of the depressive position, in which babies develop a capacity for concern and come to understand that they have the power to affect their mothers' emotional states.

Stern's contention that young babies have the capacity to understand that their mothers have an internal subjective world has a significant implication for the notion of empathy. Typically when early experiences are considered, the focus rests on mothers and their capacity to provide adequate empathy for their offspring. Stern's concept of the existence of a rudimentary capacity for empathy in young babies opens up the possibility that mutual empathy between mothers (or mothering persons) and babies is not only possible but essential for the development of a healthy, coherent sense of self and self-in-relationship.[14]

Stern's concept of attunement, an essential part of the domain of self-development that he calls the sense of a subjective self, is particularly significant in therapeutic relationships. Patients bring to the therapeutic relationship certain expectations of being or not being matched and of needing to attune to the therapist. By carefully observing these expectations, therapists can help patients make inferences about the nature of their experiences as preverbal infants with their mothers. In helping patients understand how their sense of self evolved, therapists focus, for example, on the implications of a mother–baby duo in which the feeling state of the baby was never accurately matched, or in which the baby was compelled to attune to the feeling state of the mother upon threat of abandonment (through the withdrawal of mother's attention or through mother's fragmentation). Therapists and patients rely not only on their conscious verbal exchanges but also on shared subjective experiences that occur without language. Nonverbal shared subjective experiences may be thought of as a kind of communication between the unconscious (outside of language) psyches of therapist and patient that can help access and understand the layers of the psyche that are neither part of consciousness nor encoded in language.

The fourth domain, emerging in the second year of life, is *the sense of a verbal self.* In Stern's view, language has the advantage of being a new form of relatedness but the disadvantage of moving relatedness away from the personal, immediate level onto an impersonal abstract plane. With language, babies gain entrance into a wider cultural world, but at the cost of losing the force and wholeness of the original experience.[15] Stern notes that the "word" (e.g., language) is "discovered" or "created" by the infant: The thought or knowledge is already there in the mind ready to be linked up with the word.[16] The mothering person gives the word to the infant, but there is a thought ready in the infant for the word to be given to.

In Stern's view, language is a neutral tool. It can be used to communicate inner experience, to describe a private self that is not shared with others, or as Winnicott might put it, to further entrench a False Self and widen the gulf between that False Self and the realm of the True Self that remains unarticulated in language.[17] Stern contends that language will operate initially in a patient–therapist duo in the same way that it operated for the infant–mother or infant–father duo. If the therapeutic relationship progresses effectively, the use of language broadens to encompass realms of previously unarticulated inner experience and to communicate subjective experience more effectively.[18] At the same time, language can preclude access to experience that cannot yet be encompassed symbolically. *Consequently, therapists and patients must continue to pay attention to states of being, feelings, and intuitions that do not lend themselves readily to formulations in language.* For example, patients who are retrieving memories of early abuse may benefit from work with sandtrays, paint, or clay to represent experiences nonverbally before using words.

Therapists and patients must be careful not to assume automatically that words have the same meaning to each of them. Giving language to experience that has not been represented conceptually and using language with care are especially important in understanding specific areas of primary vulnerability in patients and therapists. For example, Dr. K.'s inability to allow Lynn to experience intense feelings in his presence precluded aspects of her experience from being represented in language. Analogously, when Dr. L. raised Ann's fee and insisted on the raise against her protests instead of exploring its meaning to her, the opportunity was lost to represent in a shared language her experience of vulnerability in the present and its origins in the past.

In a chapter on clinical implications, Stern lists the parameters of a sense of a core self that account for individual differences: the degree of formation of a sense of core self, maintenance needs, and lability. These are parameters with which most human beings as well as therapists are familiar. Most therapists have worked with patients who lack a well-formed and differentiated sense of self, who require considerable support from a human environment to maintain a stable and cohesive sense of self, and who manifest a wide range of self-states. These are patients who, until inner and outer psychological connections to self and others are established in therapy, live on the edge of the realm of primary vulnerability and are in constant jeopardy of falling into it. At the other end of the continuum are individuals who have a well-developed and coherent sense of self, whose needs related to maintaining a stable sense of self are well-defined and manageable, and who experience manageable fluctuations in self-states. These patients may have adaptive mechanisms that protect them from falling into areas of primary vulnerability, but when they fall, the experience may terrify them.

In my opinion, two of the parameters that Stern names—lability and maintenance needs—are at least in part constitutionally determined or innate. We arrive in the world at birth with different thresholds of tolerance for outside stimulation. These thresholds of tolerance are difficult to modify through human interaction, although significant relationships can contribute to the negative effect of these innate characteristics. For example, an infant who cannot tolerate much stimulation and needs a preponderance of quiet, private time can be shaped to avoid human contact by a mothering person who insists upon interaction. Similarly, the same infant can be made to feel inadequate by parents who overvalue extroversion and activity. Therapists who observe these characteristics in a patient—an aversion to engaging with others or a sense of humiliation and inadequacy about being introverted or shy—can make inferences about the nature of the patient's early parent–infant interactions that caused the patient to form enduring and perhaps problematic and unnecessary self-representations.

Stern, implicitly postulating how areas of primary vulnerability originate, asserts that psychopathology derives less from a single traumatic event than from recurrent problematic experiences that go on beyond infancy and that disrupt the sense of self in the different domains. He claims unequivocally that there are no mental disorders in infants, only disorders in the relationships in which infants participate. As noted in the preceding chapter, when babies and caretakers become rigidly fixed in repetitive relational modes, areas of vulnerability are formed.

Stern gives examples of problems that arise in each of the four domains of a sense of self: Problems in the first domain (emerging self) range from learning disabilities to a fragile sense of self; problems in the second domain (core relatedness) lead to primitive agonies (Winnicott's term) about actual disruptions in ongoing functions needed to maintain essential interpersonal states; in the third domain (intersubjective relatedness), nonattunement may lead to a sense of cosmic loneliness, or selective attunement may allow a parent to shape a child's subjective and interpersonal life (Winnicott's False Self); in the fourth domain (verbal self), language can reinforce the False Self as well as the disavowal of direct experience.

Studies of Mother–Infant Interaction

Just as Stern does a yeoman's job of organizing infant research studies in order to conceptualize how an infant's subjective sense of self evolves, Beebe and Lachmann organize findings from a number of mother–infant interaction studies to evolve a conceptualization of how these interactions are represented presymbolically by infants.[19] They focus on how infant and caretaker are mutually influenced, and how, as a result of their interactions, an infant's representations of self and other evolve. They studied the intricacies of mother–infant interaction in microanalyses of film and videotapes and summarize their findings.

Like Stern, their research indicates that we tend to underestimate the capacities of infants. Infants are capable of organizing a representational world even before their capacity to symbolize (language) emerges. They can represent expected, characteristic interaction structures in terms of recurring distinctive temporal, spatial, and affective features. By the end of the first year, these representations of interaction structures are abstracted into generalized prototypes to form the basis for later symbolic forms of self- and object representations.

Beebe and Lachmann, like Stern, emphasize that the organization of experience is not solely the property of the infant, but is also the property of the dyadic system. The quality of the mother–infant interaction, whether interactions are "matching" or "derailed," affects the emerging organization of the infant's experience.[20] Failures to elicit needed responses from the mother are called "interactive errors." If these mismatched interactions lead to an experience of "interactive repair," infants learn that they can succeed in eliciting necessary responses from the human environment. Infants who experience such reparative interactions are likely to view failed interactions as fixable and to attempt to fix them. Repeated experiences of interactive errors that are not repaired lead infants to withdraw from social interactions, to form a belief that they are not able to shape the responses of others, and to experience negative affect states. These findings support Winnicott's emphasis on the importance of the maternal–infant unit as well as the contention of the Stone Center[21] that an individual's sense of self evolves in relationship to significant others. They also implicitly support the view that states we label psychopathological are located not within an individual person as an autonomous entity but in the relational experiences that gave rise to a particular sense of self-in-relationship. The modification of pathological states of being and of pathological behaviors is most likely to occur in the context of a relationship in which they can arise, be named and understood, relinquished, and mourned.

Infant researchers have developed a scale that measures affective engagement between mother and infant based on videotapes of interactions.[22] The scale ranges from positive engagement, to decreasing engagement, to a neutral midpoint, through negative attention, to inhibition of responsivity. Through statistical analysis, Beebe and Lachmann found that mother–infant pairs were mutually responsive, matching the direction and timing of affective change but avoiding an exact match of level on the scale. Through this interlocking responsivity, or matching, a psychological representation of "being with" another person is organized. Similar matching of mother–infant vocal patterns have also been documented, where mother and infant automatically match pauses between their individual turns at vocalizing. Studies of mother–infant kinesic interactions, where kinesic refers to movement or changes in orientation, gaze, and facial expression, indicate that mothers and infants influence each other. As one partner's movement becomes longer, the other partner is influenced to shorten her movement, and vice versa, so that partners compensate for changes in the other. What would we see if we transposed the scale for mothers and infants to observed patient–therapist dyads in order to assess the level of attunement and engagement and the degree of subtle mutual influence that occurs outside the conscious awareness of both individuals? For example, a young, energetic patient who meets with an older therapist might subdue her level of energy in response to therapist (the epigraphs to Chapter Four seem particularly apt in this context).

What can be inferred about the subjective experience of mothers and infants from these observations? What does the fact that mothers and infants are exquisitely attuned to one another's behavior mean? Beebe and Lachmann suggest that through matching one another's temporal and affective patterns, mother and infant recreate in themselves a subjective state similar to the other's. These subtle and automatic interactions constitute the basis for the capacity for mutual empathy. Additionally, these authors suggest, experiences of matching and being matched become represented in a presymbolic form as an expectation, like the RIG of breastfeeding. The representation of "being matched" is of crucial importance because it serves as one component of an infant's representation of self, other, and the interactive process itself. Specifically, matching experiences constitute a positive state, whereas mismatching experiences can be said to accompany negative states. A RIG of good matching may contribute to a positive sense of self and other and of interpersonal relations. Similarly, a RIG of mismatching may lead to a sense of self as ineffective in influencing others and as unable to elicit soothing responses from others.

The finding that expectations of self in relationships are formed early in development and operate to shape ensuing relational interactions may be transposed to therapeutic relationships. For example, impasses that involve power struggles often arise from a patient's unacknowledged attempt to empower herself and to have an impact on the therapist. A therapist with firm, definite ideas about what is right for a patient can keep a patient who is accustomed to being with more powerful others in a disempowered state. In one situation (see Chapter Thirteen, the case of Eileen), a patient refused to promise to call her therapist if she felt suicidal because she felt that the therapist, by insisting upon a call, was being intolerant of her feelings of despair and forcing her to inauthentically promise to "feel better." The therapist continued to insist on the telephone call; his concern for his patient obscured his capacity to recognize the patient's healthy wish to have all her feelings tolerated. Similarly, the patient's wish to be assertive and authentic obscured her capacity to see the therapist's concern. Consultation in this case was useful in helping the patient and therapist recognize the disavowed aspects of one another.

Beebe and Lachmann's studies of mother–infant interactions where there was misattunement reveal how infants cope. Mother and infant continue to influence each other in such mismatched interactions, but their degree of attunement is compromised. The infant's attention, affect, and arousal state are not optimally regulated. In an attuned relationship, the mother deescalates engagement in response to the baby's withdrawal. Beebe and Lachmann make inferences regarding the mother and infant's subjective experience. The misattuned mother can be said to have difficulty tolerating the infant's disengagement, while the infant does not have the experience of being calmed, and develops an expectancy (RIG) of misregulation, with a concomitant sense of an inability to regulate states of arousal. Correspondingly, the mother may develop a subjective sense of herself as an inadequate, rejected mother with her infant. Research evidence that early interaction patterns predict cognition, attachment, and interaction measures at one and two years attests to the enduring power of these early representations of interactions.

We can infer that these early representations contribute to the later subjective experiences of being known and understood by others and. transpose the finding to therapeutic relationships. Dr. K.'s yearning to be known and understood was answered by his patient Lynn. Her yearning to be psychologically held through a vulnerable time elicited what Beebe and Lachmann might refer to as a disengaging response, a "chase and dodge sequence of behavior," from Dr. K. Subjective experiences of being known and understood emerge in a therapeutic relationship, offering patient and therapist the opportunity to become aware of and to name the experiences, and, if useful, to modify the patterns of attunement.

Studies currently being conducted on the interactions of disabled mothers and their able-bodied infants highlight the intricacies of their mutually responsive adaptations. Megan Kirshbaum, in her article "Parents with Physical Disabilities and Their Babies," summarizes her observations of ten disabled mothers with their infants.[23] She found that babies are able to adapt as early as one month of age to their disabled mothers, thus allowing the disabled mothers to care for them in highly individualized ways. For example, a paraplegic mother invented a way of lifting her one-month-old infant so that she would not fall from her wheelchair:

> she would signal him by tugs on the front of his clothes, pause while estimating his readiness by his physical response, and lift him by his clothes. At one month of age he would adapt by curling up like a kitten and remaining very still and compact during the lift. One month later, when he was physically more capable, we documented that when drowsy during the lifts he didn't do his job as effectively. . . . His mother explained and demonstrated how he needed to be roused to cooperate.[24]

Other examples from Kirshbaum's observations of older babies demonstrate other unique reciprocal adaptations:

> One mother with multiple sclerosis, using toys initially to entice, successfully teaches a crawling baby to consistently come to her when called. An active and mischievous toddler lies still during a long diapering by her blind father, but is resistant and struggling at the outset with her sighted mother. Another toddler distinguishes between the safe home environment where some teasing and testing may be done, e.g., lying flat on the floor so it's difficult for a parent in a wheelchair to get him—and public places, where the child cooperates by consistently staying close to the parents, e.g., holding his or her hand.[25]

Work with both able-bodied and disabled infants and parents documents the extent to which mothers and babies will adapt to each other in order to ensure that the babies receive essential physical and psychological care. Despite physical disability and with adequate relational support, these mothers can sustain a psychological and emotional parental presence for their babies. Adaptation remains mutual. This mutuality is significant because one-sided adaptation to the needs of others, if it becomes an entrenched relational mode, puts an individual at risk of problems arising later in life.

We can see from these studies of infant development how central early mother–infant interactions are to the evolution both of a sense of self and other and of a sense of self-in-relationship. Expectations that are represented by infants presymbolically endure and shape future attachments and cognition. Our sense of self takes its shape in the context of significant early relationships, particularly within the maternal–infant matrix. The opportunity to modify an entrenched sense of self, like the opportunity to modify an entrenched relational mode, also occurs in the context of relationships, especially in therapeutic relationships. *Therapists, in order to address these early issues, must be prepared to deal with the primordial anxiety that arises when existing components of one's sense of self and one's sense of self-in-relationship are relinquished so that new ones can form as part of the process of change.*

Implications for Psychotherapy

Therapy patients are as vulnerable to the influence of their therapists as infants are to mothers. They imbue the therapist with an importance analogous to that which the mothering person has for an infant. They seek psychotherapy with the hope of modifying something in themselves that causes suffering. We can label the elusive "something" that patients want to change as their entrenched representations of self, other, and relationships. Patients also hope to identify and alter constricting relational modes.

In order for these representations and relational modes to be modified, patient and therapist must first identify them. Because they were formed early in life, before cognition developed sufficiently for language, they operate outside of consciousness, outside the sphere of language. Patients and therapists, relying on a variety of capacities for processing information that includes feeling and intuition as well as thinking, must work to identify them as they emerge in the interactions that occur nonverbally. Patients behave in relationship to therapists in accordance with well-established interaction patterns, which they must eventually relinquish in the service of modifying them.

As the process of relinquishing familiar modes of behavior occurs, the therapist has in the present the same powerful effect as the mothering person had in the past in influencing the establishment of new representations of self and other. The therapist, in light of the power and authority invested in her through the patient's trust in allowing vulnerabilities to surface, thus has at once an unusual opportunity to facilitate positive change, an enormous responsibility for the well-being of her patient (just as a mother has for her infant), as well as an unavoidable possibility of causing harm. The latter possibility, once it is openly acknowledged, can be mitigated with an awareness of the concepts that have been discussed.

For therapy to be effective at the deepest level, patients need to find the various paths of access to their areas of primary vulnerability. A secure therapeutic relationship in which a patient feels unconditional positive regard from the therapist, a strong alliance and sense of trust can facilitate the emergence of areas of vulnerability. Ironically, being wounded by the therapist also evokes the personal vulnerability of the patient. An experience of wounding provides the catalyst patient and therapist may use to go beyond cognitive understanding of and insight into the realm of primary vulnerability. The experience of living through the vulnerability enables transformative change to occur.

To work with patients who fall into the treacherous territory of the realm of primary vulnerability, therapists need to be able to tolerate being, or being perceived as, a source of either safety or wounding. Theirs is the challenge of bearing the difficulties that either role entails and of trying not to mitigate the degree of wounding or rush to heal it, but to bear witness to it, as Balint emphasized in his discussion of the basic fault. *If they are regarded as the source of wounding, they must bear responsibility long enough for the patient to reach a state of being able to locate that source more diffusely, at first in the complex interaction of self, other, and self-in-relation, and then as an inherent part of the human condition.* At the same time, therapists have the task of carrying the hope, temporarily unavailable to the floundering patient, that the anxiety related to the primary vulnerability will eventually be channeled constructively and creatively.

Because our sense of self and of self-in-relationship first arises within the context of human relationships, we seek an understanding of them within the context of a human relationship. Because anxiety related to primary vulnerabilities also arises in the context of a human relationship, we seek the capacity to bear it in that context. Individuals will thus continue to seek therapy, despite the difficulties inherent in a pioneering and continually evolving field. The unique structure of the therapeutic relationship, in which one individual devotes concentrated attention to another in the inviolable physical setting and temporal space of the hour enables issues in the realm of primary vulnerability to surface with special intensity. The hope for understanding and healing that is awakened in a working therapeutic relationship provides fertile ground for disappointment and failure as well as for positive change.

When therapeutic relationships end in disappointment with a sense of failure, patients have the task of managing a mixture of intense and difficult feelings. These affect states, described in Chapter

Eleven, arise from the rupture of the vitally important attachment bond that therapy patients form to their therapists. Its significance parallels in importance the attachment bond that infants form to their caretakers. But because the attachment bond is often obscured by the distressed behaviors of patients and therapists who are caught in impasses, it is often overlooked. The following chapter highlights the importance of the attachment bond, returning it to a central place in the therapeutic relationship.

CHAPTER TEN

❖ *The Centrality* ❖ *of the Attachment Bond*

This concept of the secure personal base, from which a child, an adolescent, or an adult goes out to explore and to which he returns from time to time, is one I have come to regard as crucial for an understanding of how an emotionally stable person develops and functions *all through his life.*

—JOHN BOWLBY[1]

That attachment behaviour in adult life is a straightforward continuation of attachment behaviour in childhood is shown by the circumstances that lead an adult's attachment behaviour to become more readily elicited. In sickness and calamity, adults often become demanding of others; in conditions of sudden danger or disaster a person will almost certainly seek proximity to another known and trusted person. . . . It is therefore extremely misleading for the epithet "regressive" to be applied to every manifestation of attachment behaviour in adult life. . . . To dub attachment behaviour in adult life regressive is indeed to overlook the vital role that it plays in the life of man from the cradle to the grave.

—JOHN BOWLBY[2]

The Nature of the Attachment Bond Between Therapist and Patient

The centrality of the *attachment bond* that patients form with therapists has been underemphasized in our thinking about the therapeutic dyad. Some therapists do not acknowledge the existence of a real relationship with patients separate from transference. Other theorists do emphasize the significance of the "real" or nontransference-based relationship between therapist and patient. For example, as Loewald[3] and Settlage[4] emphasize, the therapist ideally serves as a new and different kind of object for the patient, or in the terminology of the preceding chapter, as a developmental object. Greenson[5] stresses the necessity for a positive relationship, as a precondition for a working therapeutic relationship. However, with the exception of relatively recent work by the Stone Center on Self-in-Relationship,[6] the quality of the real relationship, although explicitly named by theorists of diverse perspectives as a central factor in the healing potential of therapy, fades into the background instead of remaining on center stage with such concepts as transference and countertransference or resistance and defense. The special aspect of the real relationship that can properly be called "attachment" has only been labeled, but not emphasized, except by theorists, predominantly located in England, who have been significantly influenced by Bowlby's work.

In addition to the significance of a positive, real relationship between therapist and patient, one that includes the vitally important positive therapeutic alliance, *the continuity and durability of the attachment bond* that forms between patient and therapist are significant ongoing dimensions of the therapeutic relationship. Yet in spite of our knowledge of the critical role that the nature of a secure attachment plays in the mother–infant relationship, in spite of the many parallels that have frequently been drawn between the therapeutic relationship and the mother–infant relationship, and in spite of British psychoanalyst John Bowlby's explicit and repeated emphasis on the role of the therapist as an important attachment figure, the significance of the nature of the attachment bond in the patient–therapist relationship continues to be underemphasized in the professional literature, relative to its other facets. The underemphasis occurs despite the knowledge patients and therapists share: *The attachment bond formed by adult patients in therapy to their therapists can become as central to them as the attachment bond formed by infants to their primary carepersons.* The attachment bond, like Winnicott's "environment mother," operates invisibly, at best enabling patients and therapists to take the risk of including formerly split-off, hidden, or nascent and undeveloped aspects of self in the relationship, and at worst causing acute states of panic and anxiety when the durability and continuity of the attachment bond are put at risk by an impasse.

The Nature of the Patient's Attachment

The formation of a strong attachment bond from patient to therapist, like the positive therapeutic alliance, is a precondition for the formation of working therapeutic relationships. Patients who seek therapy often do so because they have experienced significant problems in their primary attachment relationships, usually to their mothers and fathers, but also to spouses, lovers, siblings, or friends. As the preceding chapters on the formation of specific areas of primary vulnerability indicate, patients seek therapy because the vulnerabilities have been shaped, much as flowing rivers wear patterns in rocks over time, through cumulative experiences of violations, betrayals, abandonments, and repeated disconnections in their significant attachments. Patients are left with primary vulnerabilities that manifest in problematic representations of self and self-in-relationship and in their tendency to sacrifice aspects of themselves in the service of preserving important relationships. Patients seeking therapy risk the destruction of hope that they can find new ways to relate to others and to themselves. Through new tributaries from the river of the therapeutic relationship, they hope to carve different patterns on the shape of their sense of self. Only in a secure attachment will these new and more flexible modes of self-representation and being-in-relationship evolve.

Unless a strong attachment bond forms between patient and therapist, therapy that engages the areas of primary vulnerability formed by faulty or destructive self-representations and inflexible or coerced modes of relating cannot take place. When therapist and patient are mismatched, formation of an essential attachment bond is blocked. When collusions occur, patients and therapists are stuck in an entrenched mode of relating because of their fear of disrupting the attachment bond. Primary vulnerabilities are shaped around the necessity of preserving an essential attachment bond, such as that between mothers and infants. When patients *and* therapists are catapulted into areas of primary vulnerability, the attachment bond between them is inevitably put in jeopardy.

The attachment to a therapist, like an infant's attachment to the mother, represents not only an *outer* but an *inner* attachment: Both mothers and therapists serve as mediators for the infants' and patients' connection to their feelings, thoughts, and reactions to experience. The dual nature of the attachment bond—as a connection both to one's self and to the other—underscores its importance.

Bowlby's Theory of Attachment

British psychoanalyst John Bowlby has been the primary spokesperson for the vital importance of attachment bonds to caretakers for infants, adults, and therapy patients. Bowlby spent thirty years exploring the bond between infants, children, and mothers. From his research efforts, he evolved a theoretical model that explains attachment behavior.[7]

When viewed from within the framework of Bowlby's theory of attachment, the distressed responses of patients and therapists to impasses and ruptures are readily understandable. Seen from the perspective of the loss of a significant attachment, the intense affective reactions of patients and therapists no longer appear extreme.

Bowlby comments on the intensity of the emotions individuals experience in relation to their attachment bonds. His observations are directly relevant to the anguish that patients experience after the sudden loss of therapists to whom they have formed strong attachments:

> A feature of attachment behaviour of the greatest importance clinically, and present irrespective of the age of the individual concerned, is the intensity of the emotion that accompanies it, the kind of emotion aroused depending on how the relationship between the individual attached and the attachment figure is faring. If it goes well, there is a joy and a sense of security. If it is threatened, there is jealousy, anxiety, and anger. If broken, there is grief and depression. Finally there is strong evidence that how attachment behaviour comes to be organized within an individual turns in high degree on the kinds of experience he has in his family of origin, or if he is unlucky, out of it.[8]

Bowlby, basing his framework on an ethological perspective (the scientific study of animal behavior), conceives of attachment behavior and parenting behavior as having biological roots.[9] In essence, infants arrive genetically programmed to attach themselves to carepersons who will nurture and protect them. Correspondingly, parents are programmed to provide this care—witness the instinctive cuddling new mothers and fathers give their infants. Powerful emotions accompany attachment and parenting behaviors, perhaps because of the genetic basis for them. The specific forms that attachment and parenting behaviors take in a given individual are determined by past and present experiences, particularly those occurring in childhood.

In a statement that has far-reaching implications for therapy theory, Bowlby emphatically declares that concepts of dependency and regression have pathological connotations and should be replaced by concepts of attachment and caregiving. He asserts that the need for attachment is necessary for human survival. Rather than representing a state that children should leave behind in favor of autonomy, as the word "dependency" implies, attachment needs are inherently human and are never outgrown. Nor are they regressive even though they are perhaps more clearly in evidence during childhood. In fact, as Bowlby puts it, "the capacity to make intimate emotional bonds with other individuals, sometimes in the careseeking role and sometimes in the caregiving one, is regarded as a principle feature of effective personality functioning and mental health."[10]

Our theories of therapy have stressed the importance of mastering or relinquishing infantile dependency needs. Consequently, patients who rely on their therapists as caretaker/mentor figures often feel troubled by their "regressive" needs. The bias against allowing for and valuing attachment capacities in both directions has many implications for therapy as it is currently practiced. To give only one example, patients whose therapists leave on vacations most often try to grit their teeth and endure the absence. If they need to resort to calling a back-up therapist, they feel ashamed and weak, as if they cannot survive on their own. If our conception of attachment as healthy and valuable and necessary were to replace our contempt for dependency, patients who have had problematic experiences with attachment figures might seek out back-up appointments or engage the help of auxiliary therapists feeling empowered rather than ashamed. Although an attachment bond cannot automatically be transferred to another person, patients who perceive themselves to be legitimately attached to their therapists and as taking good care of themselves by utilizing other relational supports when their therapists are away, have the possibility of a good experience of separation from their primary therapists rather than of barely tolerable anguish. When a patient requests an appointment with another therapist for the time the primary therapist plans to be away an impasse may lie in wait if the primary therapist interprets the patient's behavior as stemming from an infantile need or from a resistance to facing the reality of the separation. This is a not uncommon source of impasse. Most patients have had abundant experiences of painful separations, but they are unlikely to have had the experience of being empowered to find alternative relationships that can provide support for them during the absence of their primary therapist. More often than not, merely the availability of another therapist and the permission to rely on her reduces patients' need for it or empowers them to attend to their needs.

Bowlby uses fellow researcher Mary Ainsworth's concept of "a secure base" to refer to the fact that all human beings, and children in particular, require a secure attachment to another clearly identified individual who is seen as better able to cope with the world. All human beings in difficult circumstances seek comfort and support from others; such desires are inherently human and are therefore not merely childish or regressive. The availability and responsivity of the caretaking person enable the attaching individual to feel safe and free to move out into the world to explore. An inner urgency to explore the world, like attachment, has biological roots. The availability of a secure base to which an upset or frightened person or an adventurous and free-spirited person can return enables these individuals to venture forth and take risks. A therapist optimally serves as the psychological caretaking person for the adult therapy patient, providing the secure base from which she can explore her inner world—the representational models she uses to describe herself, significant others, and the relational patterns that are most familiar to her—and her outer world of relationships and activities.

Within Bowlby's framework, the separation anxiety that may occur in the context of an increased risk of losing the caretaking person becomes an appropriate, not pathological, response to a perceived threat. Bowlby writes: "As responses to the risk of loss, anxiety and anger go hand in hand. It is not for nothing that they have the same etymological root."[11] Patients who are in a state of impasse with a therapist to whom they had once felt securely attached are likely to experience acute separation anxiety, bearing in mind that the separation refers not only to separation from a person in the outer world, but also from a connection to a part of the self the therapist mediates for the patient. *Therapists mediate the patients' connection to themselves by holding for them a vision of their potential and a sense of their coherence and complexity.*[12]

Instead of looking at human development as proceeding through specific phases, Bowlby utilizes the concept of developmental pathways proposed by the biologist C. H. Waddington.[13] In this framework, individuals have available to them at any point in the lifespan a number of possible pathways from which to choose. The ones an individual follows are chosen as the result of an interaction of the individual (as she has developed up to that point) and the present environment. The specific developmental pathway of attachment behavior in a given individual is largely influenced by the way the parents have responded to her. Parental responses contribute to the construction of representational or "working models" of self, other, and the quality of the attachment-relationship that can occur. (The term "working model" is also used by Daniel Stern and is analogous to the concept of internal objects used by the "object relations" theorists such as Klein, Winnicott, Fairbairn, and Guntrip.) These representational models tend to persist unmodified at an unconscious level; that is, they function automatically and outside of awareness.

Children form working models or representations of how relationships operate during the first few years of life, as infant research studies discussed in the preceding chapter document. These models become established as influential psychological structures or organizing principles that persist over time. Bowlby delineates three patterns of children's attachment to caretakers, based on research by Mary Ainsworth conducted in 1971: secure attachment, anxious resistant attachment (where parents have been inconsistently available), and anxious avoidant attachment (where the individual anticipates rejection). Children who do not form secure attachments, in addition to clinging or avoiding attachment, display a serious breakdown of communication with their mothers. While securely attached children may be observed to express the full gamut of emotions to their mothers, ranging from distress to contentment, children with problems in attachment fail to express either their emotions or their desire for comfort and reassurance.

Children who have secure attachments proceed along healthy pathways, while those with insecure attachments are apt to develop along problematic pathways, because the choice of pathway is determined by the interaction of the child and the human environment available to respond to her. Because the course of development is not fixed, changes in the human environment elicit changes in the path a person takes. As Bowlby succinctly puts it:

> Change continues throughout the life cycle so that changes for better or for worse are always possible. It is this continuing potential for change that means that at no time of life is a person invulnerable to every possible adversity and also that at no time of life is a person impermeable to favourable influence.[14]

Therapeutic relationships, according to this model and as emphasized in preceding chapters, thus provide both a danger and an opportunity. The danger resides in the potential for patients to be wounded or traumatized by their therapist in ways that are similar to prior experiences with their parents. If the dangerous outcome occurs, patients are as vulnerable as they were in childhood because as adults they have risked hoping to have a healing, reparative, and insight-oriented experience in therapy and they have assumed, with reason, that their therapist would be different from their parents.

A patient in therapy, in addition to having the possibility of a new experience of attachment, also has an opportunity to allow entrenched representational models of self, other, and self-in-relationship and familiar modes of relating—for example, as subjective, coerced, or developmental objects—that operate outside of awareness to emerge into consciousness. Once in consciousness, the modes of relating and representations of relationships can be identified and evaluated by patient and therapist in terms of their origin and their necessity in the individual's present life context. Therapeutic relationships that provide positive caretaking responses that were not available to the patient as a child open up the possibility of a new sense of security, and, consequently, provide infinite opportunities for new exploratory behavior in the patient's inner and outer world.

The Nature of the Therapist's Attachment Bond

Therapists who offer themselves as vehicles for change in a therapeutic relationship optimally have already traversed the terrain that their patients are embarking upon. In the context of an attachment bond with their patients, therapists also continue to work on personal areas of vulnerability through ongoing efforts to help their patients, even though the profession has not yet explicitly emphasized or acknowledged the personal work that therapists continue to accomplish. The collective emphasis has remained on working with countertransference responses that might impede the therapeutic work. Because therapists become attached to patients, and because therapists' personal vulnerabilities also become engaged in the therapeutic relationship, the threat of a rupture may be as anxiety-producing for therapists as it is for patients. The attachment bond to patients operates differently for therapists because they are primarily in the caretaker rather than careseeker position. Nevertheless, a rupture in the attachment bond for therapists can challenge their connection to themselves, particularly to their sense of a competent professional therapist-self, as well as to their patient, whom they have cared for.

Bowlby does not speculate in detail about the experience of the caretaker when the attachment bond is threatened. One reason why therapists have insisted on an exclusive relationship with their patients may have to do with a fear that the attachment bond cannot withstand, or will be diminished by, the presence of another attachment figure. Other attachment figures may include a consultant to the relationship in times of difficulty or an auxiliary therapist who is available to meet with the patient either in the primary therapist's absence or in addition to the primary therapist. Therapists may also feel envious of or competitive with other caretakers or rely unconsciously on patients as the caretakers of their professional selves. If we make the attachment bond central to therapeutic relationships and raise questions about the necessity for an *exclusive* attachment between therapist and patient, we not only arrive at new understandings of therapeutic impasses that jeopardize the attachment bond, but we open up new options for positive therapeutic experiences.

Although Bowlby alludes to a healthy need to be a caretaker, he does not speculate further about what the psychological underpinnings of this need might be.[15] While all human beings need relational connections, whether to other human beings, religious entities, or to themselves, the need to *be* a caretaker for others can have complicated origins. For example, one source of the need to be a caretaker may be to locate a channel for generative, nurturing energy. The helping occupations such as teaching, health services, and parenting are examples of channels for generative energy. But the need to be a caretaker may also arise from a need for secure attachments that will endure over time. Individuals influenced by the need for secure, unbroken attachments may seek attachments to careseekers, who, because they are dependent, are unlikely to leave the relationship. A therapeutic relationship begins with the therapist in the caregiver role and the patient in the careseeker role, but the balance shifts as the relationship is underway. Just as mothers and infants in optimal circumstances are able to shift relational modes fluidly, therapists and patients optimally shift relational modes in the service of mutual development, even though our professional focus highlights the development only of the patient. Therapists who resist allowing patients to be caregivers in order to maintain the attachment bond and patients who fear relinquishing the role of careseeker are liable to become entrenched in a fixed and psychologically limiting relational mode. When either participant in the dyad attempts to make a shift, an impasse can arise that puts the attachment bond in jeopardy. Therapists need to be particularly conscious of their own needs for secure attachments in order to allow their patients the freedom of movement in relationships they have never had and now dare to seek.

When the Attachment Bond Is in Jeopardy

Many therapeutic relationships provide patients with an opportunity for healing and reparative work and therapists with a sense of accomplishment and gratification as well as a potentially expanded sense of self. But there are also therapeutic relationships that take the dangerous path at the fork in the road and end up in impasses that are anxiety-producing and stressful for both participants. My experience doing consultations in situations where therapeutic relationships are at risk indicates that these relationships have undergone *two* levels of wounding. The two levels of wounding may not be readily apparent to either the therapist or patient because of the intense emotions that are evoked. Therapists and patients often have difficulty sorting out the components of these two levels of wounding without outside assistance.

The first level of wounding consists of the behavior or interaction that wounds the patient such that the primary vulnerabilities that originated in the context of significant attachments are activated. The wounded patient attempts simultaneously to express her feelings about the wound and at the same time to preserve the relationship to the therapist, who has now become as potentially dangerous as prior attachment figures. The excruciating dilemma the patient faces—being wounded in areas of primary vulnerability in relationship to a significant attachment figure whom she hoped would be different from the original attachment figures with whom the vulnerabilities were formed—often leads the patient to lash out at the therapist in anxiety, grief, and anger.

A second level of wounding can then be created, often unwittingly, by the therapist's problematic responses to the patient, who is now behaving in markedly upsetting ways. The therapist, thrown off center by the feelings and behavior of the patient, reacts to preserve her sense of a competent therapist-self. The therapist's problematic responses thus compound the first level of wounding and also prevent the patient from working psychologically with the nature of the primary wound. More importantly, the second level of wounding not only puts the relationship at risk but may be powerful enough to sever it.

On the basis of personal experience and consultations I have participated in, therapeutic relationships that are at risk of rupture are characterized by these two levels of wounding. The case of Ann and Dr. L discussed in Chapter Five provides us with an example of the two levels of wounding. The first level of wounding—the original behavior on the part of the therapist that wounds the patient in her personal area of primary vulnerability—consisted of Dr. L. raising his fee in the last stage of Ann's pregnancy and prior to a long separation due to his vacation and the birth. The sudden shift in the direction of the attachment bond, in which Dr. L. had been the caretaker and Ann the careseeker, at a particularly vulnerable time for Ann, who had dared to hope that she could count on Dr. L. to be a reliable, dependable caretaker, threw her into a state of acute anxiety.

The original level of wounding was then compounded by a second level, comprised of the therapist's responses to the patient following the patient's reaction to the initial trauma. Instead of remaining focused on Ann's experience and working with the acute anxiety state that she experienced, Dr. L. responded in a cold, unfeeling, and unyielding manner to her plea that he set aside the fee raise until after the birth of her baby. He insisted on making Ann the caretaker by demanding in a coercive manner that she pay a higher fee. His cold, stern demeanor evoked in Ann earlier feelings of being coerced to behave in required ways or else risk losing the attachment. Dr. L.'s continuing inability to function as a therapist and conceptualize the relational experience in terms of Ann's vulnerabilities in attachments ultimately caused the therapeutic relationship to rupture.

When a patient reacts to the therapist's wounding behavior by expressing feelings of disappointment, criticism, or anger, as Ann did, the therapist, like Dr. L., may be unable to accept, receive, or welcome the patient's distressed feelings. Therapists may be unable to empathize with patients' responses to their behavior and to recognize these responses as legitimate from the patients' perspective, however unjustified the therapists may perceive them to be. Therapists may also be unable to place the responses in the context of their patients' personal areas of primary vulnerability and to help them examine their reactions in relation to early experiences with their first caretakers. Instead of accepting their patients' needs and feelings as comprehensible both in the current therapeutic relationship and in the context of significant past relationships, therapists may fend off negative feelings and remain focused primarily on their own needs in relation to the patient. Allowing the therapeutic relationship to end at this pivotal juncture, as Dr. L. did, without as full a conscious understanding as possible of the primary vulnerabilities that are engaged, adds a devastating abandonment—the rupture of an essential attachment bond—to the original and secondary level of wounding.

Why do highly trained, experienced, well-intentioned, and self-reflective therapists behave unempathically and create a second level of wounding that puts the attachment bond at risk? The patient's reaction to whatever the therapist did to cause the original wounding trips off anxiety in the therapist. *The therapist's anxiety about the breach of the secure attachment to the patient pushes her into a personal area of primary vulnerability* related to her significant early attachment relationships. A therapist who is in jeopardy of being catapulted into an area of primary vulnerability involving significant attachments will respond self-protectively. These responses may manifest in behaviors that differ superficially, but that serve the same function of preserving a stable sense of self. Dr. L. behaved in a cold, distant manner, as if he did not care whether Ann remained his patient or not. In another case, a therapist alternately behaved toward her patient with warmth and affection in one session to preserve her sense of self as a compassionate person and then erupted in anger in the next session in an effort to establish her separateness.

When psychological energy is directed toward preserving a stable self-state, the therapist is often unable to focus on understanding, attuning to, and empathizing with her patient. Consequently, a crucial underpinning of the patient's responses to the wounding the therapist provokes is overlooked: *The patient is desperately trying to stay in relationship to the therapist and to restore the connection to the therapist that the original wounding has imperiled, even when the patient's destructive impulses have been unleashed and are being directed at the therapist or the relationship.* Because the patient may be expressing anger and anxiety in destructive ways, her underlying wish to restore and maintain the critically important relationship to her therapist may be overlooked by a therapist who is preoccupied with preserving her self-state. Consultation in separate meetings with the patient and therapist at this pivotal juncture often effect an immediate and dramatic change by helping the therapist see how attached the patient is and by helping the patient see how hard the therapist is trying to restore a stable sense of a professional self. Because a consultant looks at the impasse from a different perspective, she is often able to perceive the context of the wounding, and its origins in the patient's history. Consequently she can help both the patient and therapist recognize the opportunity that resides in the painful interaction. (See the case of Josie and Dr. M. in Chapters Two and Thirteen.)

The secondary level of wounding can take a variety of specific forms. Responses experienced by the patient as harmful may come in the form of retaliatory or intrusive interpretations. Returning to the case of Lynn and Dr. K. for an example of a retaliatory interpretation, we recall that in their last contact, a telephone call, after Lynn had begun expressing angry feelings for the first time, Dr. K. made the interpretation that Lynn was fearful of driving him crazy as she feared she had driven her mother crazy and that she needed him to withstand her attempts to do so. Lynn experienced the interpretation as an unhelpful conception for understanding the relational dynamic and restoring an alliance, but also as an assault that located all responsibility in her. In another example, a patient who had been wounded in an area of primary vulnerability by his therapist found himself in a rage. Past interactions in the therapeutic relationship took on new meaning to the patient when he looked back at them from the vantage point of his present disillusionment. Responses that had seemed helpful or benign at the time now seemed to the patient to be the therapist's means of keeping himself in the role of an authoritarian expert and infantilizing the patient. Distraught at the new perspective, the patient shared it with the therapist. The fact that the patient was for the first time able to see things from his own point of view, rather than automatically being compliant and obedient as he had had to be to maintain his parents' affection, was actually a sign of progress in the therapy. But the therapist, whose professional self-esteem was being challenged, was pushed into an area of personal primary vulnerability that threatened his formerly secure sense of attachment to his patient. Unable to receive the initial onslaught of his patient's unmodulated feelings, he reacted by retaliating with an interpretation: "You're trying to avoid facing your own role in our interaction by focusing on me, externalizing the responsibility the way that you did with your family." The patient, who had been focused on the therapist's behavior in the present and who could not immediately recognize the defensive aspect of the interpretation, regardless of its accuracy, was reduced to a state of incoherence and confusion.

Another response that patients experience as harmful occurs when therapists defensively distance themselves for protection from the anxiety generated by the threatened attachment, either by retreating into silence or by not being present emotionally to respond empathically to feelings the patient is attempting to express. Dr. K. withdrew from his patient Lynn when she went into a crisis of anguish after her younger sister Alice was injured in an automobile accident. Dr. K. was alarmed by the sudden change in his patient and how out of control she seemed to be. Fear that he could not calm her down, that she was out of control, obscured for Dr. K. the opportunity carried in her new state of being. Lynn had always been compelled to control her emotions in order not to burden her parents, whom she accurately perceived to be overwhelmed by their financial responsibilities and their worry about Alice. For the first time in her therapy, Lynn had the opportunity to yield to her feelings in relation to Dr. K. and to be held symbolically by her therapist's presence. Dr. K.'s inability to withstand her anguish created a retraumatizing experience for Lynn instead of a healing opportunity.

Therapists in like situations, whose sense of security in the attachment bond to their patients is in jeopardy, risk losing sight of the effort patients make both to be authentically themselves and to stay connected to their therapists. By reacting personally to their patients' feelings instead of to the fact that their patients are managing to express feelings in the context of the relationship bond, therapists miss the forest for the trees. For example, a therapist may perceive an angry patient as fully alive, as passionately filled with powerful energy, rather than only as hostile and attacking. A therapist may perceive a wounded patient as sharing her hurt and struggling to be authentically herself rather than as keeping her hurt hidden and sealed off from consciousness because she fears it will injure the therapist or drive the therapist away. To the extent that a goal of therapy is conceived to be a new experience of psychological and emotional wholeness in the context of a significant relationship, a wounded patient able finally to express herself is actually making progress. But therapists who struggle with anxiety over the loss of connection to themselves and their patients (conceiving of attachments as having both an internal and external component) are not free to recognize progress in the midst of turmoil.

A third form of harmful response is pathological labeling of patients, another reason why I prefer the label "primary vulnerability" to "psychotic or borderline core" or even "basic fault." Diagnostic labels entail a categorizing that necessarily obscures the fullness and complexity of individual human beings, in addition to having judgmental connotations. In some circumstances, labels serve a defensive function for the therapist, regulating her self-state by restoring her self-esteem and confidence. Labeling a patient as being in a borderline state may enable the therapist to be less frightened of the patient's behavior and to function more effectively. A therapist may also use a label as a shorthand way to communicate to a consultant: A "borderline" patient is one who has trouble perceiving the therapist as both "good" and "bad" and tends to "split" the therapist into one or the other. Although such uses of diagnostic labels may seem innocuous, they nonetheless embody and perpetuate the split in attitude whereby the patient is ill and the therapist is healthy. It might be more accurate to say that the therapist is warding off a "borderline" state that might be evoked by the behavior of the patients.

Another damaging category of response by the therapist occurs when the therapist is so anxious that she becomes a volatile rather than a stable, reliable, consistent object for the patient. An anxious, insecure therapist may be warm and caring in one session and withdrawn and defensive at the next. The therapist's fluctuating demeanor results from her unsuccessful efforts to manage the anxiety and distress she experiences in the face of her patient's behavior and from her distressed and sometimes floundering efforts to restore the relationship to solid ground. Patients in an impasse are best helped by a reliable, consistent presence on the part of therapists until they can organize their own version of the impasse. Fluctuations in demeanor of the therapist make the patient's task more difficult. Therapists have the challenge of maintaining enough stability in their personal sense of self to allow them to be relatively reliable, consistent figures for patients. When this becomes difficult, consultation with another therapist is often useful in providing a "holding environment" within which a therapist can restore her endangered or fragmented sense of self.

Once a secondary level of wounding has become engaged, the therapeutic relationship is inevitably in jeopardy. To move it from precarious ground to a new and more secure foundation, a shift must be made by the patient and/or therapist. Consultation helps to create the necessary psychological *space (or distance) between* the patient and therapist that will facilitate a shift. Winnicott used the term "potential space," elaborated on in Chapter Eleven, to give substance to the otherwise invisible psychological distance between two individuals in relationship to each other. Ogden uses the expression "collapsing into" the three different relational positions he describes (see Chapter Seven), referring to a loss of the "space between." Sometimes the patient or therapist can find some means of stepping out of troubled relationship in order to reflect upon it. Either the patient or the therapist can use the psychological distance to shift the balance, functioning in the moment as the therapist to the relationship. Most therapists have had the experience, when they feel utterly hopeless about the relationship with a patient, of seeing the patient come to a session in a completely altered mood, bringing with them clarity and insight that had seemed forever out of reach only a session before. Most patients have had the analogous experience of feeling certain that their therapeutic relationship is a harmful one from which they must extricate themselves, only to find that the therapist has put together an astute and accurate conception of what is transpiring in their work together.

But a certain number of therapeutic relationships, perhaps more than we have acknowledged openly, come to a painful, abrupt end when the secondary level of wounding spirals out of control. *All therapists, no matter how sensitive, empathic, experienced, and intelligent, are vulnerable to wounding patients and to bringing about a secondary level of wounding that causes the relationship to rupture.* Participants in a therapeutic relationship that ends painfully and abruptly are each left with a complex set of feelings to manage that can obscure the positive function of anger and of separation. Because the relationship is more central to the patient than to the therapist, and because most patients do not have access to the supports that therapists have in place through their ongoing therapy, consultation, and collegial relationships, the patient's task is more difficult and complicated. But both therapists and patients who have endured ruptured terminations have been abandoned and isolated by our profession until now.

The following chapter discusses the aftermath of a ruptured therapeutic relationship from the perspectives of patient and therapist. Naming the experiences that ensue from ruptured terminations is the first step in giving a voice and place to therapists and patients who have experienced attachments and ruptures in therapeutic relationships.

CHAPTER ELEVEN

❖ *The Mourning Process* ❖
When Therapeutic
Relationships Rupture

For example, a new light is thrown [by attachment theory] on the problem of separation anxiety, namely anxiety about losing, or becoming separated from, someone loved. . . . When separation anxiety is seen in this light, as a basic human disposition, it is only a small step to understand why it is that threats to abandon a child, often used as a means of control, are so very terrifying. . . . Not only do threats of abandonment create intense anxiety but they also arouse anger, often also of intense degree. . . .

—JOHN BOWLBY[1]

Grieving should no longer be regarded as a "weakness," but as a psychological process of the greatest importance to the health of a person. For who is spared loss? And if we do not actually have to deal with the death of someone we love, life affords partings enough, and these can bring about loss reactions similar to those which occur when we lose a loved one.

—VERENA KAST[2]

The Loss of the Attachment Bond

Impasses in therapeutic relationships that cannot be worked with constructively are liable to cause the relationship to rupture irretrievably, leaving patient and therapist alone in accompanying states of anguish. Patients are left with a contradictory mixture of intense feelings that are difficult to bear: loss and grief, disappointment and disillusionment, anger that can border on a murderous rage, overwhelming despair and hopelessness, perhaps coupled with relief and a sense of being powerful. Therapists are left with feelings that range from relief, loss, self-doubt, guilt, shame, and anxiety about their professional adequacy to concern for the patient's well-being. When

193

the therapeutic relationship terminates in a rupture, these feelings must be managed by each participant separately, outside the context of the attachment bond that has been forged during the course of the relationship.

Therapists can help patients who have experienced ruptures in important therapeutic relationships to work with the turbulent aftermath by familiarizing themselves with the emotional terrain that must be navigated. Familiarity with the intensity of affect states that patients are apt to experience will reduce therapists' need to distance themselves defensively from patients or to pathologize the affect states that patients bring to them to contain. Patients who familiarize themselves with the emotional terrain they may have to traverse will be less apt to fear the intensity of their feelings or to pathologize themselves.

Unfortunately, the prevailing theories and practices guiding the profession of psychotherapy and prescribing the structure of the relationship leave patients and therapists vulnerable to intense emotional responses to impasses and ruptures. Prevailing theory sanctions the exclusivity of the therapist–patient dyad by insisting that patients rely only on their therapists and avoid soliciting outside perspectives either from friends or other professionals. Prevailing theory also tends to pathologize or criticize patients and therapists for their responses to impasses and ruptures instead of providing them with vital supportive relational contexts. The situation of early childhood, in which patients as children were literally dependent for survival upon caretakers, without other options, is thus re-created. Unless therapists begin to hold a different stance, patients are at risk of being trapped once again in the worst aspects of an isolated nuclear family. They both have to keep secret what happens in the family, and the parental truth supersedes their own.

Patients rely on therapists because they expect them to provide a better facilitating environment for psychological growth than their parents or early caretakers offered. Unfortunately, therapists who rely on theories that advocate neutrality and the frustration of infantile needs at the expense of understanding and working through the relational issues (as if these needs can ever be fully outgrown) are often unable to offer what patients need. Even therapists who are willing to participate in flexible, empowering relationships are affected by the limitations of life and of being merely human. No human being can completely satisfy the legitimate needs of another. Consequently, both patient and therapists are caught in a double bind. They are placed in a relational context that encourages dependency in a state of isolation, discourages them from seeking help outside the dyadic relationship, and then pathologizes patients as dependent and strains the empathic capacities of the therapist. Weakness and dependency may be attributed to patients who look for auxiliary therapists upon whom they can rely. Inadequacy or inexperience may be ascribed to therapists who seek consultation that includes both patient and therapist. We face the challenge of creating new models that support patients and therapists in being able to revive early relational patterns and self-other-relationship representations and to preserve the attachment bond that then forms. At the same time, we need models that empower patients as the adult individuals with adult capacities that they are and that permit therapists to have vulnerabilities and limitations.

Patients' Experience of a Ruptured Therapeutic Relationship

As ruptures in therapeutic relationships are rarely talked about openly, therapists and patients struggle with the feelings they arouse virtually alone or with one or two close colleagues or friends. Little exists by way of adequate collective support in the form of written material for either patients or therapists. The descriptions that follow of the subjective experience of patients whose therapeutic relationship was abruptly severed in a state of impasse constitutes a beginning attempt to fill in the existing vacuum.

Panic and Anxiety

As patients sense that the attachment bond to their therapists is in jeopardy, they are apt to feel acute panic and anxiety that in itself is terrifying because it seems out of proportion to feelings that are ordinarily part of professional relationships. Patients generally lack an understanding of their normal and in fact desirable solid attachment to their therapist. Consequently, they are apt to be frightened by the intensity of their need for the relationship and to perceive themselves in pejorative terms, such as overly dependent or regressed. In a culture that continues to value strength and independence and to perceive dependency as a weak and infantile state to be outgrown, negative perceptions on the part of therapists and patients are inevitable and take conscious effort to correct.

The plight of patients is often made worse by the response of therapists to their acute anxiety. Therapists may be alarmed by the intense affect states that patients display in response to wounding or to the *threat of loss* of the therapist. If the therapist neglects the context of threatened loss in which such responses arise, she may perceive them as extreme and call them pathological. Therapists, like patients, may overlook or pathologize the nature of the attachment their patients develop in the therapeutic relationship.

The intense feelings that are part of the aftermath of a ruptured therapeutic relationship for patients stem from sudden loss of the important attachment bond that patient and therapist forge. When the therapeutic relationship ends abruptly, the loss of the relationship with the therapist as a person and as the container of the patient's sense of wholeness and cohesion leaves the patient in a state of extreme anxiety. Children who have been subjected to temporary separations from their mothers suffer acutely from the loss. As Bowlby's research documents, their separation anxiety manifests in a range of behaviors such as protest, despair, agitation, and, ultimately, detachment. Patients in therapy respond in analogous ways to the loss of their therapists.

Mourning, Grief, and Loss

Within Bowlby's attachment framework, mourning is a normal response to a loss.[3] To the patient who, as a consequence of a rupture, loses the therapeutic relationship altogether, the simple and explicit acknowledgment by others that she is in an expectable state of mourning comes as an enormous relief. Bowlby reminds us that mourning in healthy adults lasts far longer than the six-month to one-year period thought to be true in the 1950s.[4] Moreover, responses that once were regarded as pathological are now found to be common in most adults: anger at the lost person, at one's self and third parties; disbelief that the loss has occurred (to be distinguished from denial that it has occurred); and a tendency to search for the lost person in the hope of a reunion.[5] Reactions of a patient who has experienced an abrupt loss of a therapeutic relationship because of failure on the part of the therapist are not pathological when perceived from the perspective of an individual who has suffered a significant loss, internally and externally, and who is therefore in a normal human state of mourning.

The loss takes on even greater significance when we recognize that most patients seek therapy because they have experienced unsatisfactory attachments to their original caretakers, usually the parents. They are taking a risk in trying once again, going against the grain of their actual experience, to establish an enduring attachment, to provide themselves with an essential, secure relational base from which they can face the primary vulnerabilities that are the legacy of their early attachments. Some adult patients must overcome a long-entrenched block against feeling or expressing their natural need, in Bowlby's language, for "a close, trusting relationship, for care, comfort, and love—which I regard as the subjective manifestations of a major system of instinctive behavior."[6] When a failure then occurs, patients are thrown back into a state of despair that is actually worse than the state in which they began therapy. Adult patients have taken a substantial risk in allowing the awakening of attachment needs (as opposed to having regressed to a state of dependency). They have dared to form an attachment against objections from the part of themselves that walled off and rejected attachment needs as futile and dangerous. Consequently, adult patients who have dared to hope for a good experience in risking attachment and who suffer a painful and disillusioning termination may be likely to refuse to try therapy again.

Patients whose therapeutic relationships terminate abruptly in an impasse have difficulty talking about their feelings openly because they fear that their grief will seem overly intense and extreme to others. One patient who came for consultation reported missing her therapist as acutely as if he had died. He was literally as inaccessible to her as if he had perished. Shortly after her final session, she wrote an anguished letter to him, communicating all the feelings that could not be expressed directly because they were no longer meeting in person. But even with the help of the letter she wrote, her grief did not completely dissipate. It seemed to well up from a limitless source until she learned to live with it and became better able to distract herself. Ultimately the passage of time placed the feelings of grief at a distance.

Shame and Humiliation

Patients whose therapeutic relationships end in a rupture are left, in addition to grief, with feelings of shame and a sense of failure that take a long time to abate. These are also feelings that are particularly difficult to talk about openly. The severing of the therapeutic relationship is experienced subjectively as a failure, even though, when examined closely from both perspectives, it may ultimately lead to personal growth. Shame and humiliation inhibit us from disclosing our more difficult experiences, whether as patients or as therapists. But patients are especially vulnerable to feeling that they have failed because they conceive of the therapist as an expert, well qualified to help them. They expect that therapists will have worked through their vulnerabilities and problems so that any difficulties that arise interpersonally in the therapeutic relationship are necessarily their fault.

Patients worry about what others will think of them for having had failure experiences as patients. They fear that others will see a core of vulnerability in them that they are unable to see in themselves, or that others will be amazed that they had difficulty with their therapist. Patients are well aware that when they talk about painful experiences, their stories are apt to be analyzed by others in different ways. They worry about the pathological formulations that others might create about the ending of their therapy. One patient announced, "I can't tell you the name of my therapist. He's so well known that you won't believe a word I say. You'll think that I made the therapy fail, that I can't be helped."

Rage

Alongside feelings of shame and failure, a sense of murderous rage often coexists, so powerful that at times patients report feeling that it might actually destroy them. A letter written by a patient to her therapist after a rupture shows how long such anger can endure. It was written in response to what the patient considered to be an inappropriate intrusion of the therapist into her life after the therapy had ended.

During her therapy sessions, the patient had frequently talked about her peer consultation group that met weekly at the same restaurant. A year after her therapeutic relationship terminated in a rupture, the therapist appeared at the restaurant on one of her meeting days and was seated at a nearby table. The patient was extremely distressed by her therapist's invasion of her privacy and intrusion into her territory. She felt he should have remembered that she met regularly at that restaurant and been conscious of the upsetting effect that his presence might have. The patient understood that the therapist had every right to choose whatever restaurant he wanted or that he might have forgotten. But she felt strongly that his lack of awareness of his impact on her was part of the same inability to empathize with her that had pervaded their therapeutic relationship. Writing the letter represented a way for the patient to preserve her integrity. Here is an excerpt from the letter which she wrote and then chose not to send:

> In view of your knowledge of the importance of my meetings at the Bay Street Restaurant, I find your appearance there last Thursday

both unconscionable and personally painful. You are demonstrating the same lack of capacity to focus your attention on my needs and the same self-gratification at my expense that pervaded the years of therapy with you.

I certainly have every reason not to want any reminder of my damaging experience in therapy with you. I feel it is enough to have to bear my rage and anguish at the psychological and emotional energy (not to mention the financial drain) that I invested in the therapy relationship and which you in no way deserved or earned.

No doubt you will be as unable to grasp my feelings now as you were during the course of our therapy relationship. However, it is important to me to make my feelings known to you, and for you to be aware that I intend to do what I can to protect my separate space and personal boundaries.

For patients who have had therapeutic relationships end in a rupture, intense anger at their therapists can rise to the surface as if the experience happened only yesterday. Because the anger cannot be fully experienced and contained in the relationship until it is integrated, patients are left to manage their rage on their own. Without an empathic relational context to absorb it, rage, like grief, continues to well up at times as if from an unquenchable, limitless source, even years after the original failure.

Disbelief and a Sense of Betrayal

Along with shame, humiliation, and rage, patients often experience a profound sense of betrayal and disbelief. How could their therapists have allowed such damaging terminations to occur? Patients who are also therapists are certain that they would never allow a patient to leave them in such a state without making a concerted effort to preserve the relationship. In fact, patients who are enraged with their therapists often feel that they are loathsome and unlovable because they are so angry. When their therapists are able to tolerate being with patients in an enraged state and to search for its psychological origin, the patients' experience of being accepted, even with feelings that they perceive to be destructive, becomes profoundly meaningful. One man whose therapy ended abruptly in an impasse when his therapist "terminated him" expressed his feelings:

I still can't believe he just announced that we couldn't work together any more. I'd complained that he'd stopped functioning as my therapist and had become too much of a friend, which I believe he had, but I wanted him to get back on track. I didn't want the therapy to end. He just took it away from me without any warning. I asked him to give me some time to get used to the idea of stopping, but he said that I was right, he had become more of a friend than a therapist, and that it wouldn't be ethical for him to keep seeing me. I went from being a person that he cared about to being absolutely nothing. I still can't believe that he got rid of me like that.

Therapists who feel that the therapeutic relationship has become impossibly derailed certainly need to be able to end the relationship. But an awareness of the impact that an abrupt termination has on patients may help the therapist manage the termination and facilitate a transition to another therapist.

Hopelessness

One of the worst feelings that may haunt patients after painful terminations is an unshakable belief that they must be beyond help. The belief persists even after they have become cognitively aware of their therapists' psychological vulnerabilities and deficiencies and their own. Even when patients' perceptions of their therapists' limitations are accurate, they nonetheless feel that an unlovable core in them has been exposed and has caused their therapists to flee. Often patients resist attempting another therapeutic relationship because they believe that if they stay in any relationship long enough, their unlovable core will eventually be exposed and will drive even the most stalwart therapist away. These feelings are most difficult for patients who were abandoned in similar ways in early childhood.

One patient described her thoughts:

I've exposed the insatiably hungry me, the vulnerable and dependent me, the rageful scalding-hot me, the lonely and abandoned me, the worthless and rejected me, the selfish and entitled me, the engulfing and devouring me, the despairing me who is unable to bear being alive and is afraid to die, the me that dares once more to love. And I've been pushed away as intolerable, as I will be if I dare to expose these "me's" ever again to anyone else.

Sharing these feelings with me in my role as consultant ultimately provided her with an essential transitional relationship that empowered her to take the risk of pursuing therapy once again.

The Invisible Power of the Therapist and Patient

Therapists occupy a position of power and authority that is encouraged by prevailing theory, like the place parents occupy in their children's psyche. At a primitive emotional level, most patients imbue the therapist with a power and authority that eclipses their own, even in the face of rational understanding. But many patients are unaware of the power they assign to their therapists. They are often unaware of the extent to which they disavow their personal experience and doubt their own judgment and authority. Consequently, patients whose therapeutic relationships end in disillusionment often express shock, when they achieve some distance from the relationship, at the enormity of the power and faith they placed in their therapists, the importance they attributed them, and the power to wound them that their therapists had.

Because patients feel weak and vulnerable, having located the power and authority in the therapist, they are often unaware of how powerful they are to their therapists. More often than their patients realize, therapists are intimidated by the intensity of their patients' feelings, particularly rage and grief. Patients who give voice to their intense feelings in a therapy session may be completely unaware that they are intimidating their therapists and are consequently mystified when the therapists back away psychologically. Unaware of how weak and vulnerable the patients feel inside because their patients' behavior is so intimidating and powerful, therapists are consequently unable to give feedback about how powerful the patients seem.

Managing feelings of rage and grief in a relationship requires solid relational skills on the part of therapists, if they are to help patients develop these skills. The necessary relational abilities include a capacity to listen from the other person's point of view, to withstand fear and anxiety, to perceive the invisible vulnerability underlying the affect, to delay impulses to act, and to reflect on the psychological meaning of intense affect states. Yet the development of these capacities is rarely a central focus of training programs in psychotherapy, although it hopefully takes place along the way as therapists embark on therapeutic relationships with the support of supervision.

Sense of Incompleteness

Patients whose therapeutic relationships terminate abruptly and painfully often feel the frustration of having their "deep pocket" issues opened up but left exposed rather than worked through and integrated. To use an applicable metaphor from medicine, patients may feel as if a trusted and respected medical doctor had begun to operate on them, had made an incision, reached the source of the problem, and then suddenly departed the operating theater leaving the patient on the operating table. Beyond feeling abandoned by their therapists, patients may also be saddened, frustrated, and angered at the amount of time, money, energy, and risk taking they invested in their therapeutic relationships in order to arrive at their central issues. Patients then know they will have to repeat the same emotional investment in order to arrive at the same stage with another therapist. Worse, even if they invest time, money, and energy in establishing a relationship with another therapist, they are concerned that they might not gain access to the same issues again. Even if core issues are engaged in a subsequent therapy, the pathway to them will necessarily be different. When a therapeutic relationship ends in a rupture, an opportunity has been lost.

The incompleteness of the ending process in painful terminations can also augment the sense of damage with which patients are left. When patients and therapists are able to experience an ending phase in which the readiness to terminate arises organically, both of them have time to assess what was and was not accomplished within the therapy. Patients and therapists are able to separate psychologically from each other gradually. But when terminations are abrupt and painful, patients may feel as if parts of themselves were literally left behind in their therapists' offices. Not only do they feel that their most vulnerable and shameful aspects were exposed and magnified, but that valuable capacities were left behind: the capacity to be open, trusting, hopeful. Patients are left to handle the process of reclaiming these facets of themselves on their own. The reclamation process, like the separation process, may take a long time.

The Potential Space in Ruptured Therapeutic Relationships

D. W. Winnicott's concept of potential space provides a way of thinking about the subjective experience that patients have of leaving aspects of themselves behind in the once valued and now lost therapeutic relationship. Winnicott developed the concept of potential space to refer to "the hypothetical area that exists (but can also fail to exist) between the baby and the object (mother or part of mother) during the phase of the repudiation of the object as not-me, that is, at the end of being merged in with the object."[7] To paraphrase Winnicott's words, the potential space is neither inside the individual nor completely outside, but rather exists metaphorically *between* two people. When a baby or therapy patient feels confidence in the reliability and devotion of the mother or therapist, they paradoxically feel as if the mother/therapist exists as an extension of them (the subjective object) and have the illusion of omnipotence such that what they need from the mother/therapist magically appears, as if they have created it. The baby or therapy patient also has a growing awareness of the mother/therapist as a separate person (an object objectively perceived) existing outside of their control.

Winnicott posits a hypothetical or potential space that exists between the two experiences of being merged with an important object and being separate from it. He views the potential space as the source both of playing and of creativity. Within the safety of a well-established therapeutic relationship, patients can experiment with bringing forth new facets of themselves, creating or playing in the potential space between themselves and the therapists. New facets of patients and therapists emerge and develop in the potential space between patient and therapist.

In terminations that arise organically in the relational context, patients have the opportunity to establish a sense of an autonomous self in the presence of their therapists and then to terminate. When impasses arise and lead to an unexpected severing of the relationship, patients are apt to feel as if they left behind new facets of self that were not given the chance to be fully assimilated.[8] Patients may also feel that they have left aspects of themselves with the therapist, now experienced as a dangerous and unreliable person who still maintains power and control over the patients. Many patients consequently fear retaliation from their therapists and feel unsafe even though regular meetings have been discontinued. One patient left her therapist abruptly when she realized that she was caught in an unhealthy collusion that repeated the earlier controlling, domineering behavior of her father. She became temporarily afraid to answer her telephone, fearful that her therapist was going to call to rebuke her. Her decision to leave the therapist was an expression of a new and healthy assertiveness, which she feared would be annihilated by her therapist's punitive response.

Rethinking the Relationship

When patients have experiences of impasses and painful endings to therapeutic relationships, they are compelled to undergo a lengthy process of rethinking the entire course of the relationship. Customary ways of thinking about the therapist and the relationship are called into question because of the painful termination. For example, after a painful ending, patients may wonder whether their positive feelings for their therapist were genuine or existed only because they were projected onto the therapist out of a need to block out or disavow problematic aspects of the therapeutic relationship. One patient who came for consultation told me, "I need you to help me find and hold onto what was good about the therapy. I know that the whole therapy couldn't have been worthless. I don't want to lose everything just because it ended in such a terrible mess."

Doubt: Where Did the Problem Lie?

Many patients are left wondering whether the therapy might have worked if they had tried harder or been more persistent, or whether the therapist had a limitation in capacity that was not amenable to modification. One patient reported that shortly after his therapy ended in a painful impasse, he was left in a state of confusion and uncertainty, wondering if he should have continued meeting with his therapist instead of terminating. Not long after his final session, he happened to attend a talk on storytelling given at a local conference by James Fadiman, a psychologist.[9] He realized as he listened that one of the stories captured the essence of his current difficulty: distinguishing between an impasse or limitation that can be worked with effectively and one that cannot.

The story that had been told to students in psychotherapy training by a Sufi teacher was chosen as a response to a student's question: "Can you say anything that would be of use to us in our training as psychotherapists?" Without preamble, the Sufi teacher began to talk:

> Once there was a Master who traveled through the world in which he lived, teaching. He was accompanied by a loyal Dervish, an assistant and student, who had been with him for thirty years.
>
> They came one evening to a town in which a group of drunk musicians were playing (in the Islamic culture, drinking is a terrible sin, forbidden in the Koran, and those who are drunk are the most lowly and despicable of creatures).
>
> The Master told the Dervish to ask the drunken drummer to come to him. The Dervish complied with his Master's request, and the drunken drummer shambled over.
>
> The Master said to him, "Follow me!" and the drummer

followed, with the Dervish close behind. They proceeded to the harbor on the Mediterranean.

There the teacher laid his prayer rug directly on the water and stood on it, beckoning to the drunken drummer to follow him. The prayer rug supported both their weights, and began to move slowly out of the harbor.

As it began to move out, it was clear that the Master had finished his work on this earth, and was now moving on to a higher plane.

The Dervish, the faithful disciple, was left standing on the shore. "What about me?" he called out to his Master. "What about my service to you for thirty years, my studies with you? Why am I not on the prayer rug? Why is the drunken drummer on the prayer rug with you?"

And, the Master's voice appears to the Dervish and says to him: *"You Lack the Capacity!"*

Hearing the teaching story helped the patient realize that much as he wished that his therapist had had the necessary qualities to help him, and hard as he had struggled to teach them to him, the therapist had not been able to acquire that special, essential capacity the patient needed. The patient recognized that he had finally been able to terminate the therapeutic relationship when he was able to see both himself and his therapist with increased clarity and to relinquish his hopes and illusions, even in the face of his profound wish that their relationship could have been different. Making the finely tuned discrimination between a true limitation in capacity, resistance or inexperience on the part of patient or therapist that can be modified, or a mismatch in core issues of patient and therapist is a complex endeavor that requires patience, endurance, and active effort.

Because each therapist and patient dyad is unique, leading to a relationship that cannot be duplicated, the "problem" bringing about a rupture can perhaps most accurately be located, not in either individual, but within the relationship. The vulnerabilities of each participant have been constellated in the relational context, and the explosive interaction, like chemical combustion, brings about the collapse of the reflective capacities of the participants and the resulting rupture.

Self-Betrayal of Female Patients with Male Therapists

Female patients face a dual challenge from impasses and negative endings with male therapists. They have the challenge of coming to terms with the nature of the "good father" transference they may have established with their male therapists. Women who had a good relationship with their personal fathers often try to re-create a similar form of relationship with their male therapists. Too often what seemingly constituted a good relationship with their personal fathers required the unwitting sacrifice of their unique selves. Similarly, women who did not have good relationships with personal fathers may sacrifice their individuality in a struggle to win the approval and affection from their male therapists that they could not secure from their fathers. In both cases the relationship that is created tends to be so gratifying to the male therapist, who is happy to receive admiration in return for benevolent affection, that he cannot extricate himself adequately to label the dynamic that operates with the female patient. Female patients are analogously unaware of the dynamic in which they are caught. Feelings of self-betrayal arise when female patients recognize the collusion in which they have unknowingly participated, particularly if the therapeutic relationship collapses as a consequence of their recognition.

Vulnerability of Male Patients with Female Therapists

An analogous challenge faces male patients who have become disillusioned with female therapists. Male patients who have endured impasses and ruptured therapeutic relationships with female therapists have the task of facing the "good mother" transference that may have evolved and been enacted without awareness. They are at risk of sacrificing aspects of themselves to be "good sons" or "good lovers" in relation to their female therapists. Female therapists who have the need to be experienced as good mothers or as idealized women may unconsciously perpetuate their male patients' entrenchment in the role of good sons or lovers, unwittingly preventing them from developing other capacities and restricting them to a one-sided, imbalanced developmental path.

In our culture, men are socialized to be strong and independent, to separate from their mothers, to become providers for their own nuclear families. Consequently male patients are vulnerable when they allow themselves to depend upon therapists, regardless of gender, and to feel and express yearnings for attachment and love. If the therapeutic relationship ruptures when men have dared to be vulnerable, the men are at risk of being left with a sense of having been harmed and of being defective as men.

Sudden and Abrupt Disillusionment

Patients whose therapeutic relationships end in an impasse and rupture are inevitably disillusioned, not only with their therapists and with themselves, but with the process of therapy. *Even in therapeutic relationships that end satisfactorily, patients ultimately relinquish illusions about the capacities of their therapists and about what the therapy could accomplish.* Eventually, *all* patients come to an awareness of the inherent limitations in themselves and in life. Unlike patients whose therapeutic relationships end satisfactorily, those whose therapeutic relationships end in a rupture are abruptly and profoundly disillusioned—and sometimes traumatically. These patients are the ones who have a subjective sense of having been harmed.

Patients and therapists are left to ponder the assertion of Jeffrey Masson, author of *Against Therapy: Emotional Tyranny and the Myth of Psychological Healing*, that psychotherapy is an inherently flawed and dangerous profession.[10] Therapists may wonder why they were unable to provide the positive experience they know they offer to other patients. Patients who are therapists struggle with the deprivation they feel when they are able to offer their patients the qualities that their therapists lacked in relation to them.

Therapists' Experience of a Rupture

Therapists experience the full range of feeling states that patients feel: anxiety when the attachment bond is at risk, grief and loss when it ruptures, shame and a sense of failure as a therapist, anger at or blame of the patient for being difficult. Therapists are vulnerable to feelings of self-doubt and inadequacy, as well as to feelings of having been defeated or overpowered by their patients. Those who held out hope for healing feel frustrated, disillusioned, and in personal pain over their patients' suffering. Most therapists ruminate over what they might have done differently, or how they might have been at fault. These ruminations can occur periodically over the lifetime of the therapist. Clearly termination refers only to the conclusion of in-person meetings, not to the living presence of the patient in the therapist's psyche.

Therapists have a special burden of disillusionment, wanting as they do to believe that psychotherapy is a "helping" profession and that they "help" their patients. Therapeutic impasses and ruptured endings force them to confront the potential for therapy, and for themselves as therapists, to leave patients feeling harmed rather than helped. Facing the potential to wound that a healing profession also possesses is challenging and necessary task, one that each therapist must join in taking on. Rather than demonizing psychotherapy and conceiving of it as inherently flawed, as Masson does, we can instead face consciously the power to wound and harm, as well as to heal, that is true of therapeutic relationships just as it is true of all intimate human relationships in which profound attachment bonds form.

PART III

❖ Consultation to ❖
Therapeutic Relationships:
Toward Clarity and Restitution

CHAPTER TWELVE

❖ *Consultations:* ❖
An Overview

I'm worried about the consultations you're doing. Patients come to you in a put-together state and you don't see the primitive sides of them that have emerged in their therapy. When you intervene as a consultant, you'll overlook the need for them to go back to their therapist and work through the primitive issues that have come up. You'll support their leaving the therapy.

—Dr. B.

I think there's a danger of everything getting labeled a "therapeutic impasse" now that you've hung out a shingle that you have a specialty. It's too simplistic a label, too easy for patients to write off everything difficult that happens as a therapeutic impasse and to rush for consultation with it, as if you can wave a magic wand and solve everything.

—Dr. O.

The idea of you being out there doing consultations makes me very anxious. There's one patient I ended with in a bad place and I keep imagining that she'll call you for a consultation. I wonder what you'd think of me, if you'd believe everything she said.

—Dr. M.

I know that my patient would not have come back to therapy with me if she hadn't seen you. Instead of a rupture that would have left me feeling guilty and my patient feeling like a failure, we're going to be able to keep working together. I know we've both learned from the experience.

—Dr. J.

T his chapter describes the new territory that is emerging from and contributing to my investigation of impasses, wounding, and ruptures in therapeutic relationships: providing consultation to patients and therapists grappling with these predicaments. In the form of consultation that I will describe, the consultant occupies a unique position with

specific responsibilities.[1] The consultant has the challenge of determining the intersection of vulnerabilities and defenses of each
therapist–patient dyad and describing them to patients and therapists
in the context of available conceptual languages (theories). A consultant to therapeutic dyads (even when only one participant seeks
consultation) remains in contact with the patient and/or therapist
through the turbulent time when the relationship is in jeopardy. The
consultant thus preserves the continuity of the relationship even when
patient and therapist do not meet regularly. When the continuity of the
therapeutic dyad is maintained in this way by a consultant, the dyad
has a better chance of adapting flexibly to the needs and vulnerabilities
of *both* therapist and patient. By being related to and yet remaining
outside the dyad, a consultant's self-state is not in jeopardy, leaving her
freer to use capacities for empathy, compassion, and clarity of
perception. A consultant is in a position to name, without judgment or
blame, the obstacles that are impeding essential therapeutic work.
Patients and therapists are often able to receive help from a consultant
they cannot take in from each other while in defended, vulnerable
states. Consequently a consultant can help distressed therapeutic
dyads through times of impasses and wounding, enabling the
attachment bond to be maintained and the vulnerabilities and defenses
of both participants to be brought into conscious awareness and
worked with constructively. When therapeutic relationships have
already terminated in a rupture, a consultant can help patient or
therapist reach a conceptual understanding of what occurred and
facilitate a mourning process so that the person seeking consultation
can move on. When patients or therapists are concerned about the
viability of the therapeutic relationship or about a mismatch, a
consultant can assess the situation from an outside perspective that
encompasses both participants.

Consultation with these aims, in contrast to traditional consultation typically provided solely to therapists (indispensable in its own
right), takes the therapist–patient dyad out of a state of isolation and
exclusivity by providing, in the language of the Stone Center, "*an
enlarged relational context*" to support it.[2] A consultant to therapists
and/or patients in therapeutic relationships that are at risk takes into
account the strengths and vulnerabilities of both individuals (the
therapist-in-the-patient and the patient-in-the-therapist) and locates
the problem in the complex relationship of self and other rather than in
either individual alone. For example, rather than looking at transference and counter-transference phenomena predominantly as sequential, discrete responses within patients and therapists, a consultant in
this model of consultation emphasizes the intersection of patients' and

therapists' vulnerabilities and adaptive modes. A consultant working in this model also supports the expansion and increased flexibility of the relationship through focusing on the entrenched relational modes, self-representations, and areas of primary vulnerability that originated earlier in life and that have become engaged in the therapeutic relationship. The consultant is concerned with identifying how these vulnerabilities, relational modes, and self-representations have contributed to the therapeutic dilemma. At best, the consultant provides a safe place in which the person seeking consultation and the consultant are together able to take an impersonal, objective, "birds'-eye view" of the troubled relationship, finding a way out of the maze in which the therapeutic dyad is caught (or from which the patient has already escaped, confused and distressed, leaving the therapist and patient to assess separately what went wrong).

The consultations that I have been providing represent the evolution of a new service. Consequently they may be regarded as signaling or presaging the shift in process toward an expanded paradigm of psychotherapy—one that includes the mutual relational impact of patient and therapist in addition to the model of a professional with expertise and experience providing a service to a patient.

The consultations I have been providing have evolved to meet an existing but previously hidden need. As I began to be recognized as a psychologist with a special interest in working constructively with the predicaments of mismatches, impasses, wounding, and painful terminations, I began to receive requests for consultation from both therapists and patients. Some patients were worried that they were continuing to meet with a therapist who could not help them. Some were grappling with anxiety-arousing situations of impasses and wounding that threatened to bring the relationship to an abrupt and painful end. Others continued to be troubled about prior impasses and ruptures in therapy and wanted help arriving at a perspective that made sense of their experiences. As a result of these requests, I have continued to provide consultations and to offer presentations and workshops on the topic. The consultations continue to generate an ongoing source of information about impasses, wounding, and ruptures in therapy.

My work has compelled me to overcome personal resistance derived from prevailing attitudes in the profession and from anxiety about providing a service for which we have no existing model. There is a collective belief among therapists, regardless of theoretical orientation, that patients should not go "outside" the therapeutic relationship for assistance. A patient who involves an outside consultant in the therapy risks being judged as acting out, breaking the frame, or diluting the intensity of the transference. But I have found that the patients who seek consultation[3] about ongoing or prior therapeutic relationships do so, not because they want to be destructive to themselves or to their therapeutic relationship, regardless of how self-defeating their behavior may appear, but because they want to preserve the positive aspects of the relationship and learn about themselves and about themselves-in-relationship. When the therapeutic relationship is ongoing, their deepest wish is that it survive and be restored as a helpful one. Patients who seek consultation want help in improving that relationship or in shifting it back onto a positive track. When the relationship has ruptured, patients who risk seeking consultation want help in understanding what went awry, holding onto the valuable aspects of the relationship, and mourning its loss.

I have come to wonder whether the understandable anxiety that therapists feel when patients seek consultation has led to explicit and implicit sanctions that prevent troubled patients from speaking out. As therapists, we would undoubtedly encourage children in families to speak out when they are in distress, yet patients in therapy are often discouraged or only reluctantly permitted to seek outside perspectives. Therapists are understandably concerned about the integrity and skill of the consultant, about communicating to patients that they are "too much to handle," and about abandoning and rejecting them. They are also worried about being presented in a negative or distorted way and fear that the consultant will be "overly empathic" or taken in by the patient. Patients whose therapists seek consultation have analogous fears of being too difficult or of overwhelming the therapist, as well as of being pathologized by the therapist and consultant. The anxieties on everyone's part are understandable, but they can be examined psychologically rather than managed by foreclosing a potentially useful option. Anxiety may be disruptive to one's sense of self—in the case of therapists, to a sense of a competent professional self, and in the case of patients, to the familiar but problematic sense of self to which they are accustomed. Yet disruption of an established equilibrium is an essential component of change. Perhaps we might stretch ourselves as therapists by tolerating the anxiety and disequilibrium of self that the idea of consultation to distressed therapeutic dyads arouses in order to consider managing it by other means than maintaining distressed therapeutic dyads in isolation.

In addition to personal concerns that have arisen because I have been shaped as a therapist within our existing paradigm, I also have anxieties related to each request for consultation. I am always aware of the possibility that I might make a difficult situation worse, muddying the waters further. I am well aware of the need to be accurately attuned to *both* the therapist and patient, to understand their experience of the therapeutic relationship from within their subjective worlds, and to be sensitive to the relational modes that have become established within the dyad. I also have anxieties about the potential judgments and criticism that other therapists might direct toward my efforts, just as they worry about how I might view them, as the comments of therapists at the beginning of the chapter reveal.

But overriding these concerns is a conviction, based on personal experience, that we need to create resources for patients and therapists in therapeutic relationships that are caught in impasses or at risk of rupture. Consultation to therapeutic dyads has the potential to help avert, and work constructively, with traumatic impasses, wounding, and ruptures and to help patients and therapists reach an expanded consciousness of their vulnerabilities and defenses. As long as consultations to the relationship are prohibited by collective assumptions of the profession, directly or indirectly, many therapists and patients will have to struggle on their own. Those who do provide or seek consultation in situations of impasses tend to be silent, without a forum for sharing the knowledge and addressing questions generated by their efforts. Opportunities to work with core issues that impasses, wounding, and ruptures bring up pass us by.

In addition to the prohibitions operating in the profession, other resistances to developing new models of consultation for distressed therapeutic dyads crop up. Patients and therapists are ashamed and frightened of disclosing the details of the therapeutic dilemma with which they have been struggling because they know that individual vulnerabilities will be exposed. They fear that what triggered the predicament will sound trivial to those who lack an understanding of primary vulnerabilities. In addition to their fear of being judged for overreacting to trivial provocations, patients also tend to feel that the problems in the therapeutic relationship are their fault. Moreover, they worry about whether the consultation will be helpful, or will simply confirm that a failure has occurred.

As a consultant to distressed therapeutic dyads, I have been providing a service for which there are no established rules, although therapists undoubtedly provide such consultations on an occasional basis or in response to specific requests. Extrapolating from training, experience, and intuition, I have evolved a general approach to these referrals. Some of the consultations have been to patients referred by their therapists. Although the traditional attitude in the profession might regard such a referral as the therapist's admission of defeat, or as a communication to the patient that the therapist wants to be rid of her, my experience instead indicates that patients are grateful to their therapists for actively seeking a new perspective and for acknowledging that they, too, are caught in the predicament.

When patients seek consultation from me on their own, I ask them to inform their therapists when possible. Most patients have already talked about consultation with their therapists. I have, however, encountered situations where a patient asks for a consultation when the therapist is unavailable due to vacation or illness, when an impasse has compelled the patient to interrupt the continuity of sessions by taking a break, or when a therapist offers no opinion about the patient's choice for reasons that are specific to the patient or to the therapist's theoretical model. Although professional ethics and responsibility to patients requires therapists not to begin ongoing therapy with a patient who is seeing another therapist without the patient either terminating or arriving at a mutual agreement with the other therapist first, consultation is another matter. Patients are adults who in fact are free to seek consultation regarding their ongoing therapy whether or not they have the explicit permission of the therapist. But my experience suggests that the consultation has a better chance of being useful when the therapist is aware of it and not opposed to it.

Because therapists are apt to feel anxious or defensive when patients seek consultation, they may mistakenly interpret their patients' motivation in seeking outside help as primarily hostile or critical. But patients who take the dramatic step of seeking consultation typically feel anguish at the disconnection from their therapists, to whom they are deeply attached, and rather than seeking a way out, want a bridge back. They view terminating the therapy as a last resort, to be chosen only if all else fails.

Therapists, even when they support their patients' choice of seeking consultation, are concerned about how their patients will represent them in describing the impasse. The patients I have consulted with, even when they are enraged with their therapists, are also protective of them. For example, they may withhold the name of the therapist and accurately present the therapist's point of view even when it differs from their own. They are also able to zero in on the personal vulnerabilities of the therapist, often without having let the therapist know.

I have made one rule, which is that I will serve as a consultant, but I will not replace the therapist. If the patient decides to terminate the ongoing therapeutic relationship and does so, I will make referrals to other therapists if the patient wants them. This rule has helped avoid the problem of supporting the illusion that, unlike the therapist with whom they are having problems, I can be a perfectly attuned therapist without vulnerabilities, needs, or defenses that might impinge on the relationship. But despite the worry that I would be idealized as the perfect therapist while the ongoing therapist was diminished in worth, patients who have sought consultation have wanted to make use of me only as a consultant and not as an ongoing therapist. Their attachment to their therapists and their wish to find a way to preserve the therapeutic relationship have been unwavering, even when they have been profoundly wounded and are suffering acutely from grief and rage. Not one patient has expressed the wish that I could be their therapist. Instead, they have uniformly expressed appreciation to me for helping them return to the relationship with a new orientation or to terminate the therapy with a sense of clarity.

Most of the consultations I have provided last from one to two sessions, sometimes with periodic follow-up appointments on an as-needed basis. When possible, I meet initially for a session of an hour and fifteen minutes because there is so much pertinent information to convey. In addition to describing the immediate impasse, patients need and want to tell me the relevant aspects of their personal histories and the history of the therapeutic relationship, including how they have arrived at their present dilemma and what they have been trying to accomplish.

For some therapist–patient dyads, I have remained available as a consultant in a more open-ended, longer-term arrangement (specific examples will be presented in subsequent chapters) in which therapist or patient contacts me on an as-needed basis over a period of months. For example, when I have recommended structural changes in the relationship, such as an increase or decrease in frequency of sessions, or suggested new modes of managing relationship issues, the patient and/or therapist has sometimes found it helpful to contact me periodically as the work moves forward and the relationship shifts. In these situations, I function as someone who provides an empathic holding environment while the relationship is in flux. Other therapeutic dyads that struggle with recurrent phases of hopelessness, despair, negativity, or ambivalence have been helped through precarious times by the presence of a consultant who holds a vision of the value of the difficult therapeutic relationship.

I have found that one category of patients especially profits from having me remain in place, either as a consultant to the relationship or as an auxiliary therapist. These patients are women (and, in smaller numbers, men) who are recovering memories of early childhood sexual abuse.[4] Not surprisingly, issues of trust and betrayal in their ongoing therapy surface powerfully and repeatedly. By being available to the patient, I have served as an anchor or container for both the ongoing therapeutic relationship and for the patient, who at times has difficulty knowing whether the therapist is trustworthy and will help her, or whether she is unknowingly allowing herself to be abused psychologically because abuse was so familiar in her childhood. We are only beginning to learn from such courageous patients how to facilitate the process of helping them reclaim their frightened and injured younger selves, integrate unthinkable, unspeakable experiences into their conscious adult selves and restore lost faith in the value and meaning of life. Rather than insist that these individuals fit into existing theoretical assumptions about the importance of an exclusive relationship with a single therapist, we might do well to allow the patients' subjective sense of what will help them to shape our theories.

Creating an enlarged relational network of more than one therapeutic relationship for patients who have been abused as children helps not only the patient but the therapist as well. Therapists working in isolation with patients who have been abused often carry an enormous weight of responsibility as they attempt to respond flexibly to their patients' needs for continuity of contact. For example, therapists often stretch themselves to their limit in order to be available for telephone contact in between sessions or to maintain contact during vacation breaks. Therapists of patients who have suffered the trauma of early sexual and physical abuse, like the patients, may benefit from feeling held within an extended relational context.

I believe that an expanded relational network also helps therapists work with patients who are prone to collapsing into a relational mode in which the therapist becomes a dangerous, bad object, usually like a significant attachment figure from the past. Patients who cannot receive help from the therapist while in an aversive relational mode can sometimes allow a consultant to help them differentiate the therapist from other dangerous attachment figures, determine the source of danger in the present relationship, and create enough psychological distance to allow a shift to a less negative relational mode to occur. The presence of a consultant can also help patients take the risk of returning to a therapist even with their fear of being harmed or of inflicting harm.

Consultations to Patients

In the consultations I have offered to patients, I have served a variety of functions. In some cases, patients have come to me after a therapeutic relationship has already terminated in a painful rupture. We have worked together to arrive at a perspective on the areas of primary vulnerability of both patient and therapist that were activated and contributed to the termination. The consultation has allowed the patient's residue of difficult feelings, such as rage, grief, betrayal, guilt, shame, a sense of failure, and of being beyond help, to surface fully and be experienced within a relationship rather than in isolation. Intense affect states that are felt and shared within a relational context have a different meaning from when they are endured alone. Patients who have sought consultation after a ruptured termination have been grateful for the opportunity to make peace with the therapeutic relationship that they had hoped would be healing and reparative. Instead of being doomed to depression and despair in isolation because of the experience, patients have been able to learn from the problematic ending, and eventually to hope for a productive future therapeutic relationship.

An example of a consultation where therapy ended in a rupture is provided by a patient who came for help with her feelings of rejection after her therapist abruptly terminated the therapy. He told her he did not feel they could work together because the patient was "too resistant to the process." The patient acknowledged that she had difficulty talking to the therapist and that there had frequently been long periods in her sessions when she was silent. And though she believed he was correct, that the therapy was not productive, she found that being told it must stop, and that the problem was hers, left her feeling rejected and beyond help. In the consultation session, I affirmed the patient's subjective reality—that she had been rejected and blamed for the failure of the therapy—and suggested that she nonetheless try again with a different therapist because she still wanted help with the issues that brought her to therapy in the first place. I gave her referrals to therapists who I felt would be able to form a working relationship with her and who could tolerate periods of silence. I then functioned as a transitional person for her by maintaining contact until she made a connection to a new therapist. From time to time she continues to leave me messages about her progress. I continue to occupy a position in her psyche as a helpful person alongside the more negative, rejecting figure of the former therapist.

Although the majority of consultations I have provided have had a positive outcome, in others I have only been able to listen to the patients' experience and bear witness to their pain and suffering. For example, one patient came to me in great distress. The patient's health insurance no longer provided for psychotherapy, and he had to cut back from twice to once a week. The therapist made a small reduction in the fee to enable him to continue the therapy once a week. But eventually the patient's core vulnerabilities emerged and intensified such that once a week was inadequate. He was caught, unable to stop his therapy and unable to pay for enough sessions to manage the material that was coming up. The patient was angry at the therapist for encouraging him to remain in therapy without reducing the fee enough to provide him with more sessions. The patient felt left alone with the dilemma of being too attached to the therapist and too much "in the middle of things" to leave and yet unable to stand the long wait in between sessions. He described clearly and in detail his vulnerabilities and those of the therapist. Without a solution to offer, I could only listen empathically and helplessly to his plight and acknowledge that he had to wait until he had a clear sense of what to do. I believe that recognizing a patient's suffering and sharing the experience of helplessness and frustration serve a positive function, providing a relational context for a patient who would otherwise suffer alone.

In my view, receiving a patient's painful experiences and feelings of anger and despair has value even when the situation cannot be altered. Having a consultant serve as a psychological mirror and a relational connection in times of emotional anguish helps patients maintain a connection to themselves and to the possibility of a better future.

In some consultations, I have served as a transitional person while the ongoing therapeutic relationship was in jeopardy until the patient decided whether to stay or leave, or until a new therapist could be found.[5] For example, a patient who had left her therapist in the midst of a dispute over the fee nearly a year prior to calling me came for help in deciding whether to return to that therapist or to start with a new one. She was currently in the midst of a crisis around a job change, which involved making an immediate decision. We determined that she would be better off meeting with a different therapist because of the urgency of the life decision she had to make. We concluded that the unresolved issues with the former therapist were complicated and would take time to work through. Until they were resolved, the patient would be unable to make use of the therapeutic relationship with the former therapist for help with her immediate, pressing concerns. The option of returning to that therapist still remained open to her to pursue later.

Many of the consultations I have provided have helped patients in an impasse arrive at an understanding of it and return to the therapeutic relationship, averting a rupture. These consultations have been gratifying because the mourning process is difficult when a therapeutic relationship ends in a painful rupture. In one consultation, the therapist behaved in a wounding way that left the patient struggling with anger and disappointment. When she tried to express her anger and disappointment, the therapist became defensive and refused to yield her point of view long enough to hear the patient out. The therapist's rigid stance persisted for several sessions, during which the patient became increasingly hopeless about getting through the deadlock and fearful about returning to her sessions. My role as consultant was to encourage the patient to continue to express her wounded and angry feelings, but with an awareness of how vulnerable the therapist was in relation to them. My role with the therapist, in a separate contact, was to remind the therapist of how attached the patient was and of the progress she was making in struggling to include formerly disavowed aspects of her experience in the relationship. The patient had not recognized how powerful she was as she articulated her anger. Unaware of her impact, she saw herself as helpless and weak and the therapist as the strong one. Recognizing through my feedback how powerful she must appear to the therapist, and appreciating the therapist's vulnerability, although it was disillusioning, enabled her to return to the therapy despite her anxiety. The knowledge that if the impasse continued she could return for another consultation session made her feel less frightened of what might happen in the ensuing sessions.

In another situation, the patient and therapist had gotten into a struggle over the reduced fee the patient had been paying. From the patient's point of view, the therapist's suppressed anger about the reduced fee had surfaced and had been inappropriately expressed. From the therapist's point of view, as communicated to me by the patient, the patient had been manipulative and taken advantage of the therapist's good will. The patient and therapist were at loggerheads. The patient had called the therapist to cancel her next session, but at the time the patient contacted me, the therapist had not returned her telephone call to inquire why she was canceling or to encourage her to return. As we talked, we were able to clarify exactly what had been wounding to the patient. The patient was in fact willing to pay an increased fee and felt that she had taken advantage of the therapist. What was specifically upsetting to her was her perception that the therapist no longer wanted to meet with her at all. This perception was confirmed when the therapist did not telephone her to inquire about the cancellation and to urge her to come to her session. In learning about the patient's history, I found that she was considered the black sheep of her family, the troublemaker. An unspoken family myth was that if she would disappear, the family would be a happy cohesive group. This core vulnerability had clearly been activated in the therapy. Ultimately the patient decided to telephone her therapist from my office in the safety of my presence. She left the therapist a message describing the reenactment in therapy of her family situation and explaining that she needed some assurance from him that he was willing to continue to meet with her before she could come to her session. Later on the therapist called to reestablish the canceled session with her. The patient and therapist were then able to negotiate a needed shift—the patient was ready to pay the therapist's regular fee—as well as to access and work with her central vulnerability.

As time passes and individuals I have seen in consultation contact me to let me know how they are doing, I am able to assess the long-term effect of consultation and find that they often serve as pivotal episodes in the development of the therapeutic relationship. Recently I received a message from a patient with whom I met several years ago for two consultation sessions. At the time we met, she described the rupture of a significant therapeutic relationship with a female therapist. The therapist had abruptly changed her mode of working as she learned and adopted a new method of therapy. The patient had complained about the changes and repeatedly let the therapist know that the new method was not helpful to her. The therapist had given her a choice of accepting the new "rules" or of leaving. Distraught by the no-win situation in which she found herself, the patient left the therapy. As a consultant, I affirmed the legitimacy of the patient's needs (which most patients doubt because the therapist, by virtue of her role as expert, is perceived as an authority) as well as the no-win dilemma in which she had been placed by the therapist. I also supported as positive the ongoing new therapeutic relationship in which she was engaged. More than two years later, the patient left me a message letting me know she was doing well in the new therapy and in her life. I remain in her mind as a person who holds a positive view of her potential despite the devastating breach in the first therapy.

I have rarely met conjointly with a therapist and patient who are struggling with questions about a mismatch, an impasse, or the aftermath of wounding, although I have met with patient–therapist dyads who have terminated in a rupture. I have had concerns about intruding upon the dyadic relationship. However, a colleague has suggested to me that conjoint meetings with therapist and patient would affirm the mutuality of the therapeutic relationship, while avoiding conjoint meetings to protect the sanctity of the therapeutic relationship may protect an ideal—the therapist's authority and professionalism—at the expense of grappling with difficult issues.[6] Because therapists differ in their willingness and availability to participate in a consultation, whether in separate meetings or telephone contacts with a consultant or in conjoint meetings with the patient and a consultant, consultants need to formulate a plan based on the unique needs of each dyad. *The subjective meaning of the consultation* to the patient, therapist, and consultant, in tandem with the parameters or guidelines that I have outlined, determines the optimal course of action.

Some therapists and patients request a conjoint meeting with a consultant. Other therapists and patients want the dyadic therapeutic relationship to be preserved intact, but supported by the outer relational context that separate consultation to each participant provides. Other therapists choose to have no direct contact with a consultant but have no objection to their patient seeking another perspective. Sometimes the patient and therapist have different ideas about what procedure might best help the therapeutic dyad. I have tried to respond flexibly to the needs of each therapeutic dyad rather than to presume that there is one correct approach.

The format or structure of a consultation is less important than the function it serves in assisting patients and therapists. A major function provided by consultation provides is to enable patients or therapists to have the experience of being empathically held. *The experience of being accurately seen and heard, which is the essential first step in consultation with either patient or therapist, can occur either alone or in a conjoint session. Patient and therapist are better able to see and understand each other when both of them feel their subjective reality has been accurately understood.* Empathy functions to restore psychological equilibrium so that the next step of comprehending the other person's perspective can be taken. Therapists and patients often express a concern that a consultant will take the other person's side or only see one point of view. However, when patients and therapists are held psychologically by an empathic other, they are better able to shift to an empathic understanding of each other. Consequently a consultant who provides a separate psychological mirror for the patient and the therapist need not be thought of as an adversary of the other participant. Understanding with compassion the vulnerabilities and inevitable blind spots of the therapist has been an essential part of the consultation process to the patient, whether alone or in the presence of the therapist. Similarly, helping the therapist understand the vulnerabilities of the patient from a different point of view, whether separately or conjointly with the patient, has been an essential part of the consultation process for the therapist.

Naming the Therapist

Patients who seek consultation in situations of impasses are notably reluctant to give the name of their therapists for a variety of reasons. Some patients fear that they will be discredited if they tell their story and are aware that the same therapist who wounded them might be capable of helping others. One patient commented that the therapist was so well-known and respected that she feared others would doubt the validity of her experience if his name were to be known. This fear had also held her back from seeking consultation regarding the painful termination she had endured. Many patients believe that therapists will protect one another and blame the patients for problems in the therapeutic relationship.

Because patients who feel misunderstood or wounded by therapists are also attached to them, they often wish to protect the therapists even at the cost of blaming themselves. A pervasive sense of shame and failure often leads patients to take primary responsibility for the problem in the therapeutic relationship even though they may accurately perceive the therapist's contribution.

To patients, therapists are not ordinary people. Therapists have extraordinary power, just as parents have in relation to their children. The events that transpired in the therapy may sound rather ordinary to others, but to the patients seemingly commonplace interactions can have devastating impact. When patients attempt to describe the interactions that led to an impasse or wounding, they put themselves in jeopardy of being misunderstood and injured once again. This pattern, of patients being wounded and then having their reactions to the injury misunderstood, often repeats earlier experiences with significant attachment figures.

Another reason why patients withhold the name of their therapist is subtle. If patients name the therapists who inflicted the injury, they bestow ordinary humanity upon them. By giving the therapists a name, they render them into ordinary human beings that any of us might know or meet instead of into the powerful figures in the patients' psyches that they are. A common and analogous experience each of us has undoubtedly had provides a means of understanding the phenomenon I am describing. The experience is that of having a friend describe a parent in terms that make the parent seem monstrous. But on meeting, we find that the parent seems quite normal and ordinary, even likable.

Many patients, even when they feel injured by their therapists, do not want to tarnish their therapists' image and reputation. They worry that disclosing the vulnerabilities and limitations of the therapists might be as injurious to the therapists as what the therapists have done to them. For other patients, empowering themselves to disclose the name of their therapists can be an important positive step.

In consultations, I have not insisted on knowing the name of the therapist. I have left the choice up to the patient. When I have recognized or known the identity of the therapist, I have not had difficulty understanding who the therapist has been to the patient (as opposed to imagining the therapist I know in the therapeutic relationship). I have learned that each of us as a therapist, even with adequate ongoing consultation, no matter how well respected, well trained, or experienced we are, can behave unconsciously, either because of life circumstances or because of who we are, in ways that profoundly wound our patients. The sooner we acknowledge our potential to harm as well as help, the better able we will be to become aware of our unconscious behavior and to work with it, either on our own with patients or with the help of consultation.

Categories of Wounding Behavior by Therapists

In the consultations I have provided, I have encountered a variety of specific issues that trip patients into their realms of primary vulnerability and have organized them into two broad categories.[7] One category—sexual acting out with the patient by the therapist—clearly represents an unacceptable ethical and moral violation. However, even when patients have a clear and unequivocal rational understanding of their therapist's moral breach, they are nonetheless left with a residue of shame, guilt, and failure, along with despair and mistrust of being a participant in an intimate human relationship. In some cases of sexual violation by therapists, the patient is someone who has already experienced (whether or not she is aware of it) prior sexual abuse. The therapy failure obviously constitutes a setback of considerable magnitude in the patient's attempt to heal psychologically and to dare to trust again. Whether or not there were prior experiences of abuse, the experience of a sexual encounter with a therapist nevertheless becomes a pivotal event, a lifespan issue for the patient to work with. The task in consultation with these patients has been to affirm staunchly the therapist's irreparable violation, as well as to name the residue of bad feelings the patient is left to carry alone.[8] My role has also been to hold onto hope for the patient that a new therapy with a different therapist might be reparative and facilitate healing.

Other wounding behaviors by therapists fall into the second category of a grey zone. In the grey area, the therapist's intervention that caused the impasse cannot be judged as inexcusable from a legal or formally ethical point of view, although it may have been grossly incorrect, inappropriate, immoral, dangerous, or ill advised. In other cases, the subjective meaning of the intervention for the patient gives the intervention its harmful impact. An intervention that is catastrophic to one patient in the context of that patient's issues may be inconsequential to another.

Examples of impasses in the grey area include those that arise when therapists alter their policies, especially those concerning fee increases and cancellations for illness or vacations, or when they apply their policies in specific contexts without regard for unusual circumstances. Increases in fee or cancellation policies of charging for missed appointments, regardless of the reason or amount of notice, are generally established by therapists in relation to their personal needs. These policies, often referred to as "frame issues" because they establish the ground rules and contractual boundaries of the relationship, may be experienced by some patients, or other patients at certain phases of therapy, as intolerably harsh and punitive. Whether or not the therapist alters policy in response to the patient's needs, a secondary level of wounding results when the primary vulnerability underlying the patient's experience of the policy is not identified and explored. Efforts to resolve the dilemma of conflicting needs may then lead to painful and irreconcilable power struggles between patient and therapist. In these situations, the therapist is often caught in a difficult predicament: To alter the policy in a lenient direction leaves the therapist angry and the patient fearful of the therapist's anger, yet to preserve the policy renders the therapeutic relationship too unsafe for the patient to continue. At the same time, the underlying vulnerabilities are difficult to explore as long as the impasse continues in full force.

The refusal of a therapist to alter a policy for compelling reasons can wound the patient so profoundly that the relationship ruptures. In one case, a patient who missed her session because she had a miscarriage simply could not bear to pay for the missed session, nor could she continue to meet with the therapist who had added to her already intolerable pain. In another situation, a therapist charged a patient for a session she missed because she had an emergency medical procedure. Like the first patient, she could not tolerate being charged for the missed appointment. Both therapists were unwilling to set aside their twenty-four-hour cancellation policies, and in both cases the patients felt that their therapeutic relationships ended at that moment. Even when therapists subsequently modify their policy, the fact of the initial wounding may render the relationship unworkable. *For patients who have experienced a fatal wound, a necessary illusion about the therapist has been irretrievably lost too soon.* Patients who are vulnerable and wounded, and who need to start anew with a different therapist, are not helped by being blamed, criticized, or pathologized. The therapists they leave have to bear having been a source of wounding rather than a source of help, a difficult task for those who have chosen a helping, service-oriented profession. These therapists need support for holding on to hope that the patient who has left them in a wounded state, unable to remain in relationship to a person who has wounded them in an area of primary vulnerability, will take the exposed vulnerability to a subsequent therapist.

Other impasses in the grey area arise when therapists behave according to fixed theoretical principles rather than respond flexibly to needs that arise in the therapeutic dyad. Less experienced therapists and therapists in training programs with specific theoretical orientations sometimes cling to fixed principles rather than make choices based on the unique combination of patients' and therapists' vulnerabilities and defensive modes in a given situation.[9] But experienced therapists as well can adhere to a fixed idea of what constitutes a correct intervention. Most therapists want to avoid carrying out "wild analyses" or operating without conceptual guidelines. Therapists also differ, according to temperament, defensive styles, and vulnerabilities, in how flexible they are able to be in response to their patients needs. Therapists use their discretion in discriminating between patients' needs and their own and in making choices about the optimal therapeutic response moment to moment in therapy sessions. For therapists, the process of differentiating personal needs from those of the patient and deciding on the best response is a complicated endeavor. In practice, therapists rely on the theoretical perspectives available to them and on their capacities for intuition and feeling to yield the amalgam of subjective perception and accurate assessment that informs their interventions and responses. Because our profession has valued theory and thinking above the relatively elusive capacities of intuition and feeling, information generated by the latter capacities may seem to the therapists the less reliable and trustworthy path. The challenge in understanding the art and craft of therapy resides in articulating how therapists' intuitive and feeling capacities work together with theoretical perspectives.

In one situation, a patient had gradually withdrawn his initially idealized perception of his experienced therapist as all-knowing and helpful and had come to perceive him as a peer and an equal. The patient then felt ready to terminate therapy and hoped to establish a collegial relationship with the therapist. But the therapist, who had not kept pace with the patient's changing perceptions, continued to interpret the patient's feelings as resistance and to recommend that he remain in therapy. The patient, who genuinely liked the therapist, felt caught between his needs and those of the therapist. Consultation provided a place in which the vulnerability of the therapist—who was most familiar with and comfortable in the role of being helpful to his vulnerable patient but had difficulty relating to the competent, powerful aspects of his patient—could be named. The consultation enabled the patient to return to the therapist and express appreciation for what they had accomplished together instead of expressing only anger at the therapist's misperception of him. When the therapist was no longer under attack by an angry patient, and could see that the therapeutic relationship was so important to his patient that the patient had sought consultation to keep it from ending badly, he was able to let the patient terminate without interpreting the patient's wish as resistance.

Therapeutic impasses or situations of profound wounding in the grey zone may also arise when therapists are unusually vulnerable as a consequence of special stress in their lives. For example, therapists who are grappling with death or illness in their families are often self-absorbed and unable to attend empathically to their patients' needs. In one consultation, the therapist refrained from telling the patient he had suffered a personal loss and was not as available as he otherwise might have been. The therapist was influenced by traditional training, which advises keeping one's personal life outside the therapy. The rule of thumb is a necessary and good one; patients should not be burdened with the therapist's personal problems. Yet there are exceptions to the rule. There are times when information about the therapist's life is essential to explain unusual behavior on the part of the therapist to the patient, who otherwise can only imagine that she has done something terrible to provoke the change. Because the relationship—both "real" and transference—is the medium for change, there are also less clear-cut instances when a therapist's personal response furthers the therapeutic work.

In other impasses in the grey zone, an upsurge of anxiety about the course the therapeutic relationship is taking disrupts a therapist's equilibrium. Off center, therapists seem to keep tripping over themselves, making matters worse not only through their ill-advised responses but because they precipitate an abrupt disillusionment on the part of their patients, who were accustomed to admiring and relying upon them. In one situation, the therapist deviated from her customary reserved listening stance and taught her anxious patient a relaxation technique. The patient, taken aback by the shift in the therapist's mode of relating, questioned the therapist's judgment in suddenly becoming more directive, even though the technique was useful to him. The therapist, instead of remaining available to hear the patient's complaints or acknowledging that she had made a shift in her typical stance but that she had done so because she felt the shift would be helpful, became fearful that she had made a mistake. She feared that she had fostered an illusion in the patient that she had omnipotent powers. She told her patient that it had been wrong for her to teach the relaxation technique and said it contributed to the mistaken belief that she could "fix" him. Instead of resolving the issue, the therapist's explanation aroused tremendous anxiety in the patient, who, after a series of prior unsatisfactory therapeutic relationships, had come to trust and depend on her. The patient reassured the therapist that teaching the technique had not been wrong, and insisted that he needed to believe that the therapist could help him. The therapist, afraid to continue encouraging what felt to her to be the patient's idealizing projections, responded by insisting that she believed she had made an error by changing her stance and that it was wrong for her to contribute to the false belief that she could make things better for the patient. The impasse between them worsened until the patient finally sought consultation.[10]

Ordinary human frailties provide limitless fertile ground for wounding behaviors on the part of therapists that lead to impasses and ruptures in the therapeutic relationship. Therapists inevitably will misperceive patients, from the patient's point of view, or fail to be empathically attuned. Although most failures are manageable and may even be constructive, occasionally failures have a catastrophic impact because they wound the patient in an area of primary vulnerability. Then therapists often unwittingly create the secondary level of wounding referred to earlier because the patient's reaction seems to them to be so extreme that they are caught off guard and defend themselves rather than maintain their focus on the patient's vulnerability. Consultation in these situations gives the patient a framework to organize what occurred and sometimes helps to restore the therapeutic alliance. *But even if the relationship is preserved, it is always irrevocably altered. The patient has a permanently transformed sense of self and perception of the therapist.*

Consultation to Therapists

Most therapists avail themselves of some form of ongoing consultation. Because therapist and consultant may share a blind spot, a number of therapists have requested a single consultation session with me to focus on an impasse with a particular patient. The theoretical framework described in preceding chapters—the concepts of primary vulnerability, the secondary level of wounding, and the salience of the attachment bond—has proved helpful to them in understanding and working with the impasses. Looking at the dilemma with these concepts in mind has enabled the therapists to facilitate a shift.

In situations where the therapeutic relationship is in jeopardy, therapists are as vulnerable to the loss of an important attachment bond as patients and have analogous needs for empathy. Therapists are invested in feeling helpful to their patients, and failures with patients can be devastating to their self-esteem and to their pride in their chosen career. When therapists feel amply understood, like patients, they are better able to shift perspective and look at the impasse from the others' point of view. By receiving and "holding" the difficult feelings with which therapists are struggling—helplessness, frustration, anger, defeat, despair—I can often enable them to be more reliably and consistently present with their patients, thus minimizing the destructive impact of a secondary level of wounding.

Consultation specifically for a therapeutic impasse provides a place for standing back and observing the relationship from outside the dyad. When therapists are psychologically outside the predicament and reflecting on it, they often reenter the relationship with a new attitude that sometimes facilitates a needed shift. In some cases a new attitude on the part of the therapist has no immediate or visible ameliorating effect on the patient, but it allows the therapist to tolerate the troubled therapeutic relationship without discharging anger and despair in the session.

One therapist who came for consultation had been avoiding an angry encounter with a patient by making adjustments in response to her patient's urgent needs; for example, ending sessions a minute or two late, purchasing an additional clock when the patient complained about the position of the first one, and accepting cancellations without charge when her policy with other patients was not as lenient. The therapist began feeling both controlled by the patient's needs and resentful of some of the sacrifices that the adjustments required, such as loss of income. Finally the therapist refused to make an adjustment in response to her patient's request and charged for a last-minute cancellation. The patient was predictably devastated, and the therapist was angry not only at the patient's inability to tolerate her reasonable limit but at the patient's lack of appreciation for how responsive and flexible she had been. The patient, who can be said to have collapsed into the paranoid–schizoid position described by Ogden, far from perceiving the therapist as reasonable, accused her of being an unfeeling monster. The therapist, who had gone to such lengths to shelter her patient and to provide a reparative experience in the hope of enabling the patient to hold on to the therapist's "goodness," felt discouraged and hopeless.

The stalemate went on and on, with no relief in sight. No matter how the therapist framed the stalemate in the relationship—as a conflict between their needs, as a reenactment of failures in the patient's early childhood, as a necessary experience of wounding—the patient remained convinced that the therapeutic relationship was harmful to her. As the consultant, hearing about the predicament as it persisted, I became as hopeless and discouraged as the therapist. Ultimately the therapist and I had no choice but to accept the possibility that the patient, for the time being, was going to continue to perceive herself as the victim of a heartless therapist. We had to accept that the patient had a limited capacity to regard the interaction as a vivid and real experience of what she had already experienced with her mother, no matter what helping stance the therapist took. The state of acceptance enabled the therapist to endure the sessions with her patient without unbearable anger and despair, even though the situation from the patient's point of view did not change.

Rather than conclude in the consultation that the patient was beyond help, we broadened our perspective to conclude that the therapist was providing the patient with the valuable experience of exposing and living through her woundedness in the presence of a witness rather than isolated and alone. We adopted a long-range view and saw the patient as working on her woundedness across her lifespan and accepted the possibility that the therapist was providing perhaps one piece of this lifespan work rather than trying to wrap everything up in one therapeutic relationship that could encompass only a limited number of years out of an entire lifetime. A long-range understanding, although not the objective truth of the relationship, provided the therapist with a way to stay psychologically present and available in the difficult relationship with her patient. As our profession finds ways to balance the tension between subjective meaning and objective guidelines, we will expand our capacity to tolerate, sometimes for long periods, the uncertainty and doubt that arise from the inherent difficulty in distinguishing between needs and wishes of both patients and therapists.

More than two years later, the therapist contacted me to let me know that a shift in the therapeutic relationship had finally occurred. As the therapist put it, "the change occurred when I finally understood that I, in demanding that she come to her sessions without ever giving her a break (from her perspective always holding her accountable), re-created her feeling that she could never ask for anything without being punished." Although the conceptual understanding was invaluable, significant questions remained for the therapist: "In attempting to shield the patient from injury, was I unconsciously setting up the trauma that ensued? Is it helpful for therapists to give special treatment to vulnerable patients? Could we have avoided such a devastating impasse or was it inevitable? *Simultaneously striving for understanding and preserving the questions constitutes an ongoing challenge for therapists."*

When consultation with the therapist does enable the therapeutic relationship to shift from a troubled to a more harmonious state, we may not be able to know precisely which factor enabled the shift to occur. We may only be able to name the contributing possibilities: the usefulness of the conceptual frame arrived at in consultation; the holding environment that the consultation relationship provided for the therapist's strong feelings; the shift in attitude facilitated by reflecting upon the impasse in the consultation; the passage of time enabling a shift in the patient to occur. Ultimately, consultant, therapist, and patient are each left to tolerate a certain amount of not-knowing and to allow for the inability to understand completely and rationally—in short, the mystery—of all relationships.

The following three chapters present extended examples of consultations I have provided to patients and therapists who are grappling with mismatches, impasses, wounding, and ruptured terminations. Consultation to therapeutic dyads in the dilemmas of mismatches, impasses, wounding, and rupture, like psychotherapy, can lead to insight and understanding as well as provide a relationship within which change occurs. The following examples are intended to serve both as illustrations of how consultation can help and to convey directly the kinds of problems that arise in therapeutic relationships. These problems arise despite the best intentions, training, experience, ongoing consultation, and motivation of the participants and despite the serious efforts that patients and therapists make to work with them.

The examples in the next three chapters represent only one segment of a relationship in process and are not meant to signify that a permanent happy ending has occurred, nor do they imply that all consultations are helpful. Therapeutic relationships and consultation are not like fairy tales that have a discrete beginning, middle, and end in which the princess and prince live happily forever after. Even when therapeutic relationships continue on after an impasse or wounding, new dilemmas inevitably occur, although they can hopefully be traversed with the aid of knowledge gained from past dilemmas. Even when terminations are essentially positive, unresolved and untapped areas remain and life continually presents new challenges.

CHAPTER THIRTEEN

❖ *Working with* ❖ *Mismatches and Impasses*

Indeed, these patients feel absolutely caught in an insoluble dilemma. They experience not only the intense attachment to the therapist and a terror of abandonment by him, but also the rage experienced toward him. . . . These experiences reflect the regression to early traumatic interactions with a parent to whom one was attached in an ambivalent way, *without a balancing "other" from whom the patient could gain freedom to move* [emphasis added]. When one considers this constellation, it is not surprising that a first step in the intervention could be a consultation. This approach introduces another person into the treatment with whom the patient can establish a legitimate relationship. I am not referring to a one- or two-session consultation, in which one attempts to get another opinion. Rather the consultation might be considered as an intervention covering a period of a month or six weeks.

—Irene Stiver[1]

Some patients may experience the premature use of a consultant as a verification of the frightening fantasy that they have succeeded or will succeed in destroying the therapist. It is important for both the therapist and the consultant to clarify that the decision to pursue consultation is not exclusively a response to the intensity of the patient's hostile feelings. Ideally, the implementation of this therapeutic arrangement should provide enough distance from various affects to facilitate the patient's observing and integrative abilities. This clarification speaks implicitly to the patient's pervasive guilt and shame about destructive wishes and fantasies that he or she feels are not only intolerable and misunderstood but—even more painfully—unworthy of being understood.

—Steven Cooper[2]

Consultation to Patients and Therapists with an Unmanageable Fit

When mismatches become apparent, many therapists and patients do make mutual decisions to terminate. Therapists and patients also make separate decisions about the viability of a given therapeutic relationship. But some therapeutic dyads may be helped by the intervention of a consultant. Patients who are prone to doubt their perceptions of the therapist and the relationship and to blame themselves are able to present their experience to a consultant who does not have an investment in their continuing the existing relationship. The consultant, unfettered by even a rudimentary relationship with the patient, is psychologically freer to assess the dynamics of the therapeutic relationship from a different vantage point. If the consultant feels that the patient is in a therapeutic relationship that will continue to be difficult because of a fundamental mismatch, the consultant is in an ideal position to make a referral to a new therapist based on an assessment of the patient's needs. The consultant can also be available to provide a transitional relational context while the patient manages the termination with the current therapist and makes a transition to a new one.

The consultant can also invite the participation of the therapist both in assessing the mismatch and in making recommendations. Some therapists are relieved to have a consultant involved, despite anxiety about being judged by the consultant or having an outsider interfere. The therapist is spared the dilemma of personally rejecting or abandoning the patient and is not obliged to make a difficult diagnostic decision alone. Therapists who want to empower their patients and to avoid inflicting an experience of rejection or abandonment prefer that their patients make the decision to stay in therapy or to terminate and seek a different therapist.

Deciding to Terminate: The Case of Tina

Tina and Dr. V. provide an example of a therapeutic dyad struggling with a mismatch and impasse that was helped by consultation. Tina was trying to decide whether to trust her perception that Dr. V. was not the right therapist for her and terminate, or to follow Dr. V.'s advice and persist in the relationship. Instead of accepting Tina's view, Dr. V. insisted that her negative feelings toward him were related to the problems she was seeking help with. Therapists often unwittingly put patients in a dilemma, asking them to renounce infantile wishes for perfect caretaking and bear the realities of adult life, at the same time asserting with parental authority convictions about what is best for them. Patients often unconsciously put therapists in a related dilemma by imbuing them with authority and disavowing their own perceptions.

Tina, a married woman in her mid-thirties, and Dr. V., an experienced and respected male therapist in his forties, had been meeting weekly for eight sessions and were continuing to have trouble working together. Tina repeatedly felt that Dr. V. did not understand her. The sessions seemed to her to be comprised of one miscommunication after another. She felt she would be better off working with another therapist, but she did not want to leave the relationship too soon if the problem between them was something she ought to work on. She sought consultation to help her decide.

During the consultation, Tina, the daughter of a powerful, charismatic man and a mother who "lived through him and had no life of her own," heard for herself as she told her story the extent to which she was doubting her own feelings and perceptions about Dr. V. She began to relate her self-doubt to a lifetime of substituting the opinions of others for her own. In the context she described, Dr. V.'s feedback to her about her unwillingness to tolerate disappointment and negative feelings in the therapeutic relationship seemed not only off the mark, but unnecessarily judgmental and critical.

In the consultation session, Tina began to notice that her feelings of self-doubt and lack of confidence had actually increased in the two months she had been meeting with Dr. V. She began to feel a growing sense of certainty that Dr. V. was not the right therapist for her. His attitude toward Tina's feelings about the mismatch and his failure to appreciate that Tina needed to be free to make her own choice were part of the block in the empathic connection. In the language of relational modes, Tina perceived the therapy as yet another relationship in which she would have to be a coerced object in order to preserve the connection. She ultimately decided to terminate with Dr. V.

The consultation session provided an important psychological space within which Tina could attend to, clarify, and value her thoughts and feelings. She realized that she could profit from either decision. Staying in the relationship and continuing to bring up her concerns about Dr. V.'s capacity to empathize could be useful in empowering her to pay attention to and value her reactions. Deciding to leave the relationship could also be useful in helping her modify an established relational pattern of complying (being a coerced object) in order to preserve connections. Tina was relieved to gain a perspective that took her out of a no-win situation and enabled her to think in terms of which choice would be most useful. Empowering herself to seek consultation had given Tina an opportunity to "practice" being a person with needs and desires (a subjective object) in relation to me, using me as a developmental object in the service of her needs.

In the terminology described in Chapter Eight, we could say that Tina was accustomed to functioning primarily as a coerced relational partner, first for her father and mother, and then in ensuing relationships. Her decision to seek consultation represented a positive attempt to break out of a destructive, familiar pattern to find a new mode of being in relationship. Without conscious recognition, Tina was trying to find a way to lessen her sense of responsibility for maintaining relationships and was unwilling to sacrifice aspects of herself to preserve the beginning connection to Dr. V. The impasse with Dr. V. and the experience of deciding to leave him had actually been helpful to her.

Dr. V.'s experience exemplifies the deprivation that therapists suffer when patients leave because of a mismatch. Therapists in Dr. V.'s position often cannot know the positive use to which they have been put by their patients. They are left to bear the burden of not knowing, to wonder what they might have done differently, perhaps to manage their uncertainty by blaming their patients' choice to leave on the patients' pathology or on their own inadequacy as therapists. We might say that therapists like Dr. V. have been used by patients as coerced objects, an experience that for therapists may repeat a familiar but unfortunately wounding relational mode.

Deciding to Stay: The Case of Eileen

Patients who seek consultation because they have reached an impasse in an ongoing therapy that has been positive often want help in determining whether they should stay and struggle to change the relationship or terminate. Concerned that they are masochistically perpetuating an unhealthy relationship, some patients want a consultant to help them sort out their feelings and to articulate the nature of the impasse embedded in the patient's general question of whether to stay or leave. A consultant is also free to ask specific questions from an outside perspective: Has the therapeutic relationship reached the limits of what it can accomplish? Is the relationship ready to embark upon a new phase that requires a shift in relational mode? Is the patient struggling against exposing a core vulnerability or have the vulnerabilities of both participants been activated and are they intersecting in a problematic manner?

Eileen, a nineteen-year-old college sophomore, explained in a telephone call that she had terminated abruptly with her therapist in a power struggle one week before and needed help deciding whether or not to go back. Having canceled all subsequent sessions with her therapist, she was acutely anxious and asked for a consultation appointment as soon as possible.

Eileen had been meeting with her therapist since school began in the fall, six months prior to our session. She was paying for her appointments out of a generous monthly allowance from an inheritance, but she did not want her family to know that she was getting psychological help. She sought therapy because she had serious problems with procrastination. She also was experiencing difficulty socially and felt unable to develop friendships with her peers. She tended to withdraw and become depressed rather than to take risks and approach other students for company and contact. As a result she felt isolated and alone.

When she first started therapy, Eileen was hopeful about herself for the first time in her life. She felt liberated from her family, from whom she had virtually disconnected, and optimistic about beginning a successful, independent life. She began her sophomore year with a burst of energy and did well keeping up with homework and making friends. The therapist, as Eileen described her, was directive and focused on Eileen's management of her schoolwork and peer relationships. The therapist kept the focus of the sessions on schoolwork and social relationships and continually encouraged Eileen to take constructive actions rather than to sink into depression.

Eileen's initial burst of success and hopefulness about herself after beginning the therapeutic relationship did not last. She fell back into depression and became increasingly worried about herself. She was having suicidal thoughts, and reality seemed to slip away when she could not figure things out. Missing classes, sleeping all the time, and not eating properly, she was also discouraged by lack of progress in the therapy and believed that she should have been doing better by now.

The power struggle began in their last session when the therapist wanted Eileen to promise to call her if she felt suicidal. Eileen refused to promise. They argued back and forth until the therapist said she would not continue to meet with Eileen if Eileen refused to promise to call. Eileen, worried that she would have to pretend to feel better and that the therapist was refusing to accept her if she stayed depressed, told the therapist that she would rather stop than make a promise she believed was wrong and could not honestly agree to.

The psychological underpinnings of the impasse in which Eileen was caught began to emerge. Developmentally Eileen needed to feel self-sufficient and autonomous, but in the therapeutic relationship, she found herself drawn to depending on it to help her manage her inner and outer life. Her therapist was apparently assuming a dominant, managerial stance—a relational mode that was needed yet was also at odds with Eileen's wish to be in charge. Eileen wanted her therapist to be a less obtrusive developmental object.

Because I felt that Eileen was suffering acute anxiety about the loss of the relationship to her therapist, despite the conflict between her need to feel in charge and successful managing her life and her equally acute need for the therapeutic attachment, I hoped to find a way to restore the therapeutic relationship. I said that I believed that things were not quite finished with that therapist. Eileen had formed an attachment to her in the six months they had been meeting, and the therapist probably wanted to protect Eileen as much as to coerce her into an agreement to call if she felt suicidal. The therapist's effort to keep Eileen safe could coexist with Eileen's genuine despair and her need to manage her own life.

Eileen indicated that she might try to see the therapist again next week. But she still was unsure that she felt comfortable telling the therapist all her feelings. I offered to be an anchor for Eileen while she tried once again to work things out with her therapist. "Well," Eileen said, "maybe you could be a floating anchor." She asked for another appointment time with me for the following week. We made a time to meet and I offered to be available by telephone if she felt worried about herself in the interim.

The next day I received a message from Eileen canceling her appointment with me. She told me that she had decided to return to her therapist and to agree to promise to call the therapist if she felt suicidal.

Eileen's struggle to expand her sense of self-in-relationship—to allow herself to experience her vulnerability, anxiety, and need for help within a relationship without sacrificing her sense of autonomy and competence—was one source of the therapeutic impasse. Eileen and the therapist had enacted the struggle in their conflict over Eileen's promise to call if she felt suicidal. The therapist carried the vulnerability and worry, and Eileen carried the need for autonomy and independence. Eileen was able to make use of the consultation as a bridge back to her therapist.

Shifting the Relationship:
The Case of Josie and Dr. M.

Consultation is helpful to therapeutic relationships in which the patient and therapist need to negotiate a transition to different or more flexible relational modes. For example, the harmonious and positive relational mode that characterizes the beginning phase of many therapeutic relationships is virtually impossible to sustain. Even if patient and therapist manage to protect a positive mode of relationship, life itself often intervenes to disrupt the harmony. Most of us have a wish for stability and familiarity and a resistance to drastic change in relationships. In therapeutic relationships, this resistance can lead to a locked-in, collusive mode of relating that can become stifling and constricting even when it looks positive from the outside. In a different role from the therapist, the consultant has permission to intervene with a fresh perspective and can then leave the patient and therapist on their own again, free to continue working together in a new way. Consultation may not be successful in altering the primary vulnerabilities of either patient or therapist, or in modifying the nature of the issues that are constellated and need to be addressed, but it can assist in making structural changes that protect the therapeutic relationship from a catastrophic rupture. For an example of this kind of consultation, we will return to Josie and Dr. M., discussed in Chapter Two.

Josie, a lonely court reporter, had formed an intense, positive attachment to Dr. M., her therapist. Dr. M., affected by Josie's vulnerability and need for care, extended himself to her by making available appointment times at hours that eventually became inconvenient for him. When he attempted to change the appointment times and increase his fee, Josie was devastated. Her state of blissful attachment to him ended abruptly, and Josie fell into a state of murderous rage. When the impasse not only continued but worsened, Dr. M. brought up the idea of consultation. Josie grudgingly agreed to try anything that might help, and I scheduled separate sessions with each of them.

In the first session with Josie, I listened to her story. Because she was talking to a consultant rather than to Dr. M., she was not caught in the intense states of fury and hurt in which she found herself with Dr. M. She was able to talk about the therapeutic relationship in a reflective, calm manner, occasionally becoming tearful when she focused on the loss of their blissful, warm connection. She talked lucidly about her rage, acknowledging that it was destructive anger that only led to more problems instead of to reconnection. I told Josie that I would be meeting with Dr. M. and that I would meet with her again after that session. She left feeling hopeful that I might be able to help her restore the relationship to Dr. M. that had seemed irretrievably lost, along with her hope for an intimate relationship with anyone else.

In the consultation session with Dr. M., he confirmed Josie's account of their impasse. He added that he had never experienced anger as unyielding and intense from other patients. Everything he said generated more anger. He feared for Josie's life if her despair and hopelessness about sustaining an intimate relationship were to surface fully. Josie's anger and continued attendance at sessions were a relief to Dr. M. in the context of the suicidal feelings that Dr. M. knew would come up if Josie terminated the therapy. Dr. M. was acutely anxious over the possibility of Josie stopping the therapy.

Dr. M. also felt responsible for having let the impasse escalate out of control. In retrospect, he believed that he should have found some way to stop Josie from continuing to express her anger in ways that made interacting with her impossible. But he feared that if he tried to establish limits on her means of expressing anger in the midst of the impasse, Josie would become suicidal. Despite the difficulty of the therapeutic relationship, Dr. M. was committed to working with Josie. He knew that she had taken an enormous risk in trying to tolerate intimacy after living for so many years in a state of frozen isolation, and he did not want the therapy to end with a feeling of failure on both sides.

I recommended two changes in the structure of the relationship to both Dr. M. and Josie. I felt that preserving the increase in fee that Dr. M. had sought to establish at the beginning of the impasse was important because Josie's feelings of humiliation and inadequacy were heightened by her awareness of how low her fee was. I also recommended a shift in appointment time to an early morning hour that Josie could attend without jeopardizing her employment and that would be less of a sacrifice for Dr. M. than the evening hour. I stressed the importance of helping Josie build relationships outside the therapy in order both to alter her isolated state and to deintensify her relationship to Dr. M. by locating it in a broader context. Dr. M. particularly appreciated the reminder and permission to focus on Josie's life in the outer world in addition to the inner world of defenses, vulnerabilities, and adaptive mechanisms. He was relieved that I would recommend the changes to Josie because her rage, and the despair from which the rage protected her, were blocking her capacity to receive any suggestions from him. From the vantage point of consultant to the relationship I was in a strategic position to help Dr. M. and Josie implement these changes.

In a second meeting with Josie, I explained that I had met with Dr. M. and that I had some recommendations to make that would alter the structure of their meetings. I spoke to her about the recommendations I had discussed with Dr. M., explaining that the lower fee had enabled her to meet with him more often but that it also increased her sense of humiliation and dependency. The extent and intensity of Josie's anger might be reduced if her humiliation and low self-esteem were directly addressed. Because Josie was not in a wounded and angry state in relation to me, she was able to hear and accept the recommendations.

She thought about my comments and eventually accepted the structural changes I recommended. I also worked with her on constructive ways of expressing her anger. Recognizing with me how destructive her fury could be, she agreed to make an effort to cooperate with Dr. M. if he set limits on her mode of expressing anger. Josie and I then talked about the importance of building relationships outside the therapy. Josie thought that she would volunteer in a political campaign as a way to enrich her social world.

Because Josie could be self-reflective with me, and because in the role of consultant I could be more direct and active, Josie and I were able to talk about the defenses she had erected to survive in her family. The withdrawal that had protected her in her family had also kept her out of intimate relationships as an adult. In the therapeutic relationship with Dr. M., Josie had quickly relinquished these defenses when her yearning for intimacy was revived. Her self-esteem had suffered a blow when Dr. M., for his own reasons, established a different boundary between them. The wounding that resulted, and the fear that the possibility of intimacy was lost to her forever, activated the despair that Josie had been living with since childhood and that she had warded off by avoiding relationships and trying not to hope for too much. Josie now needed to rebuild her self-esteem, paradoxically by restoring some of the problematic defenses that she had relinquished, in order to tolerate the stress of relationships and the inevitable wounding they entail. Increasing the distance between Josie and Dr. M. by fixing their meeting at a feasible appointment time and at a higher fee would help to create a buffer from additional wounding during the critical time ahead. Josie and Dr. M. needed to rebuild their therapeutic alliance and restore the jeopardized attachment bond.

At the time of the consultation, both Josie and Dr. M. were relieved that a third party had intervened in a respectful, nonblaming, nonpathologizing manner to stop the downward spiral of the therapeutic relationship. They appreciated my availability to each of them, my empathy and respect, and were optimistic as they faced the rocky road of rebuilding their therapeutic relationship. Dr. M. believed the consultation had helped crystallize the issues with which they were struggling, giving him a conceptual framework to use in helping them build an expanded mode of relationship.

Dr. M. believed that he had been given an opportunity to work with a personal issue of his own. He could see that his difficulty setting limits and his fear of wounding a sensitive patient had caused him to overlook his personal needs in the beginning of therapy. Dr. M. had welcomed the opportunity to be a "good parent" to Josie, who had been a "bad child" in her family of origin. When Dr. M. wanted to meet at a more convenient time and to raise the low fee, Josie had been catapulted back into the "bad child" relational mode, causing Dr. M. to lose the "good therapist" relational mode that was satisfying to him.

One year after the consultation, Dr. M. and I had another discussion. I learned that Josie and Dr. M. had not been able to restore a stable, positive alliance. The therapeutic relationship, although it did not rupture when the attachment bond was in jeopardy, had continued to be rocky, with Josie continuing to fall into states of rage. Sometimes in their sessions Josie would attack me, losing sight of the positive function she felt that I had served at the time of the consultation. Other times, Josie would refer to me as a saviour and denigrate Dr. M. But in spite of the continuing storms in the therapeutic relationship and Josie's difficulty in preserving Dr. M. or me as individuals with both assets and limitations, Dr. M. believed that the consultation had been valuable. Changes were made in the structure of the relationship that neither could have made on their own while they were caught up in the impasse. Josie's life outside the therapy had improved substantially. She had expanded her social network and had made changes in her family relationships. The episodes of intense rage were interspersed with longer periods of alliance, and both Josie and Dr. M. were less fearful of the rageful states. Dr. M. had been better able to set limits on Josie's manner of expressing rage. Both felt less isolated with each other because I had contact with both of them and had experienced the intensity of their distress firsthand. My involvement with each of them took the dyad out of the state of isolation and placed it within a larger context of relatedness.

While the consultation with Josie and Dr. M., did not lead to a permanent happy ending, it was significant in preserving the therapeutic relationship, averting a catastrophic rupture, and in helping restructure the relationship in essential ways. Therapists and patients alike expect more of therapy than can realistically be accomplished. Therapists necessarily hold an idealized vision of their patients' potential and patients' reawakened hopes can exceed their reach. Consultants have the advantage of being able to intervene with a perspective that acknowledges both the limitations and the gains.

Shifting the Therapy to Another Level: Judy's Story

Judy's story provides an example of how a therapeutic impasse can serve as a painful but necessary occurrence for the therapeutic relationship to shift to a different phase. The shift allows for an expanded or altered relational mode between patient and therapist to be established, facilitating for the patient a new connection to herself. Consultation to the patient in this case enabled her to tolerate the anxiety and internal tumult related to relinquishing familiar modes of being with self and other. But when Judy and I first met, neither of us could imagine how the therapeutic relationship could continue at all.

Judy had seen her therapist, a woman, for nearly five years. The therapeutic relationship had been a complex but primarily positive one until several weeks earlier, when Judy had stormed out of a session in anger. When she called me for a consultation appointment, she had not yet been able to return to her therapist. Judy felt that her therapist, in attempting to stop her from leaving, had become verbally abusive. Judy was frightened and did not feel that she could safely meet alone with the therapist.

For the previous six months, Judy had been meeting once a week with the therapist, having cut back from twice a week. The therapist had wanted Judy to continue meeting more frequently, but Judy was trying to put additional time and effort into her career and insisted on maintaining the once-a-week frequency. Judy acknowledged that she also wanted to maintain a safe distance from the therapist, that more than once a week felt too regressive and intense.

One month earlier, Judy's father had died suddenly of a heart attack and her therapist, appreciating how significant the loss was, suggested adding an additional session per week. Judy experienced the suggestion as an insult to her growing autonomy and an indication of her therapist's need to keep her dependent, a familiar aspect of her relationship with her father. Judy's response to the invitation had been sarcastic, and the therapist had impulsively made a sarcastic remark in response. Angry feelings and words between them had escalated until Judy walked out. The intensity of Judy's rage and her therapist's angry response to it had frightened her.

Judy had gone home and waited for a telephone call from the therapist, who did not call. Judy feared that the therapist was afraid of her. After several days, Judy called and told the therapist that she wanted to return to her regular session the following week, but that she wanted the therapist to apologize for her angry remarks at the previous session.

The therapist insisted that Judy come into a session to talk about what had occurred. Judy insisted in turn that she could not return until she was reassured that the therapist was willing to take responsibility for her part in their angry interaction. The therapist continued to insist that Judy come to her next appointment. In the face of the therapist's refusal to apologize or to take responsibility for having been a part of the interaction, Judy canceled her next session.

Judy understood rationally that the therapist was trying to work with their angry interaction in the weekly session rather than over the telephone. But emotionally, Judy felt afraid of the therapist and unwilling to return without a sense of safety and the knowledge that the therapist would meet her halfway.

We agreed on the telephone that Judy would call her therapist and ask her not to give away Judy's appointment time permanently. She would inform her therapist that she was seeking consultation and that she would call as soon as she felt able to return to her sessions.

When Judy and I met, we connected rather quickly, largely owing to Judy's well-developed capacity to reflect psychologically on her thoughts and feelings. She was able to link her present state of mistrust and betrayal to the worst aspects of her relationship with her father. The fact that Judy had been able to feel safe and to trust her therapist had been vitally important. Their positive connection had enabled her to feel hopeful that her capacity to love and to trust, and to be loved in return, had not been permanently damaged by her childhood experiences. The rageful, angry father had been constellated within the therapeutic relationship. What needed to happen now was for Judy to align with the therapist in confronting the rageful father rather than to locate the rageful father exclusively in herself or in her therapist.

Toward the end of our session, we composed a letter to the therapist that explained the underpinnings of the impasse from Judy's point of view, described the reenactment, identified the rageful father that had surfaced between them rather than in one or the other, and included Judy's wish to find her way back to a positive alliance.

Judy delivered the letter to her therapist's office but received a telephone call from her in which the therapist stated that she would read it only in Judy's presence. The therapist added that Judy must promise her that in future sessions she would not leave the office before the end, regardless of the intensity of their interactions. After their telephone call, Judy contacted me, not knowing what to do.

I said that both she and her therapist were struggling in a difficult situation, each trying to set forth the conditions they needed in order to preserve enough of a coherent sense of self and of self-in-relationship to continue their work. I recommended that Judy meet with her therapist and read the letter aloud. I believed that the working through of the experience of extreme mistrust was an essential experience for Judy to have, and that the risk of being further wounded by the therapist was worth taking. With me in the wings to process with her whatever might occur in the therapy session, Judy had the safety net of our relationship beneath her to catch her should the impasse continue or worsen.

Judy did decide to go to a scheduled meeting with the therapist. She also made telephone contact with me shortly after the session to talk about what had transpired. The meeting had been tense and difficult. The reconciliation and restoration of positive feeling that Judy had hoped for did not occur. Once again, I encouraged Judy to return to meet with the therapist and to have telephone contact with me as needed after the next session. We continued this arrangement for several weeks. Each passing week saw no clear improvement for Judy. She did not know whether the therapeutic relationship had become abusive like that with her father, or whether a reenactment was occurring that was worth persisting through. I, too, lost a sense of clarity about what Judy should do, but I could see that she was not being harmed by the sessions and I believed she would eventually know what course of action to take. I functioned as a companion during an extended and difficult time of uncertainty and not knowing and as the holder of hope that clarity would ultimately come. But as the impasse persisted, I too began to wonder how the therapy could possibly continue.

Eventually a small positive shift occurred, and a glimmer of light appeared in the darkness. The therapist's tone of voice had seemed to soften, and she had acknowledged her feelings of caring and concern for Judy. Several days later, Judy telephoned and told me that she had made a personal breakthrough. She had understood at a deep level how she reacts to conflict in important relationships by leaving, if not literally, psychologically. Being able to meet with me through the extended impasse with her therapist had enabled her for the first time to maintain the tie to the therapist, albeit by a fragile thread, long enough for her to look inward. Judy had never before been able to see how her father's terrorizing of her had continued on inside her long after she had stopped having actual contact with him. Most importantly, she could now separate her father from her therapist and experience her therapist as an ally, not an enemy.

The letter Judy and I had composed together had served the important function of slowing her down long enough to manage the intense anxiety aroused by the prospect of peeling back layers of her defenses. The fact that I had held a middle ground and not given an opinion as to the value of the therapeutic relationship, yet had communicated that I was "with her," had been more valuable than she could say. Judy now felt that she could continue on her own to "look inside myself in the presence of my therapist."

We can only speculate about what the outcome of the therapeutic impasse between Judy and her therapist might have been had Judy not sought consultation or made use of the consultation in the way she did. But there is little doubt that the consultation helped her tolerate the anxiety, fear, and inner tumult of the impasse with the therapist until the therapeutic relationship could resettle on new ground. Judy was able to identify an aspect of her adaptive response to her father (leaving, literally or psychologically, in the face of conflict) that had become an entrenched, inflexible, relational mode. Judy's recognition of this mode enabled her to risk attempting a new response in the therapeutic relationship. Instead of continuing to put pressure on the therapist to be different, she was able to establish a different relationship to herself.

Extricating a Therapeutic Dyad from an Impasse: Andrea and Dr. E.

Therapists whose patients seek consultation necessarily bear the anxiety that accompanies exposing their professional selves and personal vulnerabilities to another therapist. The risk they take in persisting through a difficult time with the patient is augmented by adding a new, complicated factor—the presence of an outside consultant.

An example of this risk is provided by Dr. E., a therapist who reached an impasse with Andrea by agreeing to meet regularly with Andrea's stepdaughter as well as with Andrea, the patient. Dr. E. was initially reluctant to take on the stepdaughter, who was in urgent need of therapy and who had asked to see Dr. E. as a condition of moving in with Andrea, an important and positive move for both. Dr. E. ultimately agreed to meet with the stepdaughter because the importance of supporting Andrea around the important loving bond with her stepdaughter seemed to outweigh the complications that might ensue. However, a decision that initially seemed to be in everyone's best interest shifted in meaning once Dr. E. began a therapeutic relationship with the stepdaughter. Andrea found that sharing her therapist with her stepdaughter was intolerable and she felt betrayed by Dr. E. for participating in the decision. Dr. E. was in a quandary, not knowing how she could keep from rejecting the stepdaughter, who had also become her patient, and avoid derailing the ongoing work with Andrea. She sought consultation for herself and for Andrea, convinced she was exposing a situation that could not be remedied.

Andrea, who had made considerable gain in the therapy and who was deeply attached to Dr. E., was in a state of anguish. She was distraught over her perceived loss and desperately wanted her therapist back for herself. She also labeled herself a hateful and vindictive mother for not wanting her stepdaughter to continue a nurturing, therapeutic attachment to Dr. E. She was enraged with Dr. E. for not referring the stepdaughter to another therapist. Andrea felt as if all hope was lost for preserving the two most important relationships in her life. She could not give up Dr. E., nor could she ask her stepdaughter to do so.

I met separately with Andrea and Dr. E. at intervals over a period of several months. Because each was determined to persist in their struggle, I was able to maintain separate relationships with them and to help them bear the anguish of the ensuing therapy sessions. I also provided a model of being able to work separately with two individuals who were also in relationship to each other, like Andrea and her stepdaughter. With the support of consultation, Andrea's rageful feelings were contained so that she did not act on them by precipitating a rupture with either Dr. E. or her stepdaughter. She was able to use the consultation to initiate a much-needed discussion with her stepdaughter about their experience of sharing a therapist. Andrea had dreaded talking to her stepdaughter for fear of exerting pressure on her to take care of her (Andrea) by leaving Dr. E. Eventually the stepdaughter came to her own decision to transfer from Dr. E. to a male therapist in order to work on developmental issues more immediate to her present needs. The consultation acted as a container of powerful feelings and prevented wounding in the triangle of relationships (between Andrea, the stepdaughter, and Dr. E.) that would have left each individual feeling harmed.

Some time after the difficult consultation was complete and a disastrous rupture of the therapeutic relationships and the mother–stepdaughter relationship had been averted, I received letters from Dr. E. and from Andrea. Dr. E. wrote:

> As you can see from this joint note, the patient and I have been using your legacy as "the other" well. Probably the biggest gift that ensued from our consultations with you was our not having to lose the healing we'd accomplished in a vortex of past wounds that threatened to pull us into the bath. Instead, we've been able to use the near impasse as a springboard for a great leap forward.
>
> For myself personally and as a clinician it was a chance to heal the introject that claims that all damage occurring in the borderline interstices of relationships is my fault. And I've learned in the profoundest way possible that a secure attachment (something neither the patient nor I had as children) is worth its weight in emeralds.

Therapists who are willing to work with the personal vulnerabilities that inevitably become engaged in therapeutic relationships *in which the therapist allows herself to be affected by her patient* take a considerable personal risk. When the outcome is positive, therapists enjoy a transformative, healing experience that in turn provides the foundation for a healing and transformative experience for their patients as well. Patients who seek therapy have generally never had the experience of knowing that an intimate relationship with them could be of any value to the other person.

Patients who seek consultation, with or without the support and encouragement of their therapists, are also taking a risk beyond that of the primary therapeutic relationship. They are entrusting their most vulnerable aspects to an unknown consultant, daring to hope that the therapeutic relationship will be restored to a helpful mode. When the risk has a positive outcome, the reward can be immeasurable. Andrea's letter conveys both the enormity of the venture she embarked on in seeking consultation and the inestimable benefits:

> Even though I cherish all that has come from your help, letting you know out loud is yet another terrifying, painful and exciting step in the transformation in which you've played a vital role. Writing this now requires the same kind of leap of faith I took in talking with you when we met.
>
> All of my life I've been taught to hide feelings of caring and to be ashamed of them. The point I had gotten to when I met you was that I would lose the two people [her therapist and stepdaughter] most important to me if I continued to hide. I thank you for being a woman of compassion and integrity with whom I could dare to try out a different way—to allow caring to win instead of the abyss of isolation, fear, and hatred.
>
> I still have raging battles within myself about caring and trusting and allowing me to be myself. But I now also have hope and joy and people I love in my life. I hope that you will feel free to use anything of the experience [the three of us had] which would be of value in helping others nourish the caring. I would find it a fitting tribute to the triumph of the human spirit over the confines of the darkness.

*   *   *   *   *

Under the stress of therapeutic impasses, therapists' capacity to maintain the therapeutic stance that helps patients can be temporarily lost or diminished. Under stress therapists tend to have a diminished capacity to heed the subjective reality of the patient when it differs from their own. Losing their capacity for elasticity of perspective, they slip into acting as if there were only one reality, or as if the reality of the therapist is the correct perspective. When patients continue to feel misunderstood, they struggle to maintain their point of view and fight to be heard and seen by the therapist. Their fight to be seen and heard is often positive even if it is unpleasant for therapists. Patients frequently become patients in the first place because they have been overly compliant and reactive to the needs of others instead of maintaining a connection to their own needs and desires.

Therapists under the stress of a therapeutic impasse or wounding tend to lose sight of the strength of the patient's attachment bond to them, particularly in the face of a patient's rage or withdrawal or other apparent attempts to annihilate the relationship. In every case I have encountered as a consultant, the patients have not wanted the relationship to end or to end badly, no matter how they behave or declare that they feel. Therapists who can remember, even under duress, that their patients are deeply attached to them, regardless of how the patients behave, are less apt to be wounded in a way that impels them to retaliate in anger or to withdraw. Both patient and therapist then have the opportunity of looking at their established modes of being in relationship that are self-defeating and to come to an understanding of their origins.

Therapists in a stressful therapeutic relationship tend to lose sight of or to emphasize unduly (thus underestimating the current relational impasse) the early developmental matrix (or transference context) of the therapeutic dilemma and the specific vulnerability that has been activated in both patient and therapist. Most patients are already aware that their therapist's personal issues have been activated, and they often know quite specifically what the issues are. Most patients in situations of impasses and wounding are struggling to tolerate an awareness of the therapist's vulnerabilities because it forces them to relinquish former cherished illusions that the therapist is psychologically stronger.

Therapists under stress often rigidly apply theoretical guidelines rather than tolerate the chaos and confusion that dilemmas in therapeutic relationships bring about. But those who are able to weave together rationally based theoretical principles (logos) with their intuitive-feeling capacities are more likely to maintain an alliance with patients that can enable seemingly unresolvable dilemmas to be worked with constructively.

As the profession of psychotherapy begins to balance the predominating emphasis on rational understanding and clarity with the less familiar realms of intuition and feeling, states of impasse and wounding and the painful emotions and uncertainty that they generate may be tolerated to an increasing degree within the therapist–patient dyad. Therapists and patients will then have a greater capacity to endure the dark times that are inevitable in relationships as they are in life. Therapeutic relationships have the potential to help patients (and therapists) include, along with inevitable times of suffering, the experiences that bring about what we speak of as the joy in living. They have the potential to enable patients and therapists to experience the moments of mutual and intimate attachment and connection that we speak of as the joy in loving.

The next chapter contains two examples of impasses where patients and therapists were wounded in their areas of primary vulnerability. Because secondary levels of wounding occurred, the therapeutic relationship was jeopardized, increasing the anxiety of both participants in the relationship. In one case the wounding was able to be worked through. In the second case, the relationship ultimately terminated, but a painful rupture was successfully averted.

CHAPTER FOURTEEN

❖ Working with Wounding ❖ in Areas of Primary Vulnerability

The therapist who allows the patient to establish other relationships, without jeopardizing his, prevents a repetition of the patient's relationships in a family where one person was over idealized, while the other was absent or devalued. With a second person introduced, the patient does not feel all her eggs are in one basket, and is freer to make attachments with permission and then can move out of the regressive positions to further growth and development in the course of psychotherapy.

—IRENE STIVER[1]

In some cases [in which a consultant/cotherapist was involved] the patient was able to continue to see her original therapist and the "cotherapist" became less important over time; in other cases, the introduction of the "cotherapist" made it possible for the patient to leave her original therapist with less pain and significantly less regressive behaviors. In fact, the latter resolution seems more common. The concern that such an intervention would simply intensify the regression with the encouragement of splitting, etc., has not been justified in my experience.

—IRENE STIVER[2]

Working through the Wounding and Terminating: Pat's Story

Consultation to either a patient and therapist in separate meetings, or to the patient alone, can help the therapeutic dyad negotiate the impasse that arises when the patient is wounded by the therapist in an area of primary vulnerability. Patients who are wounded, especially when the therapist defensively minimizes the nature of the wounding, are often plunged into an abyss of confusion and despair from which they may have difficulty extricating themselves. The relationship that they had hoped would help them recover from past traumatic disillusionment has suddenly and unexpectedly repeated the past trauma and then failed to relieve the patient's distress. From the patients' perspective, therapists abruptly shift from being positive developmental objects to being dangerous ones. A stalemate results in which patients are impaled by the conflict between wanting to restore the lost attachment to positive objects and wishing they could flee from the dangerous objects that have repeated a trauma. Therapists are caught in a corresponding dilemma of wishing to restore the prior positive relational mode with their patients yet needing not to deny the impact of the wounding that has occurred. Consultation with another therapist can, as Stiver's comments suggest, be liberating for the patient and a relief for the therapist.

The following case of Pat and Dr. C. provides an example of the wounding of the patient in the realm of primary vulnerability. With the help of consultation, the resulting disillusionment with the therapist ultimately led to a planned termination rather than to the abrupt severing of the relationship that might otherwise have occurred. Instead of being left alone and adrift in a state of confusion and uncertainty, therapist and patient had some opportunity to reflect together about the accomplishments and limitations of their relationship.

When she came to see me for a consultation, Pat was a divorced legal secretary with no children. She had been profoundly wounded by Dr. C., a female therapist whom she had been seeing for three years. In Pat's words, her therapist had "betrayed her in a terrible way." Although Pat hoped to find some way to get through the betrayal, she was concerned that her therapist would not be able to meet her halfway.

Pat, who had been molested by her father in childhood and subsequently was drawn into a sexual relationship with a male therapist, had carefully chosen Dr. C., a woman whom she had come to like and to trust. Dr. C. had been helpful to her thus far in working on her relationship with her parents. Dr. C. also understood Pat's issues of trust and betrayal with the therapist who began an affair with her. The devastating incident with Dr. C. had occurred several days before seeking a consultation with me.

Pat had gone with a friend to a restaurant for lunch. By chance, Pat heard Dr. C.'s voice coming from a booth in the next aisle. The person Dr. C. was sitting with seemed to be a therapist, too. They were apparently talking about therapists who have sexual relationships with their patients. Dr. C. was telling the other person about a patient she was currently seeing who had been seduced by her therapist. Pat soon realized that Dr. C. was talking about her.

Pat reported that it was bad enough that the therapist was breaking confidentiality and talking about her, especially in a public place, but it was the casual way Dr. C. talked that was most wounding.

Pat managed to sit through the lunch with her friend but was unable to share what was wrong. When she finally returned home, she called Dr. C. immediately to tell her what had happened and to ask if she could have an extra appointment. Dr. C. returned Pat's call several hours later—an eternity of waiting for Pat—and was shocked to have been overheard by Pat. She did not deny that she had talked about Pat in the restaurant and apologized for her breach of confidentiality. She made an appointment time for Pat the next day.

Dr. C.'s initial response on the telephone reassured Pat that they might be able to carry on. She felt that Dr. C. was aware of the magnitude of the betrayal, willing to apologize and take responsibility for her behavior. But when Pat arrived for her extra session, she found that Dr. C. had pulled herself together and was acting as if nothing of great consequence had occurred. Dr. C. referred to Pat's overhearing her conversation as an "unfortunate incident" and said that she and Pat needed to get on with the work of the therapy. She added that Pat was displacing her anger at the therapist who had sexually abused her onto Dr. C., who was her ally. But Pat felt that the incident had been more than a mere incident to her and that Dr. C. was no longer only her ally. Dr. C. was now an ambiguous person: an ally who could be dangerous.

Pat told Dr. C. that she did not want to pay for the extra appointment because it was Dr. C.'s fault that she had needed it. If Dr. C. had not breached the confidentiality of the therapeutic relationship, Pat would not have needed an extra session. But Dr. C. would not agree to waive the fee. Pat knew she had made an issue over paying for the extra session because Dr. C. had not fully appreciated the extent of the betrayal that Pat was experiencing.

Pat's main concern was her uncertainty that she could recover from the betrayal and stay in therapy with Dr. C. She had thought of Dr. C. as solid and respectable, completely different from the first therapist, who had been unable to preserve the professional boundaries of the relationship. Now she was not sure she could ever trust Dr. C. or anybody else ever again. Although she presented her dilemma to me in a contained, reflective manner, the depth of her hurt and pain at the loss of who Dr. C. had been to her was palpable.

I affirmed to Pat that Dr. C. was a therapist whom she had felt good about and who had helped her, and who had also betrayed her in a terrible way. In overhearing Dr. C. talk about her to a colleague, Pat had been wounded in the realm of her primary vulnerability, specifically around her deepest issues—trust and betrayal, a fact that gave what happened between Pat and Dr. C. a special intensity and meaning. I explained to Pat that when a therapist wounds or retraumatizes a patient in an area of primary vulnerability, a special set of consequences follows.

The first consequence was that the person whom Dr. C. had been to Pat, the figure she represented in Pat's psyche, had been permanently altered. Dr. C. could never be the altogether trustworthy person in Pat's psyche that she once had been. The illusion of perfect safety in the relationship had been lost. The question now was whether the relationship could be restored with the mutual understanding that it had been permanently altered.

The loss of the illusion of Dr. C. as perfectly trustworthy left Pat with the task of mourning the loss of the former harmonious relationship. Whether she could do the grieving with Dr. C., in the context of an ongoing relationship, and whether Dr. C. could acknowledge the permanence of what had been lost for Pat, I did not know. But wherever Pat accomplished it, the grieving was necessary because she had suffered a major loss in an important new relationship, one she dared hope would be different from the others.

Pat did not want to disclose her therapist's name nor did she want me to have contact with her. She wanted me to remain in place as her ally. I recommended that Pat continue to talk about her feelings and about the significance of the restaurant conversation with Dr. C. in a direct way, rather than through the argument over the payment for the extra session. I told Pat that I believed Dr. C. had the challenge of tolerating the guilt and shame arising from the breach of confidence, rather than either passing the incident off as trivial or making Pat into a borderline patient who was unable to tolerate disruptions. I acknowledged that Dr. C. would undoubtedly be defensive. Pat was going to have to tolerate seeing Dr. C.'s vulnerabilities—a difficult task for any patient.

Pat told me that she saw what I meant about her not wanting to face Dr. C.'s vulnerability. When she had left Dr. C.'s office after their session the previous week, Pat had felt a strong impulse to protect Dr. C. and make her feel better. She wanted to tell Dr. C. that she could see how hard this experience was for her, but she stopped herself. Pat realized that she did not want to take care of Dr. C. the way she took care of her mother when her father went on one of his angry alcoholic rampages. In talking to me, Pat now thought that her wish to avoid taking care of Dr. C. by comforting her and making it easy for her to "forget" about the restaurant incident was healthy and positive rather than a negative attempt to avoid feelings about the therapist who had sexually abused her or to destroy the relationship with Dr. C.

Pat decided to try to stay with her feelings and assert her needs despite Dr. C.'s resistance. She asked for another session with me, and we made an appointment for the following week, after her next scheduled appointment with Dr. C. Knowing that we had another appointment time scheduled was reassuring to Pat, giving her a place to come in case her session with Dr. C. made things worse rather than better. Dr. C. would have to face the challenge of recognizing the full extent of the wounding that had occurred, repairing the rupture it had brought about, and establishing a new relationship with Pat without the illusions attached to it that the old one had. Neither Pat nor I knew if Dr. C. would be able to meet this challenge.

Pat arrived ten minutes early for our follow-up consultation and began the session by telling me that she was doing much better. The consultation with me had been helpful, although she had also had a hard and intense week. Dr. C. had been "tripping over herself," which was distressing for Pat, but Dr. C. was not being defensive the way she had been the first day. For Pat, the experience with Dr. C. brought together all of her feelings surrounding the sexual abuse by her father and the first therapist and the abandonment and lack of protective intervention by her mother. She saw that I had been in the position of the strong, good mother who could support her in standing up for herself—a new developmental object. She had been able to return to her sessions with Dr. C. and firmly and clearly assert herself.

Pat realized that seeing me for consultation had been helpful because I had believed her—serving as the witness she never had—when she told me that something terrible had happened when Dr. C. talked about her in the restaurant. I had acknowledged that something significant had occurred, whereas when she had confronted her first therapist about his sexual abuse, he had denied that it had been abuse and had asked her to forget about it. Although Dr. C., when confronted, had at first been apologetic, she then attempted to brush off the incident as trivial and had interpreted Pat's feelings as displaced anger.

Pat went on to say that not only was her experience with me different from those with her mother, father, first therapist, and Dr. C., but also that I had not completely condemned Dr. C. What I had said to her about Dr. C.'s both helping her and hurting her had been useful. Pat had been able to feel that she did not have to choose between seeing Dr. C. as all good or all bad. In the session that took place right after the restaurant incident, Dr. C. was not remorseful—she was completely defended, talking about how Pat should not let the mishap wipe out all the good work they had accomplished. But I had made room to look at the possibility that Dr. C. might be defensive and that her defensiveness did not make what she had done trivial.

Pat reported that her perception of Dr. C. had changed drastically since the incident of betrayal in the restaurant. She told me that when she first started seeing Dr. C., Pat had thought of her as older and had not wanted to know her age. Since the restaurant incident, Pat realized that Dr. C. was actually not much older than she was. The shift in Pat's perception of her age was a metaphor for the relinquishing of illusions about Dr. C.

I commented in response that patients sometimes have to help their therapists, teaching them how to be helpful. Most patients look to therapists to provide help as experts and do not expect to have to be their teacher. I also explained that seeing her therapist more realistically, without the filter of reawakened yearnings for a perfect caretaker, was part of healthy psychological development. Just as children grow up, whether they want to or not, and need to leave home, patients have a similar experience with therapists. Pat had not had a good separation from her family when she rushed into marriage as a way to separate. I hoped she would be able to have a different experience with Dr. C., one in which she could gradually come to feel that she had outgrown her and could move on.

Pat said she had been wondering whether she should cut back to once a week and asked me what I thought. I suggested that Pat and Dr. C. discuss why Pat wanted to cut back just now—whether it was out of fear of being injured again, or because Pat was withdrawing in anger, or because she genuinely felt ready to move away.

Three weeks later, Pat called again and came in for an appointment. Her work with Dr. C. was not going well. The rupture over the restaurant mishap had been worked through, but Pat continued to feel that she had outgrown the relationship and wanted to meet with a more experienced therapist. These feelings persisted even though she also knew she felt quite fond of Dr. C. and appreciated her good intentions and efforts to be helpful.

I helped Pat see that she was having a new experience of being able to find authority in herself, to express her needs directly, and to complain about how they were not being met. Right now it seemed as if all the competence and power were located in Pat and that Dr. C. did not have any. Before the crisis in the restaurant, the balance was in the opposite direction. Pat was dependent on Dr. C. and saw her as a pillar of strength. It made sense to me that Pat give herself time to see if she was ready to move on or if she was in a phase of an important shift in the balance of the relationship.

Pat contacted me periodically over the next six months as she continued to struggle with her disillusionment in Dr. C. and with her quandary over whether or when to end the relationship. During the six months, she became increasingly able to express her needs and feelings to Dr. C. At the same time, as a consequence of the catalyst that the incident in the restaurant provided, she came to recognize Dr. C.'s limitations and to realize that she had gone as far as she could in that therapy. Eventually Pat planned and carried out a termination.

Considerable psychological work happened in the period of therapy that followed the restaurant incident. The periodic consultation sessions played a role in enabling such work to happen. Pat was able to recover from the trauma of the restaurant betrayal, to change her perception of herself and Dr. C. in the context of their relationship rather than to have an abrupt and traumatic ending, and to tolerate the disappointment and relinquishing of illusions that are part of every therapeutic relationship. Dr. C. was able to limit the extent of the secondary level of wounding and thus preserve the therapeutic attachment after the restaurant incident, in part because Pat used the consultation with me to help them both.

Working through the Wounding and Continuing with Therapy: Carol and Dr. G.

Consultation can provide a transitional holding environment for both therapist and patient when they have been wounded by each other in the area of their primary vulnerabilities. The acknowledgment of the wounding and the affirmation of the feelings that an outside participant can provide enable patient and therapist to restore a sense of self and other. From a position of coherence and clarity, patient and therapist can reengage with each other with renewed perspective and the therapeutic relationship, although irrevocably altered, can continue. If we conceptualize the therapeutic relationship as having been stretched to the breaking point like a rubber band pulled to its limit, the consultation serves to hold the relationship at each end of the stretched portion, taking the pressure off, until the rubber band can relax into a new shape.

Carol, a single woman in her late thirties, had been in therapy with Dr. G., a woman in her late forties, for three years. Carol, whose father had died when she was ten and whose mother had been overwhelmed and unavailable, was a successful attorney but lacked intimate and enduring relationships.

Carol began psychotherapy with Dr. G. hoping to work on her fear of trusting others. Over the next three years a strong attachment to Dr. G. developed. But in the third year of therapy, fate drastically changed the course of Carol's life. She was diagnosed with breast cancer and underwent a mastectomy, followed by a course of chemotherapy.

The illness made it impossible for Carol to maintain her customary reserve. She found herself relying on others out of necessity and was unable to hide her grief and terror from them. Carol's formerly distant relationships with her co-workers, male and female, and with her mother, stepfather, and siblings also changed dramatically. She was assured that she would not lose her job and was given whatever leeway she needed for her caseload and time off. People responded to her lovingly and generously and Carol responded in kind.

During this period her attachment to Dr. G. deepened. Dr. G. visited Carol in the hospital after the surgery and was psychologically and emotionally present as the ordeal of chemotherapy was under way. Carol found herself feeling love for Dr. G. and for her friends, a new openness that was both wonderful and terrifying.

Three months after the surgery and well into the chemotherapy, an incident occurred that threatened to destroy not only the relationship between Carol and Dr. G., but the entire foundation of trust and care they had established together. Carol developed a physical reaction that alarmed her after one of her chemotherapy treatments. She received instructions from her physician on how to handle the physical effects, but psychologically her anxiety persisted. In a panic, she telephoned Dr. G.

Dr. G. did not return Carol's call that day or evening, an eventuality that in itself was upsetting, but they had spoken about how Dr. G. might not be able to return telephone calls immediately. Carol called a friend instead and waited until the next day. Dr. G. still did not call. Carol then left another message and once again waited for a response. That evening, Dr. G. finally called back. Carol noticed that her therapist's voice sounded somewhat cool, but Carol went on to explain that she had gone through an anxiety attack and needed to talk to her.

Dr. G.'s response was shocking and unexpected: "Your next appointment is only two days away. This can wait."

Carol felt that she had been dealt a physical blow. Her worst fears had been realized: Her needs had overwhelmed Dr. G., who must feel depleted, tired of having to support Carol, and in fact must hate her for having been such a needy, demanding patient. Carol should never have relied on anyone to come through for her and she would never trust anyone again. Within seconds Carol withdrew inside herself and could not utter a word. She gripped the telephone receiver in silence.

From the dead silence on the other end of the line, Dr. G. realized that she had made a mistake. She attempted to apologize. She explained that she was sorry to have been so brusque, and she went on to tell Carol that she was dealing with the death of a favorite aunt who had been killed in an accident earlier that week. Dr. G. had attended the funeral that day, and had not wanted to burden Carol with her problems by telling her what had happened. She told Carol that she should have known that it would have been better to tell the truth about her situation, that she was "not herself."

But Dr. G.'s apology did not bring Carol out of her frozen state. Carol still could not utter a word but was unable to hang up the telephone either. Realizing that Carol was still hanging on the line, Dr. G. asked her to try to respond in words. But Carol remained silent. Dr. G. found herself feeling both angry and afraid: Had she driven Carol into a suicidal state? Why was Carol unable to appreciate the stress Dr. G. was under and recognize how hard Dr. G. was trying to reach her? What could she do to bring Carol out of her immobilized position? Dr. G. did not know what else to say and so she waited.

After what seemed like an eternity, Carol spoke. She told Dr. G., "You should have told me about the death in your family when you first called. Instead you attacked me."

Dr. G. acknowledged that Carol was correct. She said that she did not know why she had not said what kind of state she was in at the beginning of the call. She had been taught not to disclose personal information in order to protect patients from being burdened. Perhaps she was also reluctant to talk about a personal loss that was too recent to feel real.

Carol came back to life, not with sympathy or understanding but with anger. "I don't care if you tried not to burden me. You *did* burden me by *not* telling me. And I don't really care that something terrible happened to you. It's your job not to injure me. You of all people should know what it would mean to me to be told that I don't have a legitimate reason for asking for help."

Dr. G. was shocked by Carol's blunt, critical response, her preoccupation with herself, and her inability to perceive Dr. G. as a separate person with compelling needs of her own. She struggled not to lash out or cry. She finally told Carol that they would talk further in the next session.

But the next session was a replay of the telephone call in extended form. After that session, Carol continued to come to her sessions, but she left each one in a state of anguish. She was attached to Dr. G., the first person she had allowed herself to trust, and she could see that Dr. G. was struggling. But every time she tried to soften her stubborn resistance to letting Dr. G. back in, something stopped her. She was afraid to leave herself open to being hurt again. Carol was trapped, fearful of going to her therapy sessions and having to leave feeling worse, but she was more afraid to give up hope altogether and stay away.

During this time, Dr. G., in addition to feeling vulnerable and off center as a result of her personal loss, felt completely helpless in relation to Carol. She could do nothing right. If she urged Carol to come to her sessions, Carol pushed her away. If she suggested that Carol do what she felt was best for her and cancel a session, Carol felt abandoned. If she named the dilemma they each faced, Carol angrily accused her of being a parrot that repeated the same nonsensical sentences over and over. There seemed to be no way out of the torment. Carol was becoming angrier and more despairing as each session passed without a shift in the painful impasse.

At this critical juncture, Dr. G. asked me if I would serve as a consultant to the relationship. Carol grudgingly agreed to try anything that might help, and I set up a meeting with each of them separately. In the meeting with Dr. G., after hearing her experience of the impasse, I supported her in her endeavor to receive all of Carol's feelings. I acknowledged how difficult Carol's feelings were for Dr. G. to bear and reminded her of Carol's attachment to her. Carol was making a courageous, persistent effort to preserve the relationship even though she appeared to be only pushing Dr. G. away. Carol had never been able to grieve the loss of her father or to feel sorry for herself because she did not have a father as other children had. Perhaps the envy she had felt as a child and could not express was surfacing now toward Dr. G., who had suffered a personal loss but was at least an adult instead of a young, dependent child. I urged Dr. G. to continue to acknowledge to Carol how painful her response on the telephone had been, how it had retraumatized Carol in an area of primary vulnerability, specifically her newly developing capacity to trust and allow intimacy with others.

I then met with Carol and after hearing her story, responded to her question of whether to leave the therapy by suggesting that there was value in continuing. I urged this particularly in view of the effort I knew, from my meeting with Dr. G., that she was making to work with the aftermath of the wounding experience they had lived through. I told Carol that she had never been able to struggle openly with her mother over unmet needs, to rage at her mother or her father for their limitations so that she could also have appreciated their strengths. I repeated to Carol what I had said to Dr. G.:

> You never had the opportunity to feel sorry for yourself, to express your envy of other children because they still had fathers, or to feel angry. There wasn't any way to express your pain at all. Now you have an opportunity to grieve for yourself, not only for Dr. G.'s failure on the telephone, but for your illness, the death of your father, the loss of your mother when she remarried, and to have all your feelings in a relationship instead of having them alone. That's a new and important experience even if it's hard.

I felt Dr. G. was not only giving Carol this opportunity, but she was continuing to value Carol and the relationship even in the face of Carol's anger. Carol was having to relinquish the illusion that Dr. G. could be the perfect caretaker she never had. Dr. G., just like Carol, was vulnerable to loss. Similarly, Dr. G. had to give up the illusion that she could be a perfect mother to her unmothered patient and settle for being ordinarily human.

I learned in a follow-up check-in by telephone that a shift had taken place in their relationship. As Carol put it, "We're not caught in an impasse but I'm still struggling with hard feelings. I don't feel like I can trust Dr. G. the way I did. But I'm not freezing her out the way I was and I'm not afraid to go to the sessions any more." Dr. G. reported, "I feel like Carol isn't totally shutting me out. She lets me be helpful at least some of the time. I don't feel as helpless and inadequate anymore." Their relationship, irrevocably changed, continued. The course of working through the impasse was not simple, nor was it accomplished in a matter of weeks or months. The impasse remained alive as the relationship progressed, becoming a pivotal point in their therapeutic relationship as well as an experience that changed each of them and the relationship as well.

The therapeutic relationship between Carol and Dr. G. helps us see the larger matrix that operates invisibly yet forcefully with women patients and therapists: the mother–daughter axis. Literature in psychotherapy typically focuses on only one dimension of the mother–daughter axis; namely, the patient's transference to the therapist as mother and the therapist's maternal countertransference. But the gender identity of female patients and female therapists creates a fluidity of role that is not as likely to occur in opposite gender dyads in which each participant is an "other."[3] Patient and therapist relate to each other from the vantage points of both mother and daughter as well as sister or friend. Mothers and daughters (as well as sisters and friends) typically yearn for an enduring quality of connection, closeness, and harmony of mutual understanding that is impossible to maintain in reality, except for moments or islands in time, because despite having like bodies and the same gender (acknowledging that definitions of gender are controversial), mothers and daughters are inevitably different and unique individuals. Despite the yearning for mutuality, mothers and daughters are consequently always "other" in the sense of being separate and different. The continual shifting of relational mode discussed in Chapter Eight, in which mothers and daughters move in relation to each other as developmental, coerced, and subjective partners, occurs in female patient–therapist dyads as well. When disconnections occur in these dyads, they do so against the backdrop of a yearning for mutuality that gives the mother–daughter axis a special valence and poignancy, evoking the special pain related to the conscious reminders of difference.

When Wounding Overloads the Therapeutic Relationship

Sometimes an experience of wounding is powerful enough to overload the therapeutic relationship, destroying needed illusions prematurely to such an extent that the patient cannot recover enough of them to continue. The patient experiences a loss of energy and enthusiasm for the therapy that cannot be restored, while the therapist is left feeling frustrated and helpless.

Pregnancy of a female therapist provides one example of a life change that can be too wounding for some patients to tolerate, raising in unmanageable degree the issues of envy, abandonment, fears of destroying the therapist and the baby and of being destroyed (hated), and the reality of the separateness of patient and therapist.

A therapist's extended absences necessitated by illness or choice, may also be intolerably wounding to some patients. In one situation, a patient named Kenneth sought therapy with a man, Dr. B. Kenneth had suffered crucial losses in his life: His father died when he was eleven, his grandfather when he was fifteen, and a favorite aunt when he was eighteen and about to leave home for college. He began therapy with Dr. B. hoping to confront his issue of trusting men. Kenneth settled into the therapeutic relationship quickly and comfortably, basking in the sense of security and new hope that resulted from the attachment to Dr. B.

Unexpectedly Dr. B. faced a serious illness and took six months' leave from work. Kenneth chose to wait and resume therapy on his return rather than to begin with a new therapist or meet with someone on an interim basis.

When Dr. B. returned to work, Kenneth could not regain momentum for the therapy. As the year progressed, his interest in continuing therapy steadily waned, despite Dr. B.'s availability for and encouragement of Kenneth's feelings. Eventually Kenneth was reluctant to attend his sessions and asked Dr. B. if he should terminate. Dr. B. encouraged Kenneth to remain in therapy, conceptualizing his deadened state as part of the process of reacting to Dr. B.'s abandonment of him.

But intellectual awareness of the issues did not help to restore Kenneth's capacity to reconnect with Dr. B. Kenneth came for consultation and during the course of the session had a powerful insight. As he talked about his fear that Dr. B. might die, he found himself saying that when he began therapy with Dr. B. he felt safe and secure, as if Dr. B. would protect him from the intrusion of death and illness. When Dr. B. unexpectedly became ill, he lost irretrievably the aura of protector with which Kenneth had imbued him. Some element of the transference, a needed illusion, had been stripped away and could not be restored. At that moment, Kenneth realized that he needed to take a break from the therapy. His ambivalence and conflict dissipated and Kenneth planned and carried out a termination process with Dr. B.

Therapists can help by acknowledging the impact of the wounding on patients, by being available to receive the patients' experiences without retaliating or withdrawing, and by holding the awareness that patients may need to leave the therapy without having accomplished what they had hoped for. Patients are then better able to tolerate the wounding and the related disappointment without the additional burden of feeling that they have failed.

Consultation When Wounding Evokes Early Abuse

As I continue to acquire experience as a consultant in situations where patients are wounded by therapists in their areas of primary vulnerability, I have found that female patients who were victims of early sexual abuse sometimes profit from having the option of ongoing or periodic consultation and from the presence of an auxiliary therapist (see Chapter Twelve).[4] The availability of a consultant (or auxiliary therapist) functions to help them maintain, or return more easily to, a stable sense of self and to process the inevitable wounding that occurs in therapeutic relationships. Accessing and absorbing the horrifying memories that have hovered outside of conscious awareness is a staggering task. Patients who confront the daunting challenge often feel safer when they tell their memories to more than one therapist. The real danger of depleting or overwhelming any one person or of being abandoned by the therapist in the middle of therapy due to unexpected cancellations or vacations is vastly reduced (although the powerful issues of abandonment, envy, hate, and aggression are not diminished in intensity). A consultant can also serve collateral functions such as meeting with the patient's family conjointly should doing so be useful.

I have found that the presence of a consultant or auxiliary therapist may be particularly beneficial for patients who have responded to early physical and sexual abuse with multiple personality adaptation (disorder). Although our conventional ways of thinking about the presence of more than one therapist point to the danger of splitting (making one therapist good and the other bad), a danger that would certainly seem to be heightened in a situation of multiple personality adaptation, my experience has been that the need for safety and the need to have access to a therapist when the primary therapist is unavailable due to vacation or illness outweigh by far the danger of splitting, which if it occurs can generally be minimized and contained by pointing it out and making a discrimination between the present situation in therapy and the past situation of abuse. The presence of two therapists working cooperatively provides the patient with the new relational experience of two effective caretakers that was absent in childhood.

One female patient who had experienced a rupture in her therapy with a male therapist met for some time with me on a weekly basis as a consultant to help her manage the aftermath of the ruptured therapeutic relationship. She also met concurrently with her new primary therapist. She commented that for the first time in her life she felt she was being safely held in a network of healers. She felt secure in the knowledge that the therapists had each other for support and was less fearful that her terrible memories would deplete or exhaust any one of us. When she felt ready to relinquish regular meetings with me, we planned a termination, but I remained available as a back-up during her primary therapist's vacations.

We as yet have no existing models for primary therapists to work cooperatively with auxiliary therapists or with consultants who "hold" the primary therapeutic dyad with patients who have suffered early traumatic abuse. Yet there is an urgent need for therapists to create new models and share their experiences because increasing numbers of patients are recovering memories of abuse. If we shift from a vision of an isolated therapeutic dyad functioning in a vacuum to that of an expanded relational network, or an extended family with the presence of a godmother, new models will have a conceptual foundation.

Female patients who have been abused are especially sensitive to injuries by therapists because they have been victims at too early an age of the human potential to harm others. The disillusionment for these patients when their therapists, who have been relied upon as healing attachment figures, abandon or betray them, can be virtually intolerable. Pat, in the example earlier in the chapter, offers us one view of how devastating a wounding experience with a therapist can be. A woman named Ginny gives us another perspective.

Ginny, a happily married woman with a son, and a competent professional working in real estate, had been meeting with a female therapist, Dr. W. Dr. W. retired and moved away from the area after the therapy had been under way for seven years. In the last year of the therapeutic relationship, perhaps because the impending termination acted as a catalyst, Ginny began recovering memories of early abuse. The memories began to surface slowly, as Ginny and Dr. W. followed the trail of Ginny's reaction to certain triggers in her ordinary daily life. For example, the particular sound of a dog barking and the smell of pine on a weekend walk elicited a fear response in Ginny that initially baffled both herself and Dr. W. Eventually Ginny was able to connect the sound and the scent to the memory of being sexually molested by an uncle in the backyard of a farm during a summertime visit when she was seven years old.

Ginny and Dr. W. spent the last eight months before Dr. W.'s retirement with the difficult task of simultaneously working with her memories of abuse and anticipating the termination of the therapy. Dr. W. carefully selected a male colleague and facilitated a meeting between the colleague, Dr. P., and Ginny some months before the final session. Ginny was optimistic about being able to work with a man, even though the perpetrator of the abuse was male.

After the termination with Dr. W., Ginny began meeting regularly three times a week with Dr. P. She spent the first year mourning the loss of Dr. W., to whom she had been deeply attached. She occasionally wrote to Dr. W., who always responded to her letters. Dr. P. understood the depth of Ginny's attachment to Dr. W. and did not interfere with their contact.

In the second year of the therapy Dr. P. took a four-week vacation. Ginny, who had expected to be able to weather the long separation without inordinate difficulty, was surprised and confused to find that she felt profoundly abandoned. Suffering panic attacks and then depression, she tried to telephone the back-up therapist who was taking calls during Dr. P.'s recovery. But she did not like the stern sound of his voice and hung up without asking for an appointment. Her anxiety and panic states persisted without relief until Dr. P.'s vacation ended.

When Dr. P. returned and Ginny's regular sessions resumed, she found herself unable to reattach to him. Dr. W.'s retirement, coupled with Dr. P.'s absence, blended for Ginny into one catastrophic experience of abandonment and betrayal. Both therapists turned into unreliable, untrustworthy, dangerous figures instead of the benevolent, concerned, healing attachment figures they had been. Frightened, alone, not knowing where to turn, Ginny could not trust Dr. P. to help her, nor could she bear to leave him and start over with a new therapist.

Dr. P., familiar with my consultation work in situations of impasses involving wounding and urgently concerned that the therapy with Ginny not collapse in a rupture, asked if I could intervene immediately in their complex and volatile impasse. He appreciated the seriousness of the situation, recognizing that the loss for Ginny of both Dr. W. and himself would devastate her. He hoped that I might be able to preserve their fragile connection long enough for it to grow stronger.

Desperate for help, Ginny agreed to meet with me. She found that she felt comfortable talking to me. My demeanor and way of being with her reminded her of Dr. W. I asked Ginny how Dr. P. and I could help her through her frightening experience that Dr. P. had abandoned and betrayed her and enable her to rebuild enough trust in the therapeutic relationship with him to tolerate the ups and downs. Ginny decided that she would like to meet weekly with me and continue her three weekly sessions with Dr. P. until she felt safe meeting only with him. Dr. P. and I were worried that we might become polarized into a good therapist (me) and a bad therapist (Dr. P.), but we decided not to act on our concerns and to trust that when Ginny no longer felt she needed regular appointment times with me, she would stop.

While Dr. P. and I struggled with anxiety and worry about our unconventional arrangement, Ginny flourished. When Dr. P. went on vacation again, I was available to her. When I was away, she had Dr. P. She used the time with each of us in whatever way she needed. Sometimes she would recover and relive a memory with Dr. P. and then she would come and tell me about the experience, reflecting upon it as if from a distance. The reexperiencing of the trauma with Dr. P. and absorbing or integrating it with me seemed particularly effective for Ginny. Perhaps a single therapist might have facilitated both experiences—remembering and integrating the memory—but in the context of the abandonment constellated by Dr. P.'s vacation, Ginny clearly felt safer working therapeutically with both of us.

As the work progressed and more terrible memories accumulated, we three were able to see that Ginny was certain the experiences she had survived were too terrible for a single therapist to bear. She felt safer sharing the experiences out among the three of us and was comforted by the knowledge that Dr. P. and I had each other for support. Indeed, Dr. P. and I were comforted by having each other to talk with about the events that had been a buried part of Ginny's past and that were being brought into her present. In light of her childhood suffering, her certainty was not a fantasy or an exaggeration of reality. We were also relieved that during either of our absences, Ginny would be well taken care of by the other. Yet we recognized that other therapists might view our unusual arrangement with criticism and disapproval. For example, we might be perceived as yielding to an enactment of Ginny's effort to re-create a healthy family, as supporting infantile yearnings rather than naming them and helping Ginny grieve the impossibility of having them gratified. We might also be perceived to be setting up a situation conducive to splitting that could prevent Ginny from coming to terms with the good and the bad in each therapist. But our experience indicated that "splitting" is too simplistic a concept to describe the nature of the relationships that developed. Ginny came to appreciate the individual strengths, limits, and idiosyncrasies of her therapists in tandem with an increasingly differentiated view of herself.

Ginny continued meeting weekly with me for one year, and then we terminated by gradually decreasing the number of sessions until we stopped meeting regularly. She never spoke of concerns about the arrangement with which Dr. P. and I struggled. She had always asserted that she would terminate with me when she was ready and she did. She was unwavering in her opinion that she had suffered enough deprivation and loss in her life and that she did not need help in accepting suffering. She was clear that she instead needed the experience of being able to recognize and to state clearly her needs and to have her needs met to the fullest extent possible. She always had separate agendas for her sessions with us, agendas that did not pit us against each other in competition, but that were complementary as well as conducive to our cooperation. She came to know our differences and similarities and to accept them with good humor, sometimes teasing us. "You have such trouble knowing how you feel, " she would chide Dr. P. "You're just like all men!" While she complimented me on my capacity for empathy, Ginny was also quite free to let me know that there was some elusive way she felt protected by Dr. P. that she did not feel with me. Part of the therapeutic work consisted of sorting out and making sense of Ginny's different experiences of each of us, including a recognition of how Dr. P. and I functioned as the good parents that she never had.

After we stopped meeting regularly, I continued to provide back-up coverage for Dr. P. during his vacation absences. The experience of continuity over time with me provided an additional healing component for Ginny in the relational context we provided, one that eventually came to offset her harmful early childhood as well as the truncated though positive relationship with Dr. W. Ginny's hope, endangered by Dr. W.'s retirement, that her life could contain new positive relational experiences, was preserved and affirmed.

*　*　*　*　*

Once therapists and patients acknowledge that therapeutic relationships can include profound wounding that catapults both of them into areas of primary vulnerability, we are freer to explore creative ways of managing these experiences. A consultant functions to hold the relationship and the individual participants psychologically so that the relationship can either expand to include the wounding or, if necessary, end without a traumatic rupture that harms the patient. Even therapeutic relationships with positive outcomes cannot permanently eradicate areas of primary vulnerability nor ease the suffering in life. But therapeutic relationships do have the potential to expand the possibilities for what life and relationships can hold for those who participate in them.

If a therapeutic relationship does end in a traumatic rupture, a consultant can still play a vital role in helping the patient or the therapist through the aftermath of the rupture and through the ensuing process of coming to understand what happened. The following chapter provides examples of consultation to patients and therapists in situations where the therapeutic relationship has terminated in a rupture.

CHAPTER FIFTEEN

❖ Consultation: When the ❖ Therapeutic Relationship Ruptures

What's hardest for me is to accept, even three years after the therapy ended, is the fact that I'll never have a *shared* resolution with my therapist. I can only have the peace that I can make with it. And I still haven't recovered the lost ground from the rupture. I haven't been able to make a good connection to another therapist and I'm still cynical about the profession. It's ironic that the primary vulnerability, to use your term for it, that I came to the therapist for help with—the ways I was shaped in my family to expect that my feelings wouldn't be acknowledged—is also what kept me in the therapy getting hurt over and over.

—Rhea

I really don't know what would have happened to me if I hadn't heard of you. When Dr. H. threw me out of his office I felt as if I had been dropped out of a plane at 30,000 feet. Working with you was like finding a parachute that helped me reach the ground intact and continue on.

—Dee

I had no idea that I would precipitate a massive crisis in the therapy and that the patient would flee. He didn't respond to my telephone messages. I have written him a note offering to meet with him alone and also recommending that he consult with you, either on his own or in a conjoint meeting with the three of us. I hope that he is not too angry or wounded to take a recommendation from me. I don't want the therapy to be left in such a negative, painful place even if he and I can't continue to work together.

—Dr. E.

When the Therapist Terminates the Therapy: Rhea's Story

Optimally, just as children should have parental care until they are ready to function as adults, patients in therapy should have the experience of continuing in the relationship until they feel ready to move on. But therapists are sometimes compelled to terminate therapeutic relationships for personal reasons related to illness, a geographical move, or retirement. In a state of vulnerability related to a significant life passage of their own, they are liable to be less available psychologically and unable to empathize adequately with their patients than before. Even when therapists are empathic and sensitive to the impact on their patients, the impending abandonment and loss can propel some patients, and some patients at certain phases of therapy, into a state of vulnerability around abandonment and loss. The vulnerability of both patient and therapist makes fertile ground for a therapeutic impasse or severing of the attachment bond in a ruptured termination.

As a consultant, I have provided a transitional containing relationship for a number of patients whose therapists needed to end the therapy. Typically my function with the patient has been to receive the patient's feelings fully, to identify when appropriate the vulnerable state of the therapist, and to name the manifestations of the therapist's vulnerability that have been wounding to the patient. I have also functioned to affirm that the patient's response to the loss of an important attachment bond as well as to the temporary unavailability of the therapist is neither extreme nor pathological, but rather understandable. The unique meaning of the separation and loss in the context of the patient's life experiences can also be explored and held psychologically within the consultation relationship so that, when possible, it can be brought into the therapeutic relationship. With a separate relational context within which their subjective reality is understood and affirmed, patients are better able to have empathy for themselves and for their therapists. An empathic relational context enables patients to persist through the difficult aftermath of the therapist's disclosure of the impending termination of the therapy.

Therapists have difficulty raising the reality of an impending termination with their patients because they are apt to feel guilt at abandoning the relationship, in addition to other feelings related to their personal situation. When therapists know that a consultant is available to receive their feelings and those of their patient, they are often able to be more available psychologically to their patients. Consultations to patients and therapists in a variety of circumstances have repeatedly affirmed for me the vital importance to both participants of having their subjective experience fully acknowledged and understood. When patients and therapists have their experience affirmed, they are able to perceive the other with greater clarity and compassion.

Rhea, a graduate student in history, wife, and mother of a two-year-old daughter, was referred for consultation by the counseling department of her school. Her therapist had told Rhea shortly after Rhea's daughter was diagnosed with leukemia and was beginning chemotherapy treatment that he was leaving the area and would have to terminate the therapy in six months. By the time Rhea learned of my availability as a consultant and called me, only three weeks of sessions remained. She and her therapist had been suffering through an ongoing impasse for the entire six months. Rhea hoped that a consultation could ease what was turning out to be an excruciating termination.

Rhea was a young woman in her late twenties, tall and large-boned, with a sweetness to her face and a haunting melancholy in her large hazel eyes. In her words, Rhea had formed and maintained a positive transference to her therapist for the three years they had been meeting regularly. Rhea was just settling into a time of stability, managing motherhood and school, when her child's illness was diagnosed. She had taken a leave of absence from her graduate program in order to care for her daughter. Her husband had to maintain his full-time employment in order to protect their health insurance. Though the prognosis for her daughter was excellent, the treatment process and anxiety were an ordeal. In the midst of the life stress, Rhea learned that her therapist planned to move.

Rhea was distraught that the therapist did not wait until her daughter's treatment had been completed to tell her the news, even though the amount of advance notice would have been considerably reduced. She was fearful that her anger at the therapist would distract her from being able to care for her daughter effectively. Worse, she felt that she could not face the possible loss of her child and losing her therapist as well. During the first month after the therapist told her of his upcoming move, she put the fact of the termination completely out of her mind in order to focus on her child.

But the therapist continued to bring up the impending termination, although Rhea declared that she did not want to talk about it until her daughter completed the course of chemotherapy. Before long the therapeutic relationship began to unravel. The therapist made repeated blunt comments about Rhea and her denial: "You don't want to think about my leaving so you're acting as if it's not going to happen." Rhea was distressed at his insistence that she focus on the termination when her need was to put it out of her mind until after her daughter's treatment. Rhea felt that her therapist needed to talk about the termination and that it was difficult for him when she avoided dealing with the upcoming move. Instead of facing his own difficulty, he accused Rhea of denying it. Rhea and the therapist began to get into one struggle after another over the therapist's unrelenting focus upon Rhea.

Rhea described how she kept trying to hold on to her own sense of reality, and how it would seem to wash away whenever it conflicted with her therapist's point of view. Her therapist insisted that it was valuable for her to have the experience of consciously ending the therapeutic relationship. He believed that mourning the ending with the therapist present would give a special opportunity, one that she missed when her father died suddenly of a heart attack five years before.

But Rhea's subjective experience of the therapist moving away was different. To her, having to end therapy at the therapist's choice rather than her own felt unqualifiedly terrible. If she had known the therapist was going to move, she would not have chosen to begin meeting with him. But in the face of the reality that the therapist presented to her—that the experience of a conscious separation and mourning could be valuable—Rhea began to believe that she was too needy, too sensitive, or overreacting to the therapist.

When her daughter's chemotherapy treatment was over and the child began to recover, the therapist's impending move, now only four months away, loomed large. Rhea shifted into a state of raw vulnerability, unable to sleep, eat, or concentrate. She told her therapist she was afraid she was falling apart. At this point, her therapist backed away from Rhea's fears and insisted that she function as an adult. He made comments such as, "You're not falling apart—you're doing fine. You've been through a terrible time with your daughter's illness, but it's over now." Rhea felt her therapist, after insisting that she stop denying her feelings of abandonment and loss, was now blocking them. She felt that instead of appreciating the vulnerable, childlike state she had been catapulted into, he was insisting that she "be a grown-up" and stop needing him so that he could leave her without guilt.

Rhea embarked on a concentrated effort to help her therapist help her. She brought him articles on loss and on regression in therapy. But as she saw it, he responded by pathologizing her instead of empathically receiving her feelings. Rhea said to me, "If he'd only told me, 'I can see how hard this is for you,' instead of telling me that I shouldn't be feeling what I was feeling or simply not hearing me, I could have felt a bond with him and I could have linked my feelings to earlier experiences in my family. My family never allowed me to have feelings that made them uncomfortable."

As she listened to herself explain her therapist's responses, Rhea began to recognize the extent to which she had been caught in an unsuccessful struggle to get her therapist to understand her point of view. She felt utterly exhausted from her efforts to get him to change his perspective: "I've wasted so much time and energy butting my head against the wall of his defenses—what an exercise in futility."

Rhea reflected back six months to the time the therapist had first announced his plans to relocate. She wondered aloud whether she should have ended with the therapist at that moment. But she countered her worries with an awareness that she could not have handled a termination in the midst of her daughter's chemotherapy treatment. She could not have deprived herself of a major relationship at a time of such extreme vulnerability, especially when she still had hope that he would continue to be helpful to her. Rhea went on to say that she is the kind of person who commits herself to seeing things through till the end. She would not have felt good about herself if she had ended the therapy before the therapist terminated his practice.

The therapist's handling of Rhea's response to the impending loss of the therapeutic relationship created a secondary level of wounding (see Chapter Ten). Rhea needed an acknowledgment of the pain of her loss and a place to grieve. Instead, the therapist retreated from her emotionally and made interpretive statements about her from a distance, leaving himself out. Repeated power struggles that were set off in response to her efforts to communicate her experience to the therapist became another component of the secondary level of wounding. Rhea and I could only speculate that the therapist's feelings of guilt or of personal loss related to his move were causing him to be especially rigid and constrained and to miss how hard Rhea was trying to stay in relationship to him without sacrificing her needs and feelings.

When we talked about the aftermath of the loss of a primary attachment bond, Rhea told me that she was continuing to have anxiety attacks. She described feeling agitated all the time and an inability to eat or sleep. She was relieved to hear that her anxiety was a normal, expected response to the jeopardizing of an important attachment bond. Setting aside her worry about the meaning of her anxiety in the consultation session, Rhea began to feel that it might be a relief to end the therapy after the six months of agony. Once the therapy ended, she could begin the process of mourning and moving on.

We acknowledged that Rhea's sense of herself was having to change as a consequence of her daughter's serious illness and that a comprehensive reordering of a sense of self takes time. The combined loss of the reliably ongoing therapeutic relationship and of the previously-held illusion that her child would have a childhood free of suffering was overwhelming.

Rhea's final appointment with her therapist was scheduled for the following week. She decided that she no longer wanted to invest effort in helping him respond more empathically to her. She would attend the session for the sake of her sense of completion, but she would not try to change the therapist. She asked to meet with me again after her final therapy session.

Rhea and I met the following week after her last appointment. The therapist had not changed his stance in the concluding session. Rhea was still sad, but as she had anticipated, she also felt some relief that the long ordeal of separating from her therapist was over: "Now I can finally go on with my life."

Some months later Rhea called to let me know that she and her daughter were doing well and that she had made a connection to a therapist whose name I had given her. But she did not believe that she would allow herself to care about her new therapist, or to invest the amount of energy in the relationship that she had with the therapist who had moved away.

Rhea and I had contact with each other once again three years after the initial consultation. I learned that Rhea had terminated with the therapist to whom I had referred her. She felt that she was still recovering from the setback of the first therapeutic relationship. However she had not lost hope for herself and was in the process of looking for another therapist.

Terminating in an Impasse: Marsha's Story

Some therapists terminate therapeutic relationships abruptly in an impasse for reasons other than personal life changes. Therapists may come to feel, for different reasons, that they can no longer continue to work with certain patients. In these situations, even when therapists act responsibly by assessing their effectiveness, patients are left with the intense feelings that accompany the severing of an important attachment bond as well as with feelings of profound rejection. Therapists vary in how sensitively and empathically they are able to work with obstacles to the therapeutic relationship and patients vary in vulnerability. Consultation may help patients who are wounded by therapists who feel they can no longer function competently in that capacity. A consultant can confirm for patients the problematic behavior of their therapists, identify the therapists' (as well as the patients') vulnerabilities, and help the patient work with the feelings of grief, loss, rejection, disillusionment, betrayal, or of having been harmed. Consultation may also help patients arrive at a sense of completion, providing the closure that could not occur in the therapeutic relationship, particularly if the termination was handled to accommodate the therapists' needs rather than the patients'. When patients are uncertain about attempting further therapy, a consultant can serve as a transitional person or a bridge to a subsequent therapeutic relationship.

Marsha initially came for consultation in the midst of an impasse with her therapist, a woman. The therapeutic relationship had been a long and important one for Marsha. Over the course of the ten-year relationship, Marsha had developed considerably. She had changed careers from a computer consultant to a therapist and hoped to follow in her therapist's footsteps at the training institution with which the therapist was affiliated. She had worked on her problematic relationship with her mother, a personally unfulfilled woman who redirected intense feelings of self-hatred toward Marsha.

Gradually, as the therapy progressed, Marsha had relinquished the illusions she had needed to maintain about the positive mothering she had received. She faced how destructive, albeit unintentionally, her mother had been to her. Her lost illusions had been replaced by a sense of what her mother had given her, an increased personal vitality and a greater sense of self-worth and well-being.

During the ten years, Marsha's therapist had assumed increasing responsibility and stature at the professional institution with which she was affiliated. After Marsha was accepted into the advanced training program, the therapist had seemed to Marsha to treat her more like a colleague than a patient. For example, the therapist would give Marsha advice about the seminars she was taking and the supervisors she worked with. Over time, Marsha had become concerned that the therapist had abandoned her role of therapist and had become a colleague.

Marsha became increasingly angry at her therapist and had finally confronted her therapist with her feelings. The therapist insisted that her perceptions were different from Marsha's. She believed that she had not abandoned her role of therapist. She insisted that Marsha's anger at her did not come from their involvement at the same training program, but rather represented Marsha's way of behaving abusively toward the therapist, as her mother had behaved toward her. She saw herself as a symbolic good, nurturing mother, supplying Marsha with the support that had not been available from Marsha's mother. She interpreted Marsha's anger as her way of managing feelings of envy and competitiveness.

At loggerheads with her therapist, Marsha called for a consultation. Her therapist chose not to be involved, but had no objections to Marsha seeking an outside perspective. In the consultation session, Marsha recounted her story in detail. She said she was angry at the therapist, not only for abandoning her role of therapist but also for insisting that Marsha's feelings were related to the mother-transference and not to the current situation. Her anger and anxiety intensified as each therapy session failed to lead to common ground and as she began to doubt her experience of the relationship in view of the therapist's differing perceptions. Marsha had begun to anticipate her sessions with dread and foreboding.

In discussing the situation, we clarified that Marsha's capacity to recognize that her therapist had abandoned her by shifting her role in relation to Marsha from therapist to colleague was a sign of progress. When Marsha spoke aloud her personal reality, something she had been trained not to do as a child, her therapist had discounted her reality and insisted instead on the accuracy of her own perspective, wounding Marsha in an area of primary vulnerability. The therapist's insistence on being right rather than listening empathically to Marsha's perspective and her failure to appreciate the significance of Marsha's anger as healthy assertiveness created a secondary level of wounding.

I suggested that Marsha return to her therapist, report on our consultation, and maintain her view of the progress her response to the therapist represented. I hoped that the therapist would be able to respond constructively to Marsha. We made a follow-up appointment in four weeks in order to give Marsha time to work with their disagreement in the therapy.

But two weeks later Marsha called and asked for another appointment before our scheduled time. Her sessions with her therapist had gone from bad to worse. In fact, she reported that her therapy had ended abruptly earlier that day in the middle of an angry struggle. Marsha was distressed and wanted to talk to me about what had happened as soon as possible.

When we met, Marsha told me that during the previous weeks, she and her therapist had remained in an impasse. The therapist could not tolerate hearing that Marsha felt that the therapist had become too collegial in the graduate training program. She insisted that their collegial relationship did not have to interfere with the therapeutic relationship or mean that Marsha's vulnerable or primitive aspects were not welcome in the sessions. Marsha tried to point out that the therapist was abandoning her at that very moment by refusing to accept Marsha's feelings as valid. Defending herself instead, the therapist responded to Marsha's renewed efforts to be understood by abruptly announcing that in view of Marsha's feelings, they should make that session their last. If Marsha truly felt that she was no longer helpful, they needed to terminate the therapy at once. Their relationship in the training institute would continue.

Marsha was taken aback by the therapist's sudden pronouncement. She told the therapist that she had not been threatening to terminate. She wanted to restore the therapeutic relationship or at least to have a planned termination when she felt ready. The therapist said that they had come to an irreconcilable impasse and could no longer work together as therapist and patient. As long as Marsha believed that their dual relationship thwarted the therapy, they needed to terminate. Marsha reiterated that she had hoped for another outcome. But the therapist was insistent that they stop the therapy, and Marsha had no choice but to say goodbye.

We discussed the meaning of the abrupt and unexpected termination. From Marsha's perspective, in abruptly severing the relationship, the therapist was repeating behavior that Marsha was accustomed to in her relationship with her mother. Marsha believed that her therapist was aware that she had abandoned her role of therapist, was angry at herself, and was directing her anger at Marsha instead of openly acknowledging the error or taking time to explore other ways of managing the dual relationship. The therapist had precipitously preempted Marsha by making a unilateral decision to end.

Marsha was surprised to find that she did not feel devastated by the ending. The consultation had been useful in affirming her experience. She believed that her perception of her therapist's limitations were accurate, and ironically sensed that perceiving the limitations as located not in herself but in the other person was the direct result of the years of hard work in the therapy. She was sad that she and her therapist were not able to experience a termination phase together and that the therapist had not been able to receive her appreciative feelings regarding their work together.

Disavowal of Self to Preserve Relationships: Dee and Dr. H.

The following vignette describes a specific form of therapeutic impasse and ruptured therapeutic relationship that I have encountered with some female patients working with male therapists.[1] I believe that an impasse and termination of this kind helps us to see in condensed form a problem that many women live with in our Western patriarchal culture in different degrees and in diverse forms. Every woman, simply by being a woman in a culture that objectifies her—witness the high incidence of violence against women, depression, and other forms of "psychopathology"—is at risk of participating in the impasse described in the vignette.

The impasse occurs when female patients, without realizing it, become (coerced) objects for their male therapists to use unconsciously in the service of gratifying the therapists' needs. When something occurs that makes women aware of the role they have fallen into and the betrayal by their therapists that has occurred (and that in many cases repeats a prior traumatizing betrayal), a rage erupts that may disrupt their male therapists' sense of self. To protect themselves psychologically, some therapists further objectify the female patients by rendering them into dangerous objects from which they must flee. The female patients are consequently abandoned and silenced, unable to find the powerful personal voice carried by the rage and unable to hold onto their subjective reality. Through being silenced, women not only remain isolated victims, but they also disavow their subjective experience, and are left with an impoverished and weakened sense of a female self (and I refer to a sense of self that is formed in relationship).

Female patients in a culture in which women are subordinate may unconsciously serve as gratifying objects for their male therapists, often trying to elicit positive relational responses from them by shaping themselves into what they intuitively sense their therapists need or want. Female patients become such gratifying objects that their male therapists stop observing and reflecting on the relational mode that has become engaged, and a destructive impasse with explosive potential results. Male therapists are pulled off center by their unconscious needs, and female patients are objectified, blamed for having been objectified, and then abandoned.

The enactment of a sexual relationship is perhaps the most dramatic and visible example of this category of impasse. However, the same relational pattern manifests in other forms that may be less readily apparent but that are potentially painful and damaging for both participants. With an awareness of how this specific impasse arises, female patients and male therapists can transform the danger it presents into an opportunity for an altered sense of self-in-relationship.

Dee, the daughter of hard-working blue-collar parents, is a thirty-one-year-old single woman who teaches English at a public high school. She sought therapy with a male therapist, Dr. H., to get help with her difficulty establishing a successful relationship with a man. Her only relationship with a man, Ray, had ended abruptly and painfully when she became pregnant and chose an abortion despite Ray's wishes for her to have the baby.

Dee began therapy twice a week with Dr. H. She initially perceived him to be a good listener, empathic, and perceptive. He helped her to have compassion for herself for having chosen the abortion and for having survived the loss of the relationship with Ray. His understanding of her family dynamics was invaluable to her and changed her feelings about her parents and sister. She worked on her guilt at surpassing and separating from her family—being more educated, being physically healthy, and having a higher-status job than either of her parents. The critical judgments she feared and expected from Dr. H. were never forthcoming. Instead, she saw reflected in his comments her own strengths: her persistence, endurance, loyalty, and concern for others.

Dr. H., an experienced therapist nearing forty, found himself increasingly drawn to Dee. Recently divorced, Dr. H. was lonely. He felt that Dee was describing his inner state when she talked about the agony of the loss of her relationship with Ray and about having relinquished her unborn child. At times he found himself wishing he could tell her about his plight and how it matched hers. Dr. H. had no idea that he was comforting himself with Dee. He believed that he was supporting her as she confronted difficult issues and affirming the ways she tried to help herself.

Dee found herself having feelings for a man for the first time in years. She began to think about Dr. H. all the time, held imaginary conversations with him in her mind, daydreamed about becoming romantically and sexually involved with him, pictured them being together, even being married. Responding to Dr. H.'s encouragement to share her feelings when she sat in an awkward silence, blushing, Dee shyly confided her dreams and wishes.

Dr. H. came to believe that he had fallen in love with Dee. He knew about eroticized countertransference, he had had other female patients fall in love with him and had been sexually attracted to other female patients, but he felt that Dee was different. He was sure that their feelings for each other were real, that had they met in circumstances other than a therapy office, they would have come to love each other. He believed that the therapeutic relationship could end and that they could have a "real" relationship.

When Dee talked in one of her sessions about her feeling that no man would ever love her, that she was destined to be alone and childless for the rest of her life, Dr. H. told her that her feelings were unfounded and that he loved her. If they were to end the therapeutic relationship, he would want to be with her. Dee was stunned. She could not believe her good fortune. The experience of having Dr. H., a man she admired and respected, who knew her emotional wounds and psychological issues, who knew the worst about her, tell her that he loved her was an experience she never thought could be hers.

But when Dee left the therapy session, feelings of anxiety mounted. Something felt wrong. Was Dr. H. really in love with her? Could she trust him to follow through on his promise of a relationship? She confided what was happening in her therapy to Sarah, a teacher at her school who was also in psychotherapy. Sarah said that Dee was right to be worried about the relationship with Dr. H. She said that Dee should tell Dr. H. about her doubts and offered to ask her own therapist what he thought. Sarah's therapist told Sarah that he thought that Dr. H. was behaving unethically and unprofessionally. Sarah reported her therapist's opinion to Dee.

Sarah's information only confirmed what Dee had already come to feel. She wondered if Dr. H. really would have a relationship with her or whether his feeling for her would fade outside the therapy office if they were to see each other. She came to her next session and confronted Dr. H. with her concerns, adding that Sarah's therapist thought that Dr. H. was behaving unethically and unprofessionally.

Dr. H. felt as if he had been floating in a balloon that had popped. Instantaneously, in a moment of shock, he realized that Dee was correct. Dr. H. found himself overcome with panic when he realized that he might even have put himself in jeopardy of being sued for unethical behavior. He recognized the name of Sarah's therapist and could hardly bear to imagine what his colleague thought of him. Appalled at what he had done, he began to panic that if a story that he had fallen in love with a patient began to circulate through the community, he would be shamed as a professional. Thinking only of himself, no longer concerned with Dee's needs, he immediately told Dee that they could not continue to meet anymore. This meeting would have to be their last.

Dee was stunned. She had hoped that Dr. H. would reassure her and tell her that her anxieties were unfounded. They would end the therapeutic relationship and then begin a personal relationship. That way no ethical violation could be said to have occurred. She had assumed that even if he told her that they could not have a real relationship because he was her therapist, they would continue to meet regularly in her scheduled sessions. It had never occurred to her that he would take away her appointment times and refuse to see her at all. She could not fathom how he could say he loved her in one session and tell her he never wanted to see her again in the next. In a state of shock, she asked him what he meant. Surely he would allow her some time to meet with him and talk about what had happened between them and what she could do. She could not just lose him like this all at once.

Dr. H. told her that he had jeopardized his personal and professional life. He would not have any kind of further contact with her, either in his office or by telephone. She would have to meet with someone else. He would give her a referral.

Dee told Dr. H. that he must not have thought through what he was saying. How could he cut her off like this? How could she mean something special to him in one minute and then be cast away the next? Who was she? Who was he? He absolutely had to meet with her another time.

But Dr. H. would not budge. He again said he was sorry that the therapy had gotten so far off track and that he wished the best for her. He stood up and reached out to shake her hand.

But Dee did not move. Anger she did not know she was capable of feeling rose up and grew stronger. She told Dr. H., "How dare you do this to me. As a therapist, you have a responsibility to me."

Dr. H. panicked. What if she sued him for malpractice? What if he lost his license, or worse, lost joint custody of his son? In a state of panic, Dr. H. had no capacity for concern for Dee, no empathy for her needs as his patient or as a human being. He reacted only self-protectively, out of fear. From being a coerced relational partner who gratified his needs, Dee had become a dangerous person from whom he must distance himself. He struggled for composure and told her that he could no longer be her therapist.

Dee came for consultation. After hearing her story, I offered to contact Dr. H. to see if he would agree to meet with Dee and me in a conjoint session in order to have a termination process and to give Dee an opportunity to express her feelings of outrage and disappointment. Although he shared his experience of the impasse and rupture, he refused to meet conjointly. He insisted that further meetings with Dee would make matters worse. He feared that Dee would ask that her therapy continue, and he could not agree to that.

Termination sessions with Dr. H. in the presence of a consultant would have helped Dee let go of the lost therapeutic relationship, unburden herself of her anger, and preserve the aspects of the relationship that had been positive. Its abrupt severance constituted an objectification and abandonment of Dee that retraumatized her.

Dee met with me for several months in tandem with regular

sessions with another therapist, Dr. R. She described her reaction to the abrupt end of her therapeutic relationship with Dr. H. in the following words:

> It wouldn't be so awful that he used me to meet his needs if he hadn't taken away the therapy and put me out on the street. I thought I was having a relationship with a man who could see me and love me even knowing the worst about me. I trusted him. Why shouldn't I? He's a professional, trained to help women like me. I thought he knew me and cared about me. When push came to shove, he just dropped me. I mean nothing to him and now I don't know if I'll ever mean anything to anybody. He took my therapy away. The therapy was the only safe place I had. I was helpless. I had nowhere to turn. I couldn't stand being forced out of contact with him. It made me feel like I'm garbage that he put out on the street. It was an emotional rape.

More than a year later, Dee is continuing her therapy with Dr. R. Although she trusts Dr. R., a capacity she thought was lost forever, feelings of shame, anger, loss, betrayal, a sense of failure, and a persisting fear that she is unlovable return with intensity. She did not file an ethical complaint with the local state professional board because she believed that she would be portrayed as a borderline, hysterical woman. She did not want to be further injured by having her complaint rejected.

When the Patient Terminates Abruptly: Dr. E.'s Story

When a patient leaves a therapist abruptly in the midst of an impasse, the therapist as well as the patient is often left with difficult feelings to manage. Dr. E., a therapist, came for consultation because one of his patients had terminated abruptly when Dr. E. attempted to establish boundaries in the therapeutic relationship.

Dr. E.'s patient, a man named Joe, was a respected attorney, intelligent and articulate. But as soon as he began meeting in therapy sessions, his long-suppressed yearnings for empathy and perfect attunement to his needs were awakened. He quickly began to leave lengthy telephone messages on Dr. E.'s answering machine, in which he described his internal state in detail, several times a day. At first, Dr. E. listened to his messages and then brought them up in his sessions. His hope was that Joe's need to leave the messages would diminish as he became more accustomed to the therapy and reassured that his sessions would continue to occur. Instead, the telephone messages increased in length and frequency. Dr. E. encouraged Joe to meet with him more frequently, hoping that the increased number of sessions would provide sufficient time with him so that the telephone messages would no longer be needed. But Joe's need for continuity of access to Dr. E. did not diminish and the messages persisted.

As the long messages from Joe continued, Dr. E. began to feel increasingly trapped, helpless, and angry to the point where he dreaded retrieving his messages from the answering machine. He understood that the urgency of Joe's need for contact with him had roots in his early childhood. Joe was the fourth of nine children, necessarily neglected by his working-class parents who struggled to keep the family supplied with bare essentials. Joe too had worked hard throughout his life. He could not remember a time when he was not working to earn money. Dr. E. recognized that the therapeutic relationship had given Joe the space and permission to pay attention to his psychological needs, perhaps for the first time in his life. He did not want to behave in a way that Joe would experience as wounding or rejecting.

As time passed, Dr. E. became convinced that he had to bring up his need for Joe to curtail his telephone messages, knowing that doing so would thrust both of them onto treacherous ground. With anxiety, he raised the issue as gently and empathically as he could. He explained that he understood Joe's need for frequent contact with him, but that he was having difficulty managing to listen to the lengthy messages. He told Joe that he did not want to wound or reject him, but that he found it necessary to ask Joe to curtail the messages because of his needs. He told Joe he knew that the therapy sessions had awakened his yearning for an empathic connection to Dr. E. and that Joe wished to be able to contact Dr. E. when he needed, rather than to have to wait for a scheduled session. Dr. E. understood that waiting for a scheduled appointment time might be difficult and offered to meet with Joe more often. Dr. E. expressed his hope that Joe would let him know his feelings about his request, and that he would begin to use his time in their sessions to bring up the material that he had been leaving in messages over the telephone.

Despite Dr. E.'s effort to be gentle and compassionate, Joe was both humiliated and outraged. He felt angry and betrayed. Why was Dr. E. changing his rules midstream? Dr. E. had not complained about his messages before. Wasn't he obligated, even legally, to be responsive to Joe's needs in between sessions? What was Joe supposed to do if he felt suicidal? Jump off a cliff instead of make a telephone call?

Dr. E. withstood Joe's angry attacks as calmly as he could, reflecting back to him how uncared for he felt and emphasizing that these were feelings he had also experienced in his family. Dr. E. added that the therapy sessions had brought these disavowed feelings to the forefront and the two of them now had an opportunity to struggle with the feelings together. Dr. E. repeatedly told Joe that he did care about him, that he wanted to work on the issues underlying Joe's need for continuous contact, and that he was establishing a boundary that would enable him to remain in place as Joe's therapist. But Joe's hurt and anger did not diminish. In a rage, he told Dr. E. that he could not continue as his patient in view of his feelings about how irresponsible Dr. E. had been. He left the session midway through.

Dr. E. decided to seek consultation even though Joe had terminated to see if there was another way he could have managed the impasse that would have enabled Joe to remain his patient. Dr. E. was worried that he had made a grave error in receiving the telephone calls in the first place and in attempting to limit them once they became overwhelming. He also wondered if he could take some action now that might ease the situation, both for himself and for Joe.

In view of Dr. E.'s manner of conducting therapy, I could not identify anything he might have done differently. Even if he had set limits on the telephone messages at the outset, Joe might not have been able to tolerate them. I believed that Dr. E. had accurately identified and named Joe's realm of primary vulnerability, his pervasive sense of being uncared for, and his disavowed longings for attention and empathy. Dr. E. had also averted inflicting a secondary level of wounding by being gentle and compassionate in response to Joe's rage, and in his recommendation that Joe continue meeting with him.

We decided that Dr. E. had the option of writing a letter to Joe, reiterating his concern, his perception of what had transpired in the impasse and rupture, and his hope that Joe would continue on in therapy, either with him or with a different therapist. In the end, we were forced to conclude that the brief experience in therapy had catapulted Joe into his core issues too quickly, before a strong therapeutic alliance could be established, so that they became unmanageable. We were left to wonder whether Joe would push the issues out of consciousness, or whether he would work on them further in therapy, with Dr. E. or someone else.

Despite the differentiated language we are evolving to describe the complexity of therapeutic relationships, we lack a full understanding of the factors that enable some patients to persist and work with their primary vulnerabilities, while other patients flee or harbor wounds that remain unhealed. Much of what helps *and* what hurts in therapy remains mysterious.

*　*　*　*　*

Feelings of disappointment and disillusionment are an inevitable part of every termination phase and of every successful therapy. They are not experiences to be avoided but rather are valuable sources of psychological development. Disappointment can lead to valuable reassessment of one's self, the other, and the relationship, while disillusionment can lead to new clarity. *Therapy requires of the patient the capacity to create and sustain necessary illusions for as long as they are necessary and to relinquish the illusions in order to let go of and move on from the therapeutic relationship. Therapy requires of the therapist the capacity to allow necessary illusions to form and then to allow them to be withdrawn.* One woman who came for consultation about her therapy and averted a ruptured termination describes the experience of disillusionment in the following letter:

> We managed to get through the terrible impasse. I helped him [the therapist] by backing off from correcting him and he got less anxious as a result. Then he was able to see my point of view, instead of being so wrapped up in his own that he couldn't see beyond it. Once that happened, he could recognize how his personal issues had been involved and he shared some of them with me. That led to a very warm, intimate connection between us. Now I see us more as equals and I'm getting ready to terminate the therapy. We can't go back to the way things were, but I wouldn't say that where we are is bad. I'm very grateful for the consultation with you. When I came, I badly needed to be heard and understood. I was exhausted from trying so hard, without success, to get my therapist to understand me. You helped me let go, helped me see that the difficulty we were having wasn't entirely my fault. That helped me move on. I think that my therapist and I are actually going to have a "happy ending," something I wouldn't have dreamed possible when I first came to you. It's not the ending I expected I'd have, but it's not awful either. Thank you for helping us be able to have it.

* * * * *

When disappointment and disillusionment occur with unmanageable intensity, therapeutic relationships can end in a rupture. When ruptures occur because of wounding and compounding errors that are not acknowledged, and when patients and therapists are deprived of a full range of emotional communication, patients are apt to feel that they have been harmed rather than helped by the therapeutic relationship. A consultant can help these patients endure their intense feelings, affirm their validity, and provide a companion for the patient who is enduring them. In a transitional role, a consultant can facilitate a referral to an ongoing therapist and remain in place as a secure base.

In the context of the solid attachment bond to a consultant and subsequent therapist, patients can recohere a positive sense of self and renew feelings of hope. From the new vantage point, one that would be difficult for patients to reach alone, patients are able to reflect on the damaging therapeutic relationship and to make meaning of it in the context of their psychological life.

Although consultation with patients whose primary therapeutic relationship has terminated in a rupture can help identify the nature of the wound and its context in the patient's life, and can provide an empathic relationship within which healing and restoration of self can begin, an irreparable loss has occurred. The unexpected and often sudden absence of the therapist as a positive person in the patient's psyche, and the loss of the relationship as a positive experience to which the patient can return in memory, cannot be eradicated. Consultants can help patients simply by acknowledging that an irreparable loss has occurred and by comprehending its full meaning in the subjective world of the patient. Losses of any kind, openly acknowledged and mourned, are bearable. But losses that must remain hidden and grieved for in isolation remain an ongoing source of anguish.

❖ *Conclusion* ❖

Therapeutic relationships are unique. On the one hand, they are artificially constructed professional relationships with concomitant boundaries and constraints. At the same time, they are unusually intimate and personal, activating a complicated amalgam of feelings in both participants. Patients and therapists enter into the relationships with different hopes and fears. Therapists' feelings of effectiveness in facilitating and participating in psychological change, and patients' feelings of well-being and confidence in their capacity for ongoing psychological development, are at stake.

Therapeutic relationships as they are currently structured and conceived foster the awakening and re-creation of elements unique to the maternal–and paternal–infant bond.[1] Patients come to depend on the reliability and continuity of care embedded in the stable presence of their therapists just as infants rely on parents to provide these functions. The sense of security and safety in the world and the belief that one will keep going on being that are essential to the establishment of a cohesive sense of self are an integral part of therapeutic relationships just as they are an essential part of infant–mother relationships.[2] The roots of the attachment bond between therapist and patient reside in this domain.

Therapists also carry the authority, competence, and experience of the parents, qualities that patients seek and to which they yield. Patients rely on therapists' knowledge of and experience with psychological development and the terrain of psychological change just as infants rely on parents to help them learn to make their way in the world. The roots of the capacity to hold to one's unique path throughout the life cycle lie in this domain.

Within the dimensions of the parent–infant bond that is revived in therapeutic relationships, patients need therapists to hold for them a vision of what they can hope for and accomplish within the therapeutic relationship just as infants rely on parents to carry internally and reflect back to them their unfolding capacities. Therapists, like caretakers of infants, even with the feelings of envy, competition, and neediness that are part of being human, want to experience themselves as fundamentally competent and able to provide the psychological help their patients need. Patients, even with the destructive impulses and resistance to change that are part of being human, also want to be understood and helped to modify unsatisfying ways of being with themselves and others.

Therapeutic relationships, like parent–infant relationships, become vitally important to those who enter fully into them, providing fertile soil for a strong human attachment bond to grow in tandem with the circumscribed professional relationship between two adults. Within the attachment bond that flourishes in therapeutic relationships, just as within the mother–infant relationship, the patient maintains necessary illusions or beliefs about the possibilities the relationship holds. Infants, babies, and children perceive mothering persons as omnipotently powerful, embodying authority and truth, holding the infant's fate in their hands. Only gradually, as the cognitive, emotional, and physical capacities of infants, babies, and children develop, are the caretakers perceived with increasing clarity as ordinary human beings with needs of their own. Analogously, despite their rational understanding that therapists are merely human beings, patients in therapy tend to perceive therapists as all-knowing and powerful. Because therapists generally refrain from burdening their patients with information about their separate lives, patients are apt to maintain the illusion that their therapists lack ordinary human frailties, have managed to escape the suffering inherent in life, and have worked through their own problems. Patients are likely to perceive themselves as inferior to and less powerful and adequate than their therapists, and consequently expect therapists to recognize and understand their patients' psychological needs as their parents could not. Therapists are vulnerable to corresponding illusions—that they can heal their patients' wounds, repair developmental deficits, avoid failing them catastrophically, and help them fully realize their unique human potential. Like parents who carry a vision of their childrens' future, therapists invest hope in what may be an unreachable ideal for their patients.

Just as infants need to rely on idealized caretakers and are slow to perceive them as separate human beings with needs and limitations, patients are equally slow to relinquish illusions and to perceive their therapists as separate and different from them, and as ordinarily human. The necessary and developmentally appropriate process of disillusionment that enables a patient to perceive her therapist more realistically, like the process of disillusionment that occurs when an infant weans herself from the mother's breast or when a child relinquishes a cherished transitional object, optimally occurs at the patient's pace as well one that is manageable for the therapist. (Disillusionment, as I conceive if it, is a normal part of development rather than a negative, avoidable experience.) But not infrequently therapeutic impasses result in sudden and traumatic disillusionments and ruptured terminations that take a long time to understand, integrate, and repair.

When the therapeutic relationship goes well, patients and therapists experience a sense of gratification and pleasure akin to what parents and children feel at times of harmonious attunement, when what each has to offer is exactly what the other needs. Parents feel bountiful and gratified when they facilitate the unfolding of their children's essential selves. Children feel cared for, hopeful, and expansive when they receive what they need from their parents. Analogously, therapists feel pleased with their chosen profession and with the coming together of their acquired knowledge, experience, and personal psychological work when they are helpful to their patients. Patients experience a renewal of vitality and an expansion of possibilities when they are understood psychologically by their therapists. Patients and therapists meeting each other's needs as relational partners in different modes bring about new experiences of self and other and self-in-relationship that in turn enable constricting self-representations to become flexible and to stretch.

But parent–child relationships, like therapeutic relationships, do not go well all the time. When infants are difficult to parent, caretakers struggle with feelings of personal inadequacy and feelings of frustration and resentment. Infants who sense their parents' distressed response are apt to feel unlovable and difficult and to fear abandonment and rejection. When therapeutic relationships encounter difficult times, therapists and patients struggle with analogous feelings and dilemmas. Therapists who feel rejected, abandoned, or burdened by patients are apt to create distance from them in whatever ways they can. Patients who feel that the therapeutic relationship is at risk and that they are being difficult or unlovable may try to hold onto the therapist, closing the gap between them, in whatever ways they can find, or they may leave the relationship to avoid destroying the therapist or themselves. The result of the conflict in the needs of patients and therapists creates fertile ground for impasses, wounding, and ruptures in the relationship. These are especially agonizing because patients and therapists alike hold onto hope for the relationship to have a positive meaning and outcome. Both patients and therapists must bear the uncertainty that these painful predicaments inevitably constellate: Is there a way to use the impasses, wounding, and ruptures constructively, or will they linger on in memory as damaging and harmful experiences? In view of the yearning for a harmonious relationship that patients and therapists share, the illusion that therapy is successful if it is carried out "correctly," and the shame that accompanies exposing vulnerabilities, unresolvable dilemmas, and ruptured therapeutic relationships are understandably categorized as failure experiences and split off from conscious purview.

Patients and therapists also confront predicaments unique to therapeutic relationships. When they each sense that they are mismatched, they struggle with what to do. Because the relationship is not binding, the option of arriving at a mutual decision to terminate exists, but it is difficult to exercise. Patients and therapists can be left with nagging questions about what was wrong with the match and whether the problems could have been overcome. When patients and therapists are stuck in an entrenched pattern that is familiar and comfortable but unproductive, they feel uncertain and helpless. Even if ways of breaking out of the collusion were to be clearly visible to patients and therapists, the risk of change, fear of losing control and entering uncharted territory, and anxiety about relinquishing what is familiar operate to hold them back. When patients and therapists experience wounding in areas of primary vulnerability, they are catapulted into traumatically painful times. Their adaptive modes of protecting their sense of self and of preserving the relationship often intersect problematically, leading to additional wounding interactions and placing the relationship at risk.

Therapeutic relationships are especially vulnerable to impasses, wounding, and ruptures because the basic structure gives rise to illusions that are at once necessary and dangerous. Essential in enabling patients and therapists to risk establishing a therapeutic relationship, illusions also allow for disappointments and wounding that are potentially devastating. Specific illusions—that the therapist knows what to do and can respond in helpful ways and that the patient can be understood and helped—are a fundamental part of a positive therapeutic alliance and give patients a secure base from which to explore new terrain. Therapists need confidence in their capacities and in the patients' potential just as patients need to believe in their therapists and in their capacity for change. But therapists inevitably fail to understand, are unable to make meaning, and cannot always protect patients from the sometimes catastrophic impingement of their needs and vulnerabilities. Patients inevitably test their therapists' capacity to tolerate their most destructive, problematic selves. At these unavoidable junctures, impasses occur that push therapists and patients to the brink of despair where all illusions of their separate capacities and mutual progress seem irretrievably lost.

At these times we do well to remember that a basic component of expanding human consciousness, and consequently a fundamental task of therapeutic relationships, consists of tolerating paradox and holding opposites simultaneously in view. Meaning can emerge from a context of chaos and uncertainty, and understanding is borne of confusion and despair. As human beings we teeter precariously, as we search for balance between such opposites as hope and despair, illusory and tangible gains, clarity and confusion, certainty and doubt. Free from the distractions of daily life, therapists and patients face in condensed form the quintessential dilemma in human relationships of finding the shifting balance point between merger, mutuality, and separation.

When patient and therapist have an unmanageable mismatch, necessary illusions cannot jell. In collusions, necessary illusions cannot be relinquished. When wounding in the realm of primary vulnerability occurs, necessary illusions are shattered and lost. Patients in all therapeutic relationships, regardless of the therapist's skill and experience and of the patient's psychological capacities, are vulnerable to wounding that destroys illusions. Unlike scientific procedures carried out in a laboratory under carefully protected conditions, therapy takes place in the flow of real life events where intersecting personal vulnerabilities, like alchemical spontaneous combustion, can disrupt from within. Unless the catastrophic effects of disruptions are mitigated by careful work on both the therapists' and patients' part, the participants may be stripped too quickly of the illusions needed to sustain the relationship. Patients may feel damaged rather than helped. Injuries to the psyche, like injuries to our physical body, require the supports that we know are helpful as well as the passage of time for the healing capacities of the psyche to prevail. Therapists' acknowledgment of the meaning of the wounding to patients can bring about the special intimacy of having shared both loving and wounding experiences, an intimacy that goes far deeper than the connection that an exclusively loving relationship can provide. Both therapist and patient have the possibility of experiencing a rare wholeness of self, other, and relationship that can be construed as a grace because it cannot be consciously planned for or willed into existence.

Therapists and patients who seek psychotherapy have the special challenge of attempting to do psychological work in a transitional time. Our profession is in the process of moving from a belief in and reliance on the certainties (ideas about theory and technique of psychological development and psychotherapy) that have provided us with a sense of security and structure. We are acknowledging that our certainties are shifting subjective realities determined by and embedded in cultural and personal fields of influence. The profession is moving from a view of theories of psychological development and therapy as representations of objective truth about the human psyche to a view of theories as subjective representations of experience that are continually in flux.

We are in the process of bridging and holding together in conscious awareness the dualities that have both limited us and provided us with a sense of order and self-confidence: that objective truth can be separated from subjective reality, that therapists are healthy experts and patients are distressed novices, that therapy moves in a linear direction from sickness to health, and that there are correct therapeutic techniques and categories of patients that respond favorably to them. Patients and therapists face the challenge of bearing the difficulties presented by the transitional time: the difficulty of embracing opposites rather than making one pole of a duality the only possibility, of working to extract guiding principles (theoretical conceptualizations) from shared experiences and at the same time remembering that these principles are embedded in a context to which they must remain responsive.

In keeping with our human tendency to view reality in terms of dualities, we have regarded psychological health, well-being, and expertise as residing in therapists while disturbance and psychopathology remain the exclusive province of the patient. We have theorized that wounding in "successful" therapeutic relationships will occur in manageable proportions if the therapist is competent and effective and the patient is not "too disturbed." Within this model, impasses and ruptured treatment relationships become defined as the result of incompetent, inexperienced therapists or of the pathology of patients. As we move from an exclusive reliance on absolute truths and dualities toward a philosophical world view in which absolutes give way to subjective vantage points and opposites coexist simultaneously in consciousness, new conceptualizations of therapeutic relationships open up to us. Impasses, wounding, and ruptured therapeutic relationships need not be conceived of as the consequence of a deficiency in patient or therapist or of an imperfect theory, but rather as the inevitable consequence of an intimate human relationship constructed to elicit areas of the patient's vulnerability, in order for rational insight to be intertwined with new experience.[3]

When we remain within or retreat to the familiar safety and security of fixed ideas, we silence and exclude a large group of patients and therapists—those whose experiences in therapeutic relationships have been problematic, painful, and even traumatic. When therapeutic relationships founder in impasses, patients and therapists suffer feelings of failure that arise in the context of a professional collective that does not want to make room for them. These patients and therapists, in remaining silent, become part of an invisible, silenced group that, when they speak out, threaten the established principles of a profession in transition. When we include the discourse of these patients and therapists, we gain access to experiences that can provide concepts we can use to negotiate the transition in the profession, much as the discourse of other invisible groups—women, blacks, Chicanos, the disabled, the elderly—has helped expand existing culture. If we listen to the voices of patients and therapists who have endured therapeutic impasses, profound wounding, and ruptured therapeutic relationships, we have an opportunity to narrow the gap between our clinical practice and established theory and to create permeable boundaries between them. Impasses carry us to the outer border of existing theories of therapy and psychological development and open up the possibility of creating new ways of thinking that can extend our current, limited conceptions of therapeutic relationships.

As in any time of change, resistance arises in part from a fear of the chaos that threatens when familiar systems yield to the pressure of formerly silenced influences. But if we withstand the fear long enough, new order can emerge. Patients and therapists who give voice to their experiences of impasses, wounds, and ruptured therapeutic relationships have the dual challenge of pushing against the resistance that accompanies fear of change to put forth their subjective truth, and of enduring the transitional time of chaos until a new order emerges.

As we expand from a limited, fixed conception of therapeutic relationships as moving in a linear direction toward the healing of troubled patients, we open up a conception of them as infinitely fluid, changeable, resilient, flexible, and expansive, *and at the same time* oriented toward positive change for the patient. Enlarging our conception of therapy to include paradox and opposites, we can conceive of both participants in the relationship as able to shift positions and roles, allowing room for the therapist-in-the-patient and the patient-in-the-therapist. At the same time, we preserve the shared goal of helping the patient loosen rigid conceptions of self, other, and self-in-relationship, gain access to facets of self and experience that have been unavailable to conscious awareness, risk expanded relational modes, and find new capacities for being-in-life.

As we move beyond a sharp division between our theoretical concepts and our therapeutic process and relinquish the goal of a single, unified theory of therapy, we create a reciprocal and ongoing dialogue between our concepts and our practice, one that not only includes but that values our capacities for intuition and feeling along with our rational capacities for thought and language. Theoretical concepts need not remain or become reified structures that therapists strive to fit themselves into, nor fixed categories into which patients become locked, compelling both patients and therapists to disregard potentially useful aspects of themselves. We can aim for flexible, responsive concepts—clusters of beliefs[4]—that both firmly guide the interventions of therapists and also bend to fit the unique dyad to which they apply.

Rather than isolating each therapeutic dyad by conceiving of it as a solitary and exclusive relationship, a self-enclosed system operating in a self-imposed isolation, we can open up our conception of it. We have the possibility of an expanded view of the therapeutic dyad as a self-enclosed system that is *at the same time* embedded in a larger context that can include, when advisable, the psychological holding environment and new perspective provided by a consultant.

Without the constraints of a sharp separation between conscious and unconscious and between inside and outside, we may conceive of therapeutic relationships as continuing on within the psyches of the participants even after regular meetings cease and even if the relationship has terminated abruptly in a rupture. When we enlarge our conception of therapeutic relationships to include not only positive, healing encounters but also those that are profoundly wounding and disillusioning, we enable patients and therapists to claim consciously *all* aspects of their shared experiences rather than only their "successes." Our narrow conception of what constitutes success and failure itself opens up, as meaning is understood to be created within the therapeutic dyad as well as imposed from without by measuring what occurs against an external standard. Objective standards that represent a culturally limited conception of healthy functioning can be named and recognized, and can coexist with subjective positions, rather than serve as the sole determinant of what constitutes a positive therapeutic outcome. As our categories of thinking become less fixed, we can add *qualities of states of being* to the list of hoped-for outcomes of psychotherapy that currently take the form of fixed states, such as relief of symptoms and modified defenses. A list of qualities of states of being might include, for example, flexibility in relational capacities and representations of self and other, resilience when primary vulnerabilities are reexperienced, and the capacity to withstand intense affect states and change.

When we include subjective meaning alongside the abstract principles we extract from experience, we move into a grey transitional area. In that realm, right and wrong are no longer absolute discrete, separate categories into which therapeutic interventions fit, and there are no exact prescriptions for behavior that can determine a therapist's correct choice of intervention. In the transitional realm, there is no single right answer to such questions as: When is a therapist who shapes herself in response to a patient's need attuning herself as a new developmental relational partner or enacting or gratifying a patient as a coerced relational partner? How can patients distinguish therapists who use patients as coerced relational partners to preserve their sense of a competent, appreciated therapist-self from those who are willing to embark on a personal quest for psychological growth along with the patient? How can therapists and patients distinguish between each other's needs and wants, and even if they discriminate accurately, how can they know what the appropriate response might be? When a patient asks a personal question, how can the therapist know what the answer might mean or even know which answer to choose from among the many possible responses? The responses to these questions come from two sources—*the unique psychological context or field of meaning that unique patient–therapist dyads mutually create in tandem with the established concepts that have evolved over time.* Just as in geometry, where two points are necessary to determine a line, the dual vantage points of subjective meaning and the objective or outside point of view provided by our conceptual language can together determine the direction of a constructive course of action.[5]

In keeping with the evolution in psychotherapy toward an increased capacity to hold opposites in consciousness simultaneously,[6] well-matched patients and therapists who progress without unresolvable stalemates and terminate without traumatic ruptures need no longer be perceived as part of a discrete category separate from those therapeutic dyads that struggle with impasses and wounds or that end in ruptures. *Even when therapeutic relationships progress without painful impasses, profound wounding, or the threat of a ruptured ending, disappointment that leads to reassessment and disillusionment that leads to clarity are inevitable components of the termination phase.* Patients and therapists must confront the limitations of the therapeutic relationship and the impossibility of patients being transformed into their idealized or wished for selves. The most self-reflective and aware patients and therapists must continue to cope with the "ordinary misery," to use Freud's terminology, that is inherent in every life. The projections that patients fasten onto therapists, endowing them with wished-for capacities and powers, must be withdrawn, just as the hopes and idealizations therapists invest in their patients must be relinquished. Patients and therapists who have forged an attachment bond over time through shared intimate experiences must mourn and move on.

Winnicott, who has explored the significance of transitional phenomena more extensively than any other psychoanalyst, offers us a way of thinking about what remains for patients when the therapeutic process has been completed, whether the completion occurs by mutual agreement in a nontraumatic way with both therapist and patient participating, or whether the process occurs within the patient alone (or with a consultant) after a traumatic rupture. Winnicott understood transitional objects and the potential space between two individuals, a space in which psychotherapists surely belong, to reside in a realm in between inner and outer reality where their existence and meaning is never challenged.[7] For example, mothers and babies never question whether the breast full of milk appeared because the baby willed it or because the mother knew to provide it. Parents and children never question the special place that the teddy bear occupies in the child's psyche; it remains under the omnipotent control of the child until it gradually loses its meaning. Analogously, therapists and patients in the best of circumstances tacitly permit the illusion that the therapist has special healing capacities and powers until she gradually (or traumatically) loses them and becomes special in a real way to the patient. Winnicott believed that early transitional objects, when they lose their special meaning, become diffused throughout the cultural field that occupies the space between inner and outer reality. For children the realm is an area of play, whereas for adults it represents an area of creative experience that includes the arts and religion. Because human beings are never free from the strain of giving up illusions, we need the space between outer and inner reality to provide us with a resting place and a place to do the creative work of psychotherapy.

We have thought about concrete transitional objects as limited to infancy and outgrown. But such objects, even teddy bears, need not be considered infantile or as unnecessary for adults. Therapists are transitional objects for patients, and like other transitional phenomena, they eventually shift from their special meaning and emotional charge and become part of that intermediary potential space that Winnicott intuitively visualized as existing between inner and outer reality. Winnicott understood the potential space between to provide the context for creative experience as well as a temporary sanctuary from the tensions of tolerating the demands of ordinary reality. Patients who are able to hold in their psyche their intimate and infinitely textured relationship with their therapists are able to have available within them the therapist and the therapeutic relationship as a temporary sanctuary to which they can return again and again as they need.

In the best of circumstances, like an infant weaning from the breast and the young child gradually losing interest in her teddy bear, the patient is gradually able to relinquish the therapist and at a pace of her choosing, withdrawing the psychological investment and energy that she had placed in the relationship. When regular sessions are discontinued, the therapist and the therapeutic relationship endure in the patient's psyche as the temporary retreat that Winnicott esteemed, and in the therapist's psyche as an available source of meaning and satisfaction in one's life work. But because the best of circumstances are not always possible in reality, patients whose therapeutic relationships founder in impasses or wounding and terminate in a rupture are left with negatively charged territory to avoid or a gap where a sanctuary should be. Therapists are left with an experience that diminishes their sense of professional worth and the gratification in work that lends meaning to living. We need to meet the challenge of providing these patients and therapists both relational support and an opportunity to alter the painful legacy of therapeutic relationships where the positive aspects are eclipsed by traumatic impasses, wounding, and ruptured terminations.

As we move through the transitional phase toward a paradigm that makes room for the uniqueness of each patient–therapist dyad alongside the conceptual domain that encompasses all patient–therapist dyads,[8] we will be better able to prepare patients and therapists for the treacherous and rewarding relationship that lies ahead. Our training institutions can become not only strongholds of accumulated knowledge (language and theory) that is transmitted to those passive recipients who wish to become therapists, but also safe environments within which students and teachers alike can actively continue to create language for and thus gain knowledge from life experience, including distressing aspects of therapeutic relationships.

As we continue to translate the complex experiences that occur within therapeutic relationships into language and allow our language to change in response to experience, we do well to remember that there are aspects of ourselves, others, and our relationships that we can access and *know*, but that remain outside the communicable and shared domain of words and concepts. Along with the theoretical expertise and acquired experience of the therapist and the effort and reflection of the patient, the personhood and integrity of each participant in the therapeutic relationship, the intuition, feeling, and wisdom that each individual brings to bear, and the unique chemistry of the relationship that is continually being created, affect what the therapeutic relationship includes. These special and ineffable qualities of self to which we can allude, but not completely define, are the essential qualities that help patients and therapists bear the uncertainty of psychological exploration in a transitional time. Indefinable yet familiar, they are not capacities that can be fully described or taught, but we recognize them when we are in contact with them. Like steel taking shape, these qualities of selfhood are forged from all of our life experiences—including therapeutic relationships that have withstood wounding, disappointment, and disillusionment—if we choose. They are wrought from the heat of life itself, transforming the psyches of those individuals who dare to venture fully within its fiery reach.

Survey on Therapeutic Impasse and Failure

I will be giving a talk at the November 1986 Psychotherapy Institute Symposium on the topic of errors, impasses, and failures in psychotherapy. One segment of this presentation will address those impasses that are serious enough to cause an end to the work, with intense feelings of failure, rage, and disappointment on the part of either the therapist or patient. I would like to know how common this experience is within our professional community so I will have a sense of context for my talk. I would appreciate your help in completing the following questionnaire anonymously and in returning it in the stamped envelope provided. I will share the results with you at the Symposium. Thank you!

Male _____ Female _____   Therapist: Yes _____   No _____

Age: 20–30 _____   31–40 _____   41–50 _____   51–60 _____   over 61 _____

Have you been a patient in a long-term depth psychotherapy that ended in an impasse, with accompanying rage, disappointment, or sense of failure?

Once _____   Twice _____

More than twice _____   Never _____

Please put number of times for an answer if necessary:

Was the therapist: Same sex _____   Opposite sex _____

Was the experience harmful or damaging?   Yes _____   No _____

Do you feel you have resolved the experience: On your own _____

In another therapy _____   Not yet _____

Have you been a therapist in a long-term psychodynamic therapy that ended in an impasse, with accompanying rage, disappointment, or sense of failure?

Number of patients _____ (approximate)

Was the patient: Same sex _____   Opposite sex _____

(Please put approximate number of times for an answer)

Additional comments:

Results of 1986 Survey on Therapeutic Impasse and Failure

Table B.1. Number of Men and Women in Sample

Sex	Frequency	Percentage
Male	10	10
Female	90	90

Table B.2. Age Distribution of Sample

Age Range	Frequency	Percentage
20–30	1	1
31–40	52	52
41–50	34	34
51–60	8	8
Over 61	5	5

Table B.3. Therapists Who Have Had Patients Leave in Impasse

Number of patients	Frequency	Percentage
0	12	12.50
1	31	32.29
2	24	25.00
3	12	12.50
4 or more	17	17.71

Table B.4. Therapists Who Have Been Patients in Impasses

Number of Times	Frequency	Percentage
Never	46	46.46
Once	34	34.34
Twice or more	19	19.19

Table B.5. Therapists Who Experienced Harm From Impasse as Patient

Harmful	Frequency	Percentage
Not damaged	13	28
Damaged	27	58
Both damaging and not	6	13

Table B.6. Therapist's Mode of Resolution of Damaging Experience.

Mode	Frequency	Percentage
On Own	9	20
In another therapy	26	58
Both modes	10	22
Unresolved	9	17

Summary of Other Research Studies on Painful Terminations

In searching for other research studies investigating the same question, I came across two reports that contain statistics on negative terminations. Two studies are reported in a 1986 *Harvard Medical School Mental Health Letter*. The author, Henry Grunebaum, clinical professor of psychiatry at Harvard Medical School, reports the striking finding in one study that 21% of therapists in a total sample of 71 found their own psychotherapy to be harmful.[1] Grunebaum notes, "Although controlled studies show that psychotherapy helps most patients, like other medical treatments it can be harmful as well as helpful."[2]

The harmful experiences were subsequently investigated in a second study in which subjects were obtained through advertisements in newsletters of professional organizations and then interviewed. Their experiences were difficult to categorize. One group of patients felt the therapist was cold and inhuman. Another group felt the therapist had encouraged the expression of strong feelings and had then been unable to work with them. A third group suffered from sexual abuse by therapists. Another group felt there was a mismatch between patient and therapist; these patients were least likely to feel harmed. In a humane conclusion, Grunebaum recommends trusting the patient's judgment rather than that of the therapist or outside observer, because "the patient has access to information that no outsider can be aware of."[3] He also recommends that therapists ascertain how patients feel about them and accept these feelings as real: "the patient's early impressions cannot be treated merely as a transference of childhood attitudes toward their parents."[4]

Another article describes a study conducted by Jeanine Auger at the Analytical Psychology Club of Los Angeles, where members have a special interest in Jungian therapy.[5] Of the seventy responses (where the return rate was 49%), 43% report negative termination experiences. In this sample the experience of a negative termination was even more common than in Grunebaum's study.

An article by Guy and Liaboe in *The Clinical Psychologist*, a psychology journal, on the topic of the utilization and usefulness of therapy for an experienced psychotherapist, refers to a research study by Buckley, Karasu, and Charles.[6] These investigators report that 21% of the psychotherapists they surveyed reported that their previous therapy had been harmful to them in some way. The study is cited as one of the reasons why experienced therapists do not seek psychotherapy.

The article by Guy and Liaboe on the usefulness and utilization of psychotherapy by experienced therapists also addresses the psychic stress that is inherent in the profession. Failure experiences with patients is one clear cause of the psychic stress that therapists suffer: "Such negative factors [inherent in the practice of psychotherapy] are the physical and psychic isolation (Will, 1979), *repeated feelings of loss and abandonment as a result of planned and unplanned terminations* (Greben, 1975; my italics).[7] Intensive psychotherapy is a relationship in which both parties are affected for better or worse.

❖ *Notes* ❖

Introduction

1. Depth psychotherapy and psychoanalysis are elusive, ineffable processes that have been described, defined, and understood in many different ways. I will use the term "depth psychotherapeutic relationships" to refer to long-term, intensive therapeutic relationships that include the unconscious psyche of both participants and in which the central psychological issues of the patient and the therapist become engaged. The therapeutic relationship provides both the vehicle and the container within which the conscious awareness of the patient and the therapist expands. Entrenched, familiar relational modes of being with one's self and others and entrenched, familiar self-representations can be identified as they are experienced in the relationship, creating the possibility of modifying them. Other therapists would not agree with my understanding and would, for example, conceive of depth psychotherapy as engaging only the core issues of the patient rather than those of the therapist as well. For simplicity, I will use the term "therapy" throughout the book to refer to depth psychotherapy.
2. I use the word "patient" rather than "client" because its meaning derives from the Latin word *patiens*, to suffer. Patient means "capable of bearing affliction with calmness," certainly an appropriate word for a psychotherapy patient. As Alexandra Kaplan points out in a footnote to her article, "Female or Male Psychotherapists for Women: New Formulations," in *Women's Growth in Connection*, neither word seems fully satisfactory. She adds, "It is noteworthy that there is no independent word for someone who seeks psychotherapy" (p. 269). One element in our shared dissatisfaction with the nouns *patient* and *client* consists of the changing paradigm of psychotherapy: Neither the medical model nor a formal business model captures the essence of psychotherapy.
3. I will use "therapist" rather than "analyst." The word "therapist" derives from the Greek word, *therapeia*, which means "service," and from *therapeuin*, which means "in attendance." These meanings fit more closely with a paradigm of depth psychotherapy as a process to which both participants submit rather than a paradigm of depth psychotherapy in which the therapist remains detached and "does something" to the patient.
4. George E. Atwood, Robert D. Stolorow, and Jeffrey L. Trop, "Impasses in Psychoanalytic Therapy: A Royal Road," *Contemporary Psychoanalysis*, Vol. 25, no. 4 (October 1989); pp. 554–573. This article puts forth a theoretical

conceptualization of the intersubjective conjunctions and disjunctions that occur as the psychological worlds of the therapist and patient interact.

5. Hilde S. Burton points out that our difficulty holding opposites in consciousness simultaneously is an example of splitting or dissociation as part of everyday functioning (personal communication).

6. Freud, after the death of his father, experienced a painful descent that eventually led to his well-known work *Interpretation of Dreams*. Jung, after his relationship with Freud, his mentor, ended in a rupture, experienced states of being that today would be labeled psychotic. Yet he tells us in his autobiography, *Memories, Dreams, and Reflections*, that these experiences contained the seeds for his entire body of work. Melanie Klein's theories derived from her analysis of her son, Erich, and a significant paper on loneliness written late in her life was directly related to personal experience of grief, depression, and loneliness (see Grossfurth, *Melanie Klein: Her World and Her Work*).

7. By sensationalistic, I refer to the scandals surrounding Jung's treatment of his patient Sabina Spielrein; Freud's treatment of his patient Emma and the fact that he analyzed his daughter, Anna; and to Klein's analysis of her son Erich.

8. I refer to the intersubjective approach articulated by Stolorow, Atwood, and Brandschaft and to the work of Stephen Mitchell most recently apparent in the appearance of a new journal, *Psychoanalytic Dialogues: A Journal of Relational Perspectives*.

9. Looking more closely at the therapist's personal resistance to change in work with a particular patient is a relatively new idea. For the most part, the focus within the profession has been primarily on the patient's resistance to change. Joyce Lindenbaum, in a discussion of my presentation on "Therapeutic Impasses" (Northern California Chapter of Psychoana-lytic Psychology, San Francisco, CA, October 30, 1990) emphasized the therapist's effort to restore a former, familiar relationship.

10. Mary Field Belenky, Blythe McVicker Clinchy, Nancy Rule Goldberger, and Jill Mattuck Tarule, *Women's Ways of Knowing: The Development of Self, Voice, and Mind* (New York: Basic Books, 1986).

   The authors of *Women's Ways of Knowing* started from the premise that the conceptions of knowledge that have been accepted in our culture have been shaped by men. Major educational institutions were founded by men for the education of men; men have established the values and theories that provide the foundation for everyone. The authors of *Women's Ways of Knowing* write about the forms of knowing that are characteristic of women, based on their extensive and open-ended interviews of different groups of women. They chose open-ended interviews so that their preconceived ideas of what to expect would not limit what they learned from the women they spoke with, even though the analysis of data was made more complex.

   Based on data from their interviews of different groups of women, the authors delineate a hierarchy of positions of knowing. The first position is *silence,* characterized by an extreme denial of self and a dependence upon external authority for direction that is true of the most deprived group of women. The second position is *received knowledge,* which entails listening to the voices of others. The position reflects an externally oriented perspective on knowledge and truth, where authority always resides outside the individual. The third position is *subjective knowledge,* which is characterized by listening to one's inner voice, "a new conception of truth as personal, private, and subjectively known or intuited." The definition of self of some women in the position of subjective knowledge may be in a state of flux as they relinquish definitions that the culture supplies. The fourth position is *procedural knowledge,* in which the voice of reason prevails. Knowing in the position of procedural knowledge requires careful observation and analysis rather than intuition alone. The interviewers identified two forms of procedural knowledge, which they labeled *separate* and *connected* knowing. "Separate knowing" relies on impersonal reason, whereas "connected knowing" is based on the conviction that the most trustworthy knowledge comes from personal experience. Separate knowers learn through formal instruction whereas connected knowers learn through empathy. Most institutions of higher learning value separate knowing—the rational, analytic voice; the subjective voice of feeling and intuition is less valued, often relegated to the realm of the personal and private. The final position, that of *constructed knowledge,* is the position that integrates the different voices. It begins as

> an effort to reclaim the self by attempting to integrate knowledge that they [women being interviewed] felt intuitively was personally important with knowledge they had learned from others. They told of weaving together strands of rational and emotive thought and of integrating objective and subjective knowing. Rather than extricating the self in the acquisition of knowledge, these women used themselves in rising to a new way of thinking. (pp. 134–135)

Chapter One

1. Margaret Little, *Transference Neurosis and Transference Psychosis* (New York: Jason Aronson, 1981) p. 243.
2. Harry Guntrip, "My Experience of Analysis with Fairbairn and Winnicott (How Complete a Result Does Psycho-Analytic Therapy Achieve?)" in Peter Buckley, ed., *Essential Papers on Object Relations* (New York: New York University Press, 1986), pp. 447–468. The article can also be found in *International Review of Psychoanalysis* vol. 2 (1975): 145–156.
3. Stephen Kurtz, *The Art of Unknowing: Dimensions of Openness in Analytic Therapy,* (Northvale, NJ: Jason Aronson, 1989), p. 40.
4. Barbara Stevens Sullivan, "The Disliked Patient," in *Psychotherapy*

Grounded in the Feminine Principle (Wilmette, IL: Chiron 1989,) writes:

> It is not clear to me that there is anything constructive to be done about the patient who is really caught in what we could call the death instinct, in an unconscious determination not to grow . . . ultimately the therapist's power seems limited to giving the patient a rather mild nudge in a constructive direction . . . the extent to which the patient's own constructive energies will emerge cannot be predicted in advance. (p. 181)

5. Ibid., pp. 181–196.
6. Guntrip, "My Experience of Analysis with Fairbairn and Winnicott." The article was written not long after he learned of Winnicott's death and shortly before he died.
7. Ibid., p. 146.
8. Ibid., p. 156.
9. Little, *Transference Neurosis and Transference Psychosis*, p. 273.
10. Ibid., pp. 277–278.
11. Margaret Little, *Psychotic Anxieties and Containment: A Personal Record of an Analysis with Winnicott* (New York: Jason Aronson Inc., 1990), p. 33.
12. Little, *Transference Neurosis and Transference Psychosis*, p. 300.
13. Dorte von Drigalski, *Flowers on Granite: One Woman's Odyssey through Psychoanalysis* (Berkeley: Creative Arts Book Company, 1986).
14. Nini Herman, *My Kleinian Home: A Journey through Four Psychotherapies* (London: Quartet Books, 1985). Interestingly, the two book-length accounts of failed therapies that I have come across were both written by female patients (there are accounts of "successful" analyses written by male patients). Perhaps this is a reection of a cultural reality—that men as the stronger sex must not reveal vulnerabilities or disclose shameful experiences.
15. A new psychoanalytic journal was inaugurated in 1991 entitled *Psychoanalytic Dialogues: A Journal of Relational Perspectives*, dedicated to "facilitating debate among theoreticians and clinicians working within this array of relational perspectives." Included within what the editors are labeling relational perspectives are British object relations theory, Self psychology, certain currents of Freudian thought, and the empirical tradition of infancy research and child development.
16. Herman, *My Kleinian Home*, p. 63.
17. Ibid., p. 64.
18. Ibid., p. 90.
19. Ibid., p. 100.
20. Ibid., p. 103.
21. Ibid., p. 107.
22. Therapists may choose to allow relational modes to evolve without explicitly analyzing them, simply allowing them to occur, but optimally therapists strive to be conscious of relational modes and to understand their positive function in the therapeutic relationship. Herman's therapist, from her perspective, remained unconscious of the relational mode that was established and was unaware of the anxiety it aroused in her.

23. Herman, *My Kleinian Home*, p. 108.
24. Ibid., p. 115.
25. Roger Kennedy, Review of *My Kleinian Home*, in *The International Review of Psychoanalysis*, Vol. 13, P. 2 (1986), 250–251.
26. Ibid., p. 250.
27. Ibid., p. 251.
28. Two articles are Judy L. Kantrowitz, Ann L. Katz, Deborah Greenman, Humphrey Morris, Frank Paolitto, Jerome Sashin, and Leonard Solomon, "The Patient–Analyst Match and the Outcome of Psychoanalysis: A Pilot Study," *Journal of the American Psychoanalytic Association*, Vol. 37, No. 4 (1989): 893–919; and George E. Atwood, Robert D. Stolorow, and Jeffrey Trop, "Impasses in Psychoanalytic Therapy: A Royal Road," *Contemporary Psychoanalysis*, Vol. 25, No. 4 (October 1989): 554–573.
29. Atwood, Stolorow, and Trop, "Impasses in Psychoanalytic Therapy," pp. 556–557.
30. Ibid., pp. 558–559.
31. Stephen Kurtz, *The Art of Unknowing*, pp. 38–39.

Chapter 2

1. D. W. Winnicott (1960), "Ego Distortion in Terms of True and False Self," *Maturational Processes and the Facilitating Environment* (New York: International Universities Press, 1980), p. 151.
2. Sigmund Freud (1937), "Analysis Terminable and Interminable," in *Standard Edition of the Complete Psychological Works of Sigmund Freud* (Vol. 23), trans. and ed. James Strachey, with Anna Freud, assisted by Alix Strachey and Alan Tyson, pp. 211–253.
3. Ibid., p. 247.
4. Ibid., p. 248.
5. Ibid., p. 250.
6. Discussion of the False Self is based on D. W. Winnicott (1960), "Ego Distortion in Terms of True and False Self," pp. 140–152.
7. Ibid., p. 151.
8. Ibid., p. 152.
9. Judy L. Kantrowitz, Ann L. Katz, Deborah A. Greenman, Humphrey Morris, Frank Paolitto, Jerome Sashin, and Leonard Solomon, "The Patient–Analyst Match and the Outcome of Psychoanalysis: A Pilot Study," *Journal of the American Psychoanalytic Association*, Vol. 37, No. 4 (1989): 893–919. In this unusual paper for a traditionally psychoanalytic journal, the authors report the findings of a pilot study: the match between analysand and analyst is of central importance in the analytic situation.
10. C. Kerenyi, "Prolegomena," in *Essays on a Science of Mythology* (Princeton, NJ: Princeton University Press, 1973), p. 21.

Chapter 3

1. Harold F. Searles, "The Patient as Therapist to His Analyst," in *Countertransference and Related Subjects: Selected Papers* (New York: International Universities Press, 1979), pp. 380–459. A discussion of patients' inherent human need to heal their analysts just as they struggled to heal their parents.

Chapter 4

1. John Klauber, "Elements of the Psychoanalytic Relationship and Their Therapeutic Implications," in Gregorio Kohon, ed., *The British School of Psychoanalysis: The Independent Tradition* (New Haven, CT: Yale University Press, 1986), p. 204.
2. Lewis Aron, "The Patient's Experience of the Analyst's Subjectivity," *Psychoanalytic Dialogues: A Journal of Relational Perspectives*, Vol. 1, No 1 (1991): 36.
3. Jay R. Greenberg, "Countertransference and Reality," *Psychoanalytic Dialogues: A Journal of Relational Perspectives*, Vol. 1, No. 1 (1991): 52, 72.
4. Analogously, male patients with female therapists often abandon themselves in order to please a "good mother" or hold back from disclosing feelings and vulnerabilities because of the culture's insistence that boys must separate from their mothers.
5. Psychoanalyst D. W. Winnicott was unusual in his awareness of the limitations of therapists' interpretations. He understood that therapists can deprive patients of the joy of self-discovery out of their personal need to make interpretations and wrote the frequently quoted sentence, "I think I interpret mainly to let the patient know the limits of my understanding." Winnicott, *Playing and Reality* (Middlesex, Eng.: Penguin Books, 1971), p. 102.
6. Parts of the ensuing discussion of the case of Lynn and Dr. K. are derived from a previously published article by the author: "The Mother without a Face Revisited: Initiation into the Feminine," *Psychotherapy Institute Journal*, Vol. 3 (November 1986): 75–86.
7. The final report of the American Psychological Association's National Task Force on Women and Depression concludes that American women are twice as likely as men to be depressed because of the experience of *being female in contemporary culture*. The report urges that depression in women be examined in a biopsychosocial context and emphasizes that women are at high risk of depression because of the interaction of women's biology with environment. Ellen McGrath, Gwendolyn Puryear Keita, Bonnie R. Strickland, and Nancy Felipe Russo, eds., *Women and Depression: Risk Factors and Treatment Issues* (Washington DC: American Psychological Association, 1990).
8. Jean Baker Miller, *Toward a New Psychology of Women* (Boston: Beacon Press, 1986).

9. Carol Gilligan, *In a Different Voice: Psychological Theory and Women's Development* (Cambridge, MA: Harvard University Press, 1982).
10. See publications from the Stone Center, Wellesley College, and Miller, *Toward a New Psychology of Women.* Also Gilligan, *In a Different Voice,* and Mary Field Belenky, Blythe McVicker Clinchy, Nancy Rule Goldberger, and Jill Mattuck Tarule, *Women's Ways of Knowing: The Development of Self, Voice, and Mind* (New York: Basic Books, 1986).
11. C. G. Jung, *Collected Works, Vol. 9* (Princeton, NJ: Princeton University Press, 1959), par.24. The metaphor of "anima" is useful apart from Jung's conceptions of archetypes of the collective unconscious and the controversy surrounding these conceptions.
12. Ibid., par 40.
13. Marion Woodman, "Abandonment in the Creative Woman," *Chiron: A Review of Jungian Analysis* (Wilmette, IL: Chiron, 1985), p. 43.
14. Ibid., p. 41.
15. Betty Meador, "Transference/Countertransference between Woman Analyst and the Wounded Girl Child," in *Chiron: A Review of Jungian Analysis* (Wilmette, IL: Chiron, 1984), pp. 163–164.
16. Woodman, "Abandonment in the Creative Woman," p. 79.
17. See the case of Dee and Dr. H. in Chapter Fifteen.
18. Susan Griffin, *Woman and Nature: The Roaring Inside Her* (New York: Harper & Row, 1978).

Chapter 5

1. Patrick J. Casement, *Learning from the Patient* (New York: Guilford Press, 1991), p. 318.
2. Winnicott writes in "Primary Maternal Preoccupation (1956)," in *Through Paediatrics to Psychoanalysis* (New York: Basic Books, 1975):

> It is my thesis that in the earliest phase we are dealing with a very special state of the mother, a psychological condition which deserves a name, such as *primary maternal preoccupation*. I suggest that sufficient tribute has not yet been paid in our literature, or perhaps anywhere, to a very special psychiatric condition of the mother, of which I would say the following things:
>
> It gradually develops and becomes a state of heightened sensitivity during, and especially towards the end of, the pregnancy. It lasts for a few weeks after the birth of the child. It is not easily remembered by mothers once they have recovered from it. (pp. 301–302)

3. I am not referring to Jung's notion of an archetypal Self, which carries the image of wholeness in the collective unconscious stratum of the psyche, but rather to what Jung would call the ego.
4. Heinz Kohut used this example in a talk at the annual Self-Psychology Conference in Berkeley, California, shorly before his death. The example is referred to in Heinz Kohut, *How Does Analysis Cure?* ed. Arnold Goldberg, with Paul Stepansky (Chicago: University of Chicago Press, 1984), p. 213.

5. An article on the hospice appeared in the *Oakland Tribune, Parade Magazine,* November 19, 1989.
6. C. G. Jung, "The Archetypes and the Collective Unconscious," in *Collected Works,* Vol. 9 (Princeton, NJ: Princeton University Press, 1968), par. 3: Jung acknowledges that Freud "was aware of its [the unconscious'] archaic and mythological thought-forms." Information included in this section on archetypes is taken from Jung's writings in Vol. 9 of the *Collected Works,* New Jersey, Princeton University Press, 1968.
7. Ibid., par. 6.
8. Jung, "A Review of the Complex Theory," *Collected Works,* Vol. 8, par. 203.
9. See Chapter Nine on infant research and the realm of primary vulnerability for a more complete discussion of the origins of vulnerabilities in mother–child and father–child relationships.

Chapter 6

1. Heinz Kohut, *How Does Analysis Cure?* ed. Arnold Goldberg, with Paul Stepansky (Chicago: University of Chicago Press, 1984), p. 213, note 4.
2. Michael Balint, *The Basic Fault: Therapeutic Aspects of Regression* (New York: Brunner/Mazel, 1979), pp. 22–23.
3. D. W. Winnicott (1962), "Ego Integration in Child Development," in *The Maturational Processes and the Facilitating Environment* (New York: International Universities Press, 1980), pp. 57–58.
4. Kohut, *How Does Analysis Cure?* p. 49.
5. Ibid., pp. 49–50.
6. Ibid., p. 16. The concept of disintegration anxiety is also discussed in Heinz Kohut, *The Restoration of the Self* (New York: International Universities Press, 1977), pp. 104–105.
7. Kohut, *How Does Analysis Cure?* p. 16.
8. Ibid., p. 49.
9. Ibid., pp. 17–18.
10. Ibid., p. 19.
11. Ibid., p. 69.
12. Kohut, *The Restoration of the Self,* p. 171.
13. Balint, *The Basic Fault.*
14. Ibid., p. 6.
15. One highly significant function that a therapist/consultant serves for an individual who has lived through a therapeutic impasse and painful termination is that of bearing witness to the loss and participating in the mourning process.
16. *American Heritage Dictionary of the American Language,* p. 1438.
17. I do not mean to imply that the concept of psychological damage is irrelevant or useless. Patients who have been psychologically damaged by traumatic environments and experiences do seek psychotherapy.
18. Winnicott, "Ego Integration in Child Development," pp. 56–63.

19. D. W. Winnicott, "Fear of Breakdown," in Gregorio Kohon, ed., *The British School of Psychoanalysis: The Independent Tradition* (New Haven, CT: Yale University Press, 1986), pp. 173–184.

Chapter 7

1. Excerpt from Eudora Welty, *One Writer's Beginnings*, quoted in Marilyn Sewell, ed., *Cries of the Spirit: A Celebration of Women's Spirituality* (Boston: Beacon Press, 1991), p. 76.
2. Jessica Benjamin, *The Bonds of Love: Psychoanalysis, Femininism, and the Problem of Domination* (New York: Pantheon Books, 1988), p. 24.
3. D. W. Winnicott (1962), "Ego Integration in Child Development," in *Maturational Processes and the Facilitating Environment* (New York: International Universities Press, 1980), p. 57.
4. D. W. Winnicott (1960), "The Theory of the Parent–Infant Relationship," in *Maturational Processes and the Facilitating Environment* (New York: International Universities Press, 1980), p. 46.
5. John Bowlby, *A Secure Base: Parent–Child Attachment and Healthy Human Development* (New York: Basic Books, 1988).
6. I will refer to the maternal or mother–infant matrix for simplicity, with the understanding that both biological and adoptive mothers, as well as fathers and men, can serve functions that we think of as mothering. Male and female therapists can elicit yearnings for mothering. For example, Freud wistfully responded to his patient, the poet Hilda Doolittle—as reported in her book, *Tribute to Freud* (New York: New Directions, 1984) p. 147—when she asked whether other patients had, like her, a mother-transference to him, "Oh, VERY many."
7. D. W. Winnicott (1960), "Ego Distortion in Terms of the True and False Self," in *Maturational Processes and the Facilitating Environment* (New York: International Universities Press, 1965), p. 39.
8. D. W. Winnicott (1963), "The Development of the Capacity for Concern," in *Maturational Processes and the Facilitating Environment* (New York: International Universities Press, 1980), p. 75.
9. *American Heritage Dictionary of the American Language*, p. 807.
10. Thomas Ogden, *The Matrix of the Mind* (Northvale, NJ: Jason Aronson 1986), p. 180.
11. Jane Swigart, *The Myth of the Bad Mother: The Emotional Realities of Mothering* (New York: Doubleday, 1991). Swiggart emphasizes that mothering is a collective responsibility that belongs not only to the mother but to the father, extended family, and culture.
12. Christopher Bollas, *The Shadow of the Object* (New York: Columbia University Press, 1987), p. 14.
13. Ibid., p. 28.
14. Ibid., p. 21.
15. Harry Guntrip, *Personality Structure and Human Interaction* (London: Hogarth Press, 1982), p. 30.

16. Hanna Segal, *Introduction to the Work of Melanie Klein* (New York: Basic Books, 1974), p. 26.

17. Ibid., p. ix.

18. Thomas Ogden, *The Primitive Edge of Experience* (Northvale, NJ: Jason Aronson, 1989). The ensuing discussion of the autistic–contiguous, paranoid–schizoid, and depressive positions is based upon this book.

19. Bollas's conception of the mother as a *transformational object* enriches Ogden's description of the early autistic–contiguous position.

20. Ogden, *Primitive Edge of Experience*, p. 4.

21. Ibid., p. 14.

Chapter 8

1. Margaret S. Mahler, Fred Pine, and Anni Bergman, *The Psychological Birth of the Human Infant* (New York: Basic Books, 1975), p. 4.

2. Daniel Stern, *The Interpersonal World of the Infant: A View from Psychoanalysis and Developmental Psychology* (New York: Basic Books, 1985), p. 10.

3. D. W. Winnicott (1960), "The Theory of the Parent–Infant Relationship," in *Maturational Processes and the Facilitating Environment* (New York: International Universities Press, 1980), p. 39.

4. Jessica Benjamin, *The Bonds of Love: Psychoanalysis, Feminism, and the Problem of Domination* (New York: Pantheon Books, 1988), pp. 23–24.

5. I prefer to use the term "relational partner" as a substitute for the term "object," but I will use the two concepts interchangeably because the language of object relations is familiar and common.

6. Similarly, predominating theories of depth psychotherapy have tended to be unidirectional and unidimensional. Jung, who viewed patient and therapist as equally involved in depth psychotherapy, is an exception. But Jungian theory has not yet been accepted into mainstream psychotherapy. Balint, with his concept of the harmonious interpenetrating mix-up of patient and therapist during phases of regression, is another exception.

7. Michael Balint, *The Basic Fault: Therapeutic Aspects of Regression* (New York: Brunner/Mazel, 1968), p. 165.

8. Leon Grinberg, Dario Sor, and Elizabeth Tabak de Bianchedi, *Introduction to the Work of Bion* (Northvale, NJ: Jason Aronson, 1977), pp. 53–60.

9. Thomas Ogden, *Projective Identification and Psychotherapeutic Technique* (Northvale, NJ: Jason Aronson, 1982).

10. Mardi Ireland has a book in progress on *Women Who Are Not Mothers*.

11. The summary of Margaret Mahler's theory of early development is taken from Mahler, Pine, and Bergman, *Psychological Birth of the Human Infant*.

12. The brief summary and discussion of Lacan's theory is based on Ellie Ragland-Sullivan, *Jacques Lacan and the Philosophy of Psychoanalysis* (Chicago: University of Chicago Press, 1987).

13. Lacan's theory attributes specific functions to mothers and fathers in a way that discredits both mothers and fathers. Mothers can foster autonomy and

independence in babies and fathers can provide the source for a sense of primary identity.

13. I will use the term "mother" for simplicity's sake, with the understanding that a mothering person can be a man or an adoptive mother.

14. The pattern of relationship discussed is applicable not only to mothers and infants but to human relationships in general.

15. The term "developmental object" was presented in a paper given by Calvin Settledge at the annual Earl Simburg lecture at Alta Bates/Herrick Hospital, Berkeley, California, April 11, 1991.

16. For an excellent analysis of a case in which the patient's developmental needs changed and the analyst needed to shift his understanding of the patient, see Jeffrey L. Trop, and Robert D. Stolorow, "A Developmental Perspective on Analytic Empathy: A Case Study," *Journal of the American Academy of Psychoanalysis*, Vol. 19, No. (1991): 31–46.

17. Stern's observational studies of mothers and infants highlight the ways mothers and infants attune to each other, matching affect states and intensity of mood. Stern believes that these behaviors represent the beginning of awareness that internal states can be known and shared, and as such are the precursors of empathy, a capacity that requires a higher level of cognitive and affective development.

18. Martin Stanton, *Sandor Ferenczi: Reconsidering Active Intervention* (Northvale, NJ: Jason Aronson, 1991), pp. 151–164.

19. We also need to allow mothers increasingly to be subjective relational partners for their children, always with the awareness of the imbalance inherent in both roles.

20. Marshall Klaus emphasized the malleability and vulnerability of pregnant women in a presentation at Alta Bates/Herrick Hospital on May 6, 1991 when he declared, "No pregnant woman should ever be yelled at!" He described his research in which pregnant women who were supported by another woman (known as a "doula") in the last stage of the pregnancy and labor had fewer problems adjusting after birth than a control group of women who did not have the continuous supportive presence of another woman. Klaus believes that obstetrical practices in the United States will be undergoing a massive revision as information provided by research such as his is assimilated into the culture.

21. Mothers have the challenge of remembering that when they talk to their adult children, they are also talking on a psychological level to their child at other developmental levels.

Chapter 9

1. Daniel Stern, *The Interpersonal World of the Infant: A View from Psychoanalysis and Developmental Psychology* (New York: Basic Books, 1985), pp. 4–5.

2. Margaret Little, *Psychotic Anxieties and Containment: A Personal Record of an Analysis with Winnicott* (Northvale, NJ: Jason Aronson, 1990), pp. 107–108.

3. Harry Guntrip, "My Experience of Analysis with Fairbairn and Winnicott (How Complete a Result Does Psycho-Analytic Therapy Achieve?)", in Peter Buckley, ed., *Essential Papers On Object Relations* (New York: New York University Press, 1986), p. 460, 461–462.

4. D. W. Winnicott (1960), "The Theory of the Parent–Infant Relationship," in *Maturational Processes and the Facilitationg Environment* (New York: International Universities Press, 1980), pp. 51–52.

5. Both developmental psychologists and psychotherapists function in a cultural context that influences their observations and the concepts they create. Psychologist Philip Cushman critiques the work of developmental psychologist Daniel Stern from a social-constructionist perspective in his article, "Ideology Obscured: Political Uses of the Self in Daniel Stern's Infant," *American Psychologist*, Vol. 46, No. 3 (March 1991); 206–219.

6. D. W. Winnicott, "Mirror-role of Mother and Family in Child Development," in *Playing and Reality* (Middlesex, England: Penguin Books, 1971), pp. 130–138. Winnicott, without the benefit of recent observational studies of infants and mothers, drawing exclusively upon his personal observations as a pediatrician, addressed the theoretical significance of mother–baby eye contact for the baby's developing sense of self. Winnicott contended that in optimal mother–infant dyads, a baby looking into the mother's eyes would see herself reflected as if in a mirror. If the mother is unable to "see" the baby as a separate object and instead sees her own expectations reflected, the baby's sense of self will be influenced accordingly. Only those aspects of self that receive maternal attention will develop, whereas aspects of self that are ignored by mother because they are invisible to her will remain outside the organization of the developing ego-self of the baby. Winnicott understood that none of us can truly "see" other people completely as who they are, separate from our own projections. His notion of the "good-enough" mother applies to this maternal capacity as it does to all others: A mother must be able to mirror accurately at least some qualities that are intrinsic to her baby.

7. Stern, *Interpersonal World of the Infant*, p. 21.

8. Christopher Nolan, *Under the Eye of the Clock* (New York: St. Martin's Press, 1987), pp. 37–38.

9. Kim Chernin, personal communication.

10. Frances Tustin, *Autistic Barriers in Neurotic Patients* (New Haven, CT: Yale University Press, 1986), p. 197.

11. Stern, *Interpersonal World of the Infant*, pp. 67–68.

12. Cushman, "Ideology Obscured," p. 208.

13. Kim Chernin points out that Stern emphasizes the baby's activity in shaping the responses of the mothering person and underestimates the extent to which the mother acts on the infant (see e.g., Stern, *Interpersonal World of the Infant*, p. 21, for a description of how the baby controls the mothering person through visual gaze). Stern consequently stresses the baby's activity rather than its passive receptivity, which would be an important component of the experience Bollas describes (personal communication).

14. The Stone Center Self-in-Relation theory includes a concept of mutual empathy. This concept is also developed in Jessica Benjamin, *The Bonds of Love: Psychoanalysis, Feminism, and the Problem of Domination* (New York: Pantheon Books, 1988).
15. See Cushman, "Ideology Obscured," pp. 213–217, for a comprehensive and thought-provoking critique of Stern's conception of language development in the infant.
16. Stern acknowledges that he is building on Winnicott's concept of transitional phenomena. (See Winnicott, "Transitional Objects and Transitional Phenomena," in *Playing and Reality*, pp. 1–30.) The origin, function, and meaning of language is an area of lively theoretical speculation and differing views do exist; for example, that of French psychoanalyst Lacan.
17. See Winnicott (1960), "Ego Distortion in Terms of the True and False Self," in *Maturational Processes and the Facilitating Environment*, pp. 140–152.
18. See Ellen Siegelman, *Meaning and Metaphor in Psychotherapy* (New York: Guilford Press, 1990), on the use of metaphor in therapy. Siegelman provides a rich understanding of how metaphor, when revived from a concretized and deadened state, can access unarticulated inner experience, if the therapist recognizes the signals.
19. Beatrice Beebe and Frank M. Lachmann, "The Contribution of Mother-Infant Mutual Influence to the Origins of Self- and Object Representations," in *Psychoanalytic Psychology* (Hillsdale, NJ: Erlbaum, 1988), pp. 305–337.
20. Edward Tronick and A. Gianino, "Emotions and Emotional Communication in Infants," *American Psychologist*, Vol. 44, No. 2 (February 1989); 112–119. Tronick and Gianino have also carried out research that addresses the infant's subjective experience of success or failure in facilitating coordinated interactions with the mother.
21. Judith V. Jordan, Alexandra G. Kaplan, Jean Baker Miller, Irene P. Stiver, and Janet L. Surrey, *Women's Growth in Connection: Writings from the Stone Center* (New York: Guilford Press, 1991).
22. Beebe and Lachmann, "Contribution of Mother–Infant Mutual Influence," p. 314.
23. Megan Kirshbaum, "Parents with Physical Disabilities and Their Babies," *Zero to Three*, Bulletin of the National Center for Clinical Infant Programs, Vol. 8, No. 5 (June 1988); pp. 8–14.
24. Ibid., p. 11.
25. Ibid., p. 11.

Chapter 10

1. John Bowlby, *A Secure Base: Parent–Child Attachment and Healthy Human Development* (New York: Basic Books, 1988), p. 46.
2. John Bowlby, *Attachment and Loss*, Vol. 1, (New York: Basic Books, 1982), pp. 207–208.

3. Hans W. Loewald, "On the Therapeutic Action of Psychoanalysis," in *Papers on Psychoanalysis* (New Haven, CT: Yale University Press, 1980), pp. 221–256.

4. Calvin Settlage, Presentation on adult development and psychoanalysis, Annual Earl Simburg lecture, Alta Bates/Herrick Hospital, Berkeley, California, April 11, 1991.

5. Ralph R. Greenson, *The Technique and Practice of Psycho-Analysis* (London: Hogarth Press and Institute of Psychoanalysis, 1981).

6. See *Work in Progress* papers, the Stone Center, Wellesley College, Wellesley, MA.

7. Bowlby, *Secure Base*.

8. Ibid., p. 4.

9. Bowlby, *Attachment and Loss*, Vol. I.

10. Bowlby, *Secure Base*, p. 121.

11. Ibid., p. 79.

12. For an extend discussion of this point, see Loewald, "On the Therapeutic Action of Psychoanalysis," pp. 221–226.

13. C. H. Waddington, *The Strategy of the Genes* (London: Allen & Unwin, 1957).

14. Bowlby *Secure Base*, p. 136.

15. See Searles (1979) for a discussion of the psychological underpinnings of the need to be a caretaker.

Chapter 11

1. John Bowlby, *A Secure Base: Parent–Child Attachment and Healthy Human Development* (New York: Basic Books, 1988), pp. 29–30.

2. Verena Kast, *A Time to Mourn* (Einseideln, Switzerland: Daimon Verlag, 1988), p. 15.

3. Bowlby relies on the work of a colleague of his at the Tavistock Clinic, Colin Murray Parkes, for his information on bereavement. Parkes believed that mourning takes about one year to accomplish. In an interview with Robert Langs published in her book *Transference Neurosis and Transference Psychosis* (Northvale, NJ: Jason Aronson, 1981), p. 301, Margaret Little, a British psychoanalyst, comments on Parkes's findings somewhat acerbically but, from my point of view, quite accurately:

> Yes, you work through anger, self-pity, and remorse, and so on, until you arrive eventually at a relatively peaceful state of pure grief. But, I said, mourning is for life, and every now and then the original thing just jumps up and hits you again and knocks you flat, and for the time being everything else is knocked out. My letter was published by B.B.C., and I had ten letters in response to it, all thanking me and saying: "I have felt alone, and peculiar, having this happen. Other people have reproached me." . . . I had to write Dr. Parkes and tell him this, and say that . . . for everyone who wrote there would have been many more who did not write.

4. Bowlby, *Secure Base*, p. 32.

5. Ibid., p. 32.
6. Ibid., p. 55.
7. D. W. Winnicott, *Playing and Reality* (Middlesex, UK: Penguin Books, 1971), p. 126.
8. Thomas Ogden gives the concept of "analytic space" a related meaning. He writes that the termination phase of an analysis provides time for the "contraction" of the analytic space so that patients come to feel that they have that space within themselves. If the contraction of the space cannot occur, Ogden writes that "the prospect of the end of the analysis is experienced as tantamount to the loss of one's mind, or the loss of the space in which one feels alive." Thomas Ogden, *The Primitive Edge of Experience* (Northvale, NJ: Jason Aronson, 1989), p. 188.
9. James Fadiman, "Teaching Stories," copy by Tape Masters, 176 Forest Avenue, Pacific Grove, California 93950.
10. Jeffrey Moussaieff Masson, *Against Therapy: Emotional Tyranny and the Myth of Psychological Healing* (New York: Atheneum, 1988).

Chapter 12

1. Frances Tobriner proposes the concept of godmother as a model for the role of a consultant. A godmother, chosen by the parents, has the interests of the child at heart yet remains in relation to the parents.
2. Based on a joint presentation in Oakland, CA, on June 1, 1991, by Sue Nathanson Elkind, Judith Jordan, Jean Baker Miller, and Janet Surrey (Stone Center's Self-in-Relation Perspective on Women's Psychological Development, May 31–June 1, 1991). Irene Stiver is currently evolving a relational model of therapeutic impasses. See Stiver, "Developmental Psychopathology: Introducing a Consultant in the Treatment of Borderline Patients," *McLean Hospital Journal*, Vol. 13 (1988): 89–113).
3. The number of patients who have sought consultation from me obviously constitute only a small sample relative to the number of patients in psychotherapy.
4. See Chapter Fourteen for an extended example of this kind of consultation.
5. The role of a consultant serving as a transitional or "bridge" person is also beginning, as a result of clinical experience that therapists are sharing, to find its niche as a valuable resource when therapists become ill or die. See Laurel Samuels, Review of Harvey J. Schwartz and Ann-Louise Silver, eds., *Illness in the Analyst: Implications for the Treatment Relationship*, and Laura Barbanel et al. "The Death of the Psychoanalyst," *Contemporary Psychoanalysis*, Vol. 25, No. 3, in *The San Francisco Jung Institute Library Journal*, Vol. 4 (1992): 27–38.
6. Hilde S. Burton, personal communication.
7. A recent journal article contains a helpful classification of empathic failures of therapists: Edna M. Mordecai, "A Classification of Empathic Failures for

Psychotherapists and Supervisors," *Psychoanalytic Psychology*, Vol. 8, No. 3 (Summer 1991): 251–262.

8. In California, therapists are required to give patients a booklet, *Good Therapy Does Not Include Sex*, that informs them of their legal rights and the criminal and civil suits that can be filed.

9. See Jonathan H. Slavin, "On Making Rules: Toward a Reformulation of the Dynamics of Transference in Psychoanalytic Treatment," Presentation at Northern California Chapter of Psychoanalytic Psychology, San Francisco, CA., October, 1990.

10. There are certainly times when it is helpful for therapists to acknowledge errors to patients. In this situation, the underlying issue, which became concentrated in a debate over whether a mistake had been made, had to do with the shift in the therapist's way of working and the different subjective meanings the therapist and patient had attributed to the change.

Chapter 13

1. Irene Stiver, "Developmental Dimensions of Regression: Introducing a Consultant in the Treatment of Borderline Patients," *McLean Hospital Journal*, Vol. 13 (1988): 102.

2. Steven Cooper, Discussion of Stiver, "Developmental Dimensions of Regression," p. 112.

Chapter 14

1. Irene Stiver, "Developmental Dimensions of Regression: Introducing a Consultant in the Treatment of Borderline Patients," *McLean Hospital Journal*, Vol. 13 (1988): 105.

2. Ibid., 105–106.

3. I suspect that a similar matrix operates for male therapists and male patients, even though boys are socialized from the beginning to be separate and autonomous from both their mothers and fathers. As men begin to write about their yearnings for connection to their fathers, the hidden father–son axis will become increasingly visible, and as it does, the limited emphasis on the patient's father transference to the male therapist and the male therapist's paternal countertransference can be enlarged to include the same fluidity of role that characterizes mothers and daughters and female therapeutic dyads.

4. Male patients who have been sexually or physically abused as children might also profit from the presence of an auxiliary therapist. My experience functioning as a consultant or auxiliary therapist to patients who were sexually abused as children has thus far been limited to female patients.

Chapter 15

1. This form of impasse may also occur with patients and therapists of the same gender or with a male patient and female therapist. For example, a male patient might unconsciously make use of a female therapist as a gratifying, good mother as a result of his unconscious yearning. If his yearning met an unconscious need of the female therapist to *be* a good mother, she might be at risk of relying upon him as an object to gratify her need. Without an awareness of the dynamic and an ability to reflect on the relational pattern that had become entrenched, the therapist could not name the pattern so it could be worked with therapeutically. A collusive impasse would result.

Conclusion

1. I refer to maternal and paternal functions that are typically carried by women and men who parent infants. But these functions can be provided by either parent or other caretakers. Implied in this view of therapeutic relationships is a conception of a patient's transference to a therapist as an amalgam of aspects of both mothers and fathers as well as other significant caretakers.
2. D. W. Winnicott (1962), "The Child in Health and Crisis," *Maturational Processes and the Facilitating Environment* (New York: International Universities Press, 1965), p. 70.
3. To carry on the analogy to mother–infant relationships, we are currently expanding our conception of mothering to include the inevitable impasses and ruptures that occur without locating blame exclusively in the mother or in the child. We are also beginning to place mother–infant dyads in the context of an extended family that includes the father in a primary role as well as the culture at large.
4. A term used by Victoria Hamilton in a forthcoming book, *Patterns of Transference Interpretations.*
5. To the extent that subjective meaning is associated with the feminine capacities in each of us and that objective meaning is associated with masculine capacities, we are also talking about a complementarity or partnership between masculine and feminine to supplant the imbalanced dominance of the masculine.
6. The capacity emphasized by C. G. Jung.
7. D. W. Winnicott, "Transitional Objects and Transitional Phenomena," *Playing and Reality* (New York: Penguin Books, 1981), pp. 1–30.
8. The transition is parallel to the transition in conception of mothering that is occurring, in which the uniqueness of each mother–child dyad is recognized and appreciated alongside the accumulated knowledge of principles of mother/child-rearing.

Appendix C

1. Henry Grunebaum, "Helpful and Harmful Psychotherapy," *Harvard Medical School Mental Health Letter*, pp. 5–6.
2. Ibid., p. 5.
3. Ibid., p. 6.
4. Ibid.
5. J. A. Auger, "Images of Endings," *Journal of Analytical Psychology*, Vol. 31 (1986): 45–61.
6. James D. Guy and Gary P. Liaboe, "Personal Therapy for the Experienced Psychotherapist: A Discussion of Its Usefulness and Utilization," *The Clinical Psychologist* (Winter 1986): 20–23.
7. Ibid., p. 21.

❖ *Bibliography* ❖

Aron, Lewis. "The Patient's Experience of the Analyst's Subjectivity," *Psychoanalytic Dialogues: A Journal of Relational Perspectives*. Vol. 1, No. 1 (1991): 29–51.

Atwood, George E., Robert D. Stolorow, and Jeffrey L. Trop. "Impasses in Psychoanalytic Therapy: A Royal Road," *Contemporary Psychoanalysis*, Vol. 25, No. 4 (October 1989): 554–573.

Auger, J. A. "Images of Endings," *Journal of Analytical Psychology*. Vol. 31 (1986): 45–61.

Balint, Michael. *The Basic Fault: Therapeutic Aspects of Regression*. New York: Brunner/Mazel, 1979.

Beebe, Beatrice, and Frank M. Lachmann. "The Contribution of Mother–Infant Mutual Influence to the Origins of Self- and Object Representations," in *Psychoanalytic Psychology*. Hillsdale, NJ: Erlbaum, 1988, pp. 305–337.

Belenky, Mary Field, Blythe McVicker Clinchy, Nancy Rule Goldberger, and Jill Mattuck Tarule. *Women's Ways of Knowing: The Development of Self, Voice, and Mind*. New York: Basic Books, 1986.

Benjamin, Jessica. *The Bonds of Love: Psychoanalysis, Feminism, and the Problem of Domination*. New York: Pantheon Books, 1988.

Bettelheim, Bruno. *Freud and Man's Soul*. New York: Knopf, 1983.

Bollas, Christopher. *The Shadow of an Object*. New York: Columbia University Press, 1987.

———. *Forces of Destiny: Psychoanalysis and Human Idiom*. London: Free Association Books, 1989.

Bowlby, John. *Attachment and Loss*. Vols. 1 and 2. New York: Basic Books, 1982.

———. *A Secure Base: Parent–Child Attachment and Healthy Human Development*. New York: Basic Books, 1988.

Brodey, Warren M. "On the Dynamics of Narcissism: Externalization and Early Ego Development," *Psychoanalytic Study of the Child*, Vol. 20. New York: International Universities Press, 1965, pp. 165–193.

Buckley, Peter, ed. *Essential Papers on Object Relations*. New York: New York University Press, 1986.

Casement, Patrick J. *Learning from the Patient*. New York: Guilford Press, 1991.

Carotenuto, Aldo. *A Secret Symmetry: Sabina Spielrein between Jung and Freud*. New York: Pantheon Books, 1982.

Cushman, Philip. "Ideology Obscured: Political Uses of the Self in Daniel Stern's Infant," *American Psychologist*. Vol. 46, No. 3 (March 1991): 206–219.

DeAngelis, Tori. "Personal Events Pave Road to Understanding," *APA Monitor*. Vol. 20, No. 7 (July 1989).

Doolittle, Hilda. *Tribute to Freud*. New York: New Directions, 1984.

Drigalski, Dorte von. *Flowers on Granite: One Woman's Odyssey through Psychoanalysis*. Berkeley: Creative Arts Book Company, 1986.

Flax, Jane. *Thinking Fragments: Psychoanalysis, Feminism, and Postmodernism in the Contemporary West*. Berkeley: University of California Press, 1990.

Freud, Sigmund (1937). "Analysis Terminable and Interminable," in *Standard Edition of the Complete Psychological Works of Sigmund Freud*, Vol. 23, trans. and ed. James Strachey, with Anna Freud, assisted by Alix Strachey and Alan Tyson, pp. 216–253.

Gay, Peter. *Freud: A Life for Our Time*. New York: Norton, 1988.

Gilligan, Carol. *In a Different Voice: Psychological Theory and Women's Development*. Cambridge, MA: Harvard University Press, 1982.

Greenberg, Jay R. "Countertransference and Reality," *Psychoanalytic Dialogues: A Journal of Relational Perspectives*, Vol. 1, No. 1 (1991): 52–73.

Grinberg, Leon, Dario Sor, and Elizabeth Tabak de Bianchedi. *Introduction to the Work of Bion*. Northvale, NJ: Jason Aronson, 1977.

Grossfurth, Phyllis. *Melanie Klein: Her World and Her Work*. New York: Knopf, 1986.

Grunebaum, Henry. "Helpful and Harmful Psychotherapy," *Harvard Medical School Mental Health Letter*, pp. 5–6.

Guntrip, Harry. *Personality Structure and Human Interaction*. London: Hogarth Press, 1982.

———."My Experience of Analysis with Fairbairn and Winnicott (How Complete a Result Does Psycho-Analytic Therapy Achieve?)," in Peter Buckley, ed. *Essential Papers on Object Relations*. New York: New York University Press, 1986, pp. 447–468.

Guy, James D., and Gary P. Liaboe. "Personal Therapy for the Experienced Psychotherapist: A Discussion of Its Usefulness and Utilization," *The Clinical Psychologist*. (Winter 1986): 20–23.

Hamilton, Victoria. *Narcissus and Oedipus: The Children of Psychoanalysis*. London: Routledge & Kegan Paul, 1982.

Herman, Nini. *My Kleinian Home: A Journey through Four Psychotherapies*. London: Quartet Books, 1985.

Jordan, Judith V., Alexandra G. Kaplan, Jean Baker Miller, Irene P. Stiver, and Janet L. Surrey. *Women's Growth in Connection: Writings from the Stone Center*. New York: Guilford Press, 1991.

Jung, C. G. "The Syzgy: Anima and Animus," in *Collected Works*, Vol. 9. Princeton, NJ: Princeton University Press, 1959.

———. *Memories, Dreams, Reflections*. New York: Vintage Books, 1965.

———. "The Practice of Psychotherapy," in *Collected Works*, Vol. 16. Princeton, NJ: Princeton University Press, 1966, pp. 163–323.

———. "The Archetypes and the Collective Unconscious," in *Collected Works*, Vol. 9. Princeton, NJ: Princeton University Press, 1968.

———. "A Review of the Complex Theory," in *Collected Works*, Vol. 8. Princeton,

NJ: Princeton University Press, 1981, pp. 92–104.

Kantrowitz, Judy L., Ann L. Katz, Deborah Greenman, Humphrey Morris, Frank Paolitto, Jerome Sashin, and Leonard Solomon. "The Patient–Analyst Match and the Outcome of Psychoanalysis: A Pilot Study," *Journal of the American Psychoanalytic Association*. Vol. 37, No. 4 (1989): 893–919.

Kast, Verena. *A Time to Mourn*. Einseideln, Switzerland: Daimon Verlag, 1988.

Kennedy, Roger. "Review of *My Kleinian Home*," *International Review of Psychoanalysis*, Part 2. Vol. 13 (1986): 250–251.

Kerenyi, C. "Prolegomena," in *Essays on a Science of Mythology*. Princeton, NJ: Princeton University Press, 1973, pp. 1–24.

Kirshbaum, Megan. "Parents with Physical Disabilities and Their Babies," *Zero to Three*, Bulletin of the National Center for Clinical Infant Programs, Vol. 8, No. 5 (June 1988): 8–14.

Klauber, John. "Elements of the Psychoanalytic Relationship and Their Therapeutic Implications," in Gregorio Kohon, ed., *The British School of Psychoanalysis: The Independent Tradition*, New Haven, CT: Yale University Press, 1986, pp. 200–213.

Kohon, Gregorio, ed. *The British School of Psychoanalysis: The Independent Tradition*. New Haven, CT: Yale University Press, 1986.

Kohut, Heinz. *The Restoration of the Self*. New York: International Universities Press, 1977.

———. *How Does Analysis Cure?* ed. Arnold Goldberg, with Paul Stepansky. Chicago: University of Chicago Press, 1984.

Kuhn, Thomas S. *The Structure of Scientific Revolutions*. Chicago: University of Chicago Press, 1970.

Kurtz, Stephen. *The Art of Unknowing: Dimensions of Openness in Analytic Therapy*. Northvale, NJ: Jason Aronson, 1989.

Langs, Robert. *The Listening Process*. Northvale, NJ: Jason Aronson, 1978.

Little, Margaret. *Transference Neurosis and Transference Psychosis*. Northvale, NJ: Jason Aronson, 1981.

———. *Psychotic Anxieties and Containment: A Personal Record of an Analysis with Winnicott*. Northvale, NJ: Jason Aronson, 1990.

Loewald, Hans. *Papers on Psychoanalysis*. New Haven, CT: Yale University Press, 1980.

Mahler, Margaret S., Fred Pine, and Anni Bergman. *The Psychological Birth of the Human Infant*. New York: Basic Books, 1975.

Masson, Jeffrey Moussaieff. *Against Therapy: Emotional Tyranny and the Myth of Psychological Healing*. New York: Atheneum, 1988.

McGrath, Ellen, Gwendolyn Puryear Keita, Bonnie R. Strickland, and Nancy Felipe Russo, eds. *Women and Depression: Risk Factors and Treatment Issues*. Washington DC: American Psychological Association, 1990.

Meador, Betty, "Transference/Countertransference between Woman Analyst and the Wounded Girl Child," in *Chiron: A Review of Jungian Analysis*. Wilmette, IL: Chiron, 1984, 163–174.

Miller, Jean Baker. *Toward a New Psychology of Women*. Boston: Beacon Press, 1986.

Mordecai, Edna M. "A Classification of Empathic Failures for Psychotherapists and Supervisors," *Psychoanalytic Psychology*, Vol. 8, No. 3 (Summer 1991): 251–262.

Morris, William, ed. *American Heritage Dictionary of the English Language*. Boston: Houghton Mifflin, 1980.

Nathanson, Sue. *Soul-Crisis: One Woman's Journey through Abortion to Renewal*. New York: New American Library, 1989.

Nolan, Christopher. *Under the Eye of the Clock*. New York: St. Martin's Press, 1987.

Ogden, Thomas. *Projective Identification and Psychotherapeutic Technique*. Northvale, NJ: Jason Aronson, 1982.

——. *The Matrix of the Mind*. Northvale, NJ: Jason Aronson, 1986.

——. *The Primitive Edge of Experience*. Northvale, NJ: Jason Aronson, 1989.

Ragland-Sullivan, Ellie. *Jacques Lacan and the Philosophy of Psychoanalysis*. Chicago: University of Illinois Press, 1987.

Rutter, Peter. (1989). *Sex in the Forbidden Zone: How Men in Power—Therapists, Doctors, Clergy, Teachers & Others—Betray Women's Trust*. Los Angeles: J. P. Tarcher.

Samuels, Laurel. Review of Harvey J. Schwartz and Ann-Louise Siler, eds., *Illness in the Analyst: Implications for the Treatment Relationship* and Laura Barbanel, et al. "The Death of the Psychoanalyst," *Contemporary Psychoanalysis*, Vol. 25, No. 3, in *The San Francisco Jung Institute Library Journal*, Vol. 4 (1992): 27–38.

Schafer, Roy. *The Analytic Attitude*. New York: Basic Books, 1983.

Searles, Harold F. "The Patient as Therapist to His Analyst," in *Countertransference and Related Subjects: Selected Papers*. New York: International Universities Press, 1979, pp. 380–459.

Segal, Hanna. *Introduction to the Work of Melanie Klein*. New York: Basic Books, 1974.

Siegelman, Ellen. *Metaphor and Meaning*. New York: Guilford, 1990.

Stanton, Martin. *Sandor Ferenczi: Reconsidering Active Intervention*. Northvale, NJ: Jason Aronson, 1991.

Stern, Daniel. *The Interpersonal World of the Infant: A View from Psychoanalysis and Developmental Psychology*. New York: Basic Books, 1985.

Stevens, Anthony. *Archetypes: A Natural History of the Self*. New York: Morrow, 1982.

Stiver, Irene. "Developmental Dimensions of Regression: Introducing a Consultant in the Treatment of Borderline Patients," *McLean Hospital Journal*, Vol. 13 (1988): 89–113.

Sullivan, Barbara Stevens. *Psychotherapy Grounded in the Feminine Principle*. Wilmette, IL: Chiron, 1989.

Swigart, Jane. *The Myth of the Bad Mother: The Emotional Realities of Mothering*. New York: Doubleday, 1991.

Tronick, Edward, and A. Gianino. "Emotions and Emotional Communications in Infants," *American Psychologist*. Vol. 44, No. 2 (February 1989): 112–119.

Trop, Jeffrey L., and Robert D. Stolorow. "A Developmental Perspective on

Analytic Empathy: A Case Study," *Journal of the American Academy of Psychoanalysis*, Vol. 19, No. 1 (1991): 31–46.

Tustin, Frances. *Autistic Barriers in Neurotic Patients*. New Haven, CT: Yale University Press, 1989.

Waddington, C. H. *The Strategy of Genes*. London: Allen & Unwin, 1957.

Weston, Amy. "The Wounded Healer: Power and Vulnerability in the Psychotherapy Relationship," Paper presented at the Saturday Seminars Series, Berkeley, 1989.

Whitmont, Edward C. *The Symbolic Quest: Basic Concepts of Analytical Psychology*. Princeton, NJ: Princeton University Press, 1969.

Winnicott, D. W. (1956). "Primary Maternal Preoccupation," in *Through Paediatrics to Psychoanalysis*. New York: Basic Books, 1975, pp. 301–305.

———. (1956). "The Antisocial Tendency," in *Through Paediatrics to Psychoanalysis*. New York: Basic Books, 1975, pp. 306–315.

———. (1958). "The Capacity to Be Alone," in *Maturational Processes and the Facilitating Environment*. New York: International Universities Press, 1980, pp. 29–36.

———. (1960). "Ego Distortion in Terms of the True and False Self," in *Maturational Processes and the Facilitating Environment*. New York: International Universities Press, 1980, pp. 140–152.

———. (1960). "The Theory of the Parent-Infant Relationship," in *Maturational Processes and the Facilitating Environment*. New York: International Universities Press, 1980, pp. 37–55.

———. (1962). "Ego Integration in Child Development," in *Maturational Processes and the Facilitating Environment*. New York: International Universities Press, 1980, pp. 56–63.

———. (1963). "The Development of the Capacity for Concern," in *Maturational Processes and the Facilitating Environment*. New York: International Universities Press, 1980, pp. 73–82.

———. *Playing and Reality*. Middlesex, Eng.: Penguin Books, 1971.

———. "Fear of Breakdown," in Gregorio Kohon, ed., *The British School of Psychoanalysis: The Independent Tradition*. New Haven, CT: Yale University Press, 1986, pp. 173–184.

Woodman, Marion. "Abandonment in the Creative Woman," in *Chiron: A Review of Jungian Analysis*. Wilmette, IL: Chiron, 1985, 23–46.

Young-Bruehl, Elisabeth. *Anna Freud: A Biography*. New York: Summit Books, 1988.

❖ *Index* ❖